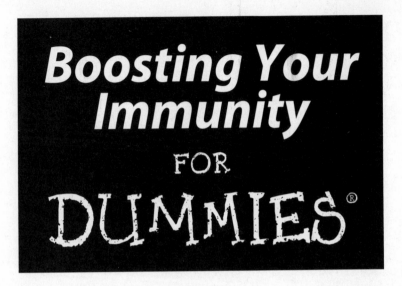

Boosting Your Immunity

FOR

DUMMIES®

by Dr. Wendy Warner and
Dr. Kellyann Petrucci

WILEY

John Wiley & Sons, Inc.

Boosting Your Immunity For Dummies®

Published by
John Wiley & Sons, Inc.
111 River St.
Hoboken, NJ 07030-5774
www.wiley.com

WILEY

About the Authors

Wendy Warner, MD, is a holistic gynecologist, educator, and writer. After receiving her BS at the University of Tennessee, she attended medical school at the University of Tennessee at Memphis and completed her residency in obstetrics and gynecology at Temple University Hospital in Philadelphia, where she served as Chief Resident her final year. She started private practice in a conventional ObGyn setting in suburban Philadelphia after residency and served as Chair of the Department of ObGyn at two hospitals.

Shortly after starting practice, Dr. Warner realized that although she was trained to do an awful lot of medicine, much of it wasn't relevant to getting and staying healthy. After training with herbalists and energy workers, she eventually became involved with the American Board of Integrative Holistic Medicine, the organization that certifies physicians in integrative holistic medicine. She served on the board of directors for ten years, two of those as president. She has been on the teaching faculty for that organization since 2002. In 2004, Dr. Warner founded Medicine in Balance, a collaborative holistic medical practice in suburban Philadelphia., In that practice, she provides conventional gynecologic care as well as holistic medical consultations for women, men, and teens.

From early on in her practice, Dr. Warner has been teaching. She has led workshops and "Mini Med School" at her office, is a frequent presenter at medical conferences about holistic medicine, has spoken to various lay groups, and was an invited guest on *The Dr. Oz Show* to discuss functional medicine. To receive periodic health information updates, sign up for her blog at www.medicineinbalance.com.

Kellyann Petrucci, DC, earned her BA from Temple University, hosted her alma mater's Department of Public Health Intern Program, and mentored students entering the health field. She earned her MS from St. Joseph's University and her DC from Logan College of Chiropractic University Programs, where she served as the Postgraduate Chairperson. Dr. Kellyann did postgraduate coursework in Europe. She studied Naturopathic Medicine at the College of Naturopathic Medicine, London, and she is one of the few practitioners in the United States certified in Biological Medicine by the esteemed Dr. Thomas Rau, of the Paracelsus Klinik Lustmühle, Switzerland.

In Dr. Kellyann's many years in a thriving nutritional based practice and consulting, she's helped patients build the strongest, healthiest body possible. She learned early on that looking and feeling amazing came down to learning simple lifestyle principles that made amazing differences in people's lives. She realized that deep nutrition wasn't about fancy powders, ancient elixirs, or the latest creams; it was about reprogramming the body to get back to the basics and eat and live in a way that naturally boosts immunity, and all else will follow. She found the principles of eating and living for superimmunity to be the key for those that get well, stay well, lose weight, and fight aging. Dr. Kellyann has seen so much success from learning these immune-boosting health principles that she feels a moral obligation to spread the message of eating real food and living in a way that moves people toward health and super immunity.

Dr. Kellyann is the coauthor for the health and lifestyle book *Living Paleo For Dummies* (Wiley). She also created the successful kids' health and wellness program Superkids Wellness and developed the PaleoSmart System and International Wellness Consulting. You can find free nutritional videos and a weekly dose of news, tips, and inspiration on her website at www. drkellyann.com.

Dedications

From Dr. Warner: I dedicate this book to my patients, who teach me every day and remind me why I became a physician. Also to my colleagues and staff at Medicine in Balance, who help make my professional dream come true. To my parents, Jim and Betty Warner, who have been wondering when I'd get around to writing a book, and to my friends and colleagues at the ABIHM, who are mentors and sounding boards and inspiration.

And mostly to my husband, Brad Hubbell: You have been supportive and patient throughout this process, and I'm always amazed to hear how much you brag about me. You make my life complex and interesting and wonderful.

From Dr. Kellyann: I deeply appreciate my boys: my husband, Kevin, and my little guys John and Michael. They manage to understand my dreams and visions and are gracious enough to do whatever they can to make them happen. I pray they will intuitively know that my greatest dreams have already been met by sharing my life with them. And for my parents, John and Ellie, who have always taught me to make character and strength a keynote in my life.

My life has been filled with the most magical of memories, thanks to my little sister Kathleen, who is the most effervescent, strong-minded person I've ever known. We've been on this wellness path together for so many years, and my respect for her runs deep. And to my brothers Joseph and John Michael, who have made every childhood memory I have one of joy and playful imagination. I am truly blessed to have brothers that bring such laughter and simple fun to my life. Also, a big hug and nod of deepest appreciation to my best friend Dr. Jennifer Bonde, who has been by my side through every trial, tribulation, and learning experience I've had for the last 20 years. Jen, I value every smidgen you've added to my crazy awesome life!

Authors' Acknowledgments

From Dr. Warner: This has been an amazing journey that wouldn't have happened without my coauthor, Dr. Kellyann Petrucci. She has amazing energy and enthusiasm, and we learned that our strengths complement each other perfectly. She juggles a *lot* of hats at once, and I deeply appreciate her ability to focus on the task at hand and do it with grace and a smile. Thank you also to our team at Wiley, each of whom gave their all to this project from start to finish and were willing to put up with our somewhat hectic schedules. Your advice and guidance were invaluable. Also, thanks to my staff, Liz and Darlene. With my attention sometimes on writing rather than practicing, they've done a graceful job of keeping things running smoothly in the office.

From Dr. Kellyann: First, a big thanks to my gifted coauthor Dr. Wendy Warner for making this collaboration such a pleasure. Her talents as a physician are matched by her truly good heart; Wendy lives the lifestyle she promotes, and you can't help but feel a sense of calm in her presence. Thanks for adding nothing but positivity to my life! I also feel deep gratitude and will be forever thankful to my agent, Bill Gladstone, of Waterside Productions, Inc., for not only motivating me but, more importantly, believing in me. And to Margot Hutchinson of Waterside Productions, who is always selflessly shepherding a deal behind the scenes. Also, thank you to my friends at Wiley: Acquisitions Editor Tracy Boggier, who always puts in 110 percent, and Project Editor Elizabeth Rea, who managed every detail to perfection.

Publisher's Acknowledgments

We're proud of this book; please send us your comments at http://dummies.custhelp.com. For other comments, please contact our Customer Care Department within the U.S. at 877-762-2974, outside the U.S. at 317-572-3993, or fax 317-572-4002.

Some of the people who helped bring this book to market include the following:

Acquisitions, Editorial, and Vertical Websites

Project Editor: Elizabeth Rea

Senior Acquisitions Editor: Tracy Boggier

Copy Editor: Jennette ElNaggar

Assistant Editor: David Lutton

Editorial Program Coordinator: Joe Niesen

Technical Editor: Jillian Finker, ND, CNS

Editorial Manager: Michelle Hacker

Editorial Assistant: Alexa Koschier

Art Coordinator: Alicia B. South

Recipe Tester: Emily Nolan

Nutritional Analyst: Angie Scheetz, RD

Cover Photos: © iStockphoto.com/ Vasilis Nikolos; Zlatko Kostic; Logorilla; Brasil2; Elena Elisseeva; camilla wisbauer; Anton Ignatenco; Elena Gaak; demypic; Mordolff; jo unruh

Cartoons: Rich Tennant (www.the5thwave.com)

Composition Services

Project Coordinator: Katherine Crocker

Layout and Graphics: Jennifer Creasey

Proofreader: Evelyn Wellborn

Indexer: BIM Indexing & Proofreading Services

Illustrators: Kathryn Born, Elizabeth Kurtzman

Publishing and Editorial for Consumer Dummies

Kathleen Nebenhaus, Vice President and Executive Publisher

David Palmer, Associate Publisher

Kristin Ferguson-Wagstaffe, Product Development Director

Publishing for Technology Dummies

Andy Cummings, Vice President and Publisher

Composition Services

Debbie Stailey, Director of Composition Services

Contents at a Glance

Recipes at a Glance

Table of Contents

Part II: What Happens When Your Immune System Gets Off Track 37

Chapter 3: Strengthening Your Allergy Defense System 39

Chapter 4: Autoimmune Disorders: Dealing with an Overactive Immune System 53

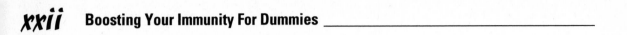

Introduction

You're probably familiar with the many diet plans, books, infomercials, and products on the market that have one goal in mind: to get you skinnier. Okay, fair. But what if you could get the same results by just getting healthy and staying healthy? What if you could look better, feel better, *and* experience fewer cold and flu symptoms or other illnesses just by making simple diet and lifestyle changes that boost your immunity? The simple truth is that when you boost your immunity, you *can* have it all.

When you begin to eat and live in a way that boosts your immunity, you naturally remove inflammatory foods as well as the foods that don't move you toward health. You begin eating true *superfoods* — foods rich in vitamins, minerals, and antioxidant power that make you feel better than you may have in years. What overall effect does boosting your immunity have in your life? You'll have reduced risk of heart disease, diabetes, cancers, colds, flus, and other illnesses. You'll have more energy, look younger, lose weight, get stronger, and sleep more soundly.

The immune-boosting plan isn't a diet in the traditional sense, although we do ask you to give up certain foods — sometimes just for a short time and, in some cases, indefinitely. Although that may sound intimidating, this book shows you the reasons you should avoid certain foods for optimal health. We also provide plenty of practical tips to make the transition as easy as possible for you and your family. From how to stock your kitchen cupboards to how to stay healthy while you travel, from reversing disease to exercising wisely, you'll find everything you need to adopt an immune-boosting lifestyle.

About This Book

Embracing a healthier paradigm may feel overwhelming at first, but *Boosting Your Immunity For Dummies* helps you understand the benefits of living an immune-boosting life. In this book, we explain the underlying science of how the immune system works and define all its parts and functions. We pay special attention to what happens when your immune system gets off track and what you can do about it.

We break down the patterns of an immune-boosting lifestyle so you know exactly where to begin, and we help you understand just what to include in your diet to reach your goals. Whether you're trying to get healthy, stay healthy, lose weight, reverse a medical condition, fight aging, or improve your energy, you'll find the information you need to succeed. We also explain the nutritional aspects of the immune-boosting lifestyle and answer your questions about superfoods, herbs, vitamins, minerals, supplements, and more.

Because boosting your immunity goes beyond the food that you put on your plate, we also explore how you can improve your sleep, enhance your cells through detoxing, and benefit from immune-boosting breathing and moving.

If you're more interested in practical application than scientific theories, we've got you covered there, too, with chapters that outline how to revamp your kitchen for boosting immunity and how to plan and stock your kitchen for the nutritionally superior immune-boosting foods.

And finally, *Boosting Your Immunity For Dummies* wouldn't be complete without plenty of delicious, satisfying recipes to help you and your family make the transition to living healthier. The recipes will keep you nutritionally fed from breakfast through dinner with healthy snacks in between and even a few dessert recipes for those special occasions when you want something a little sweeter than usual. We also share a lot of easy meal ideas that don't require a recipe at all.

Conventions Used in This Book

We use the following conventions throughout the text to make things consistent and easy to understand:

- All web addresses appear in `monofont`.
- When this book was printed, some web addresses may have needed to break across two lines of text. If that happened, rest assured that we didn't put in any extra characters (such as hyphens) to indicate the break. So when using one of these web addresses, just type in exactly what you see in this book, pretending the line break doesn't exist.
- We use **boldface** to highlight keywords in bulleted lists and the action parts of numbered steps.

Here are some specific recipe-related conventions that apply throughout the book:

- ✔ Vegetarian recipes are marked with a tomato in the Recipes in This Chapter list.
- ✔ Temperatures are all given in degrees Fahrenheit. (If you prefer working in the metric system, turn to the appendix for help converting temperatures to Celsius.)
- ✔ All eggs are large, unless noted otherwise.

What You're Not to Read

We've written this book so you can find information easily and quickly. Each chapter covers one aspect of boosting immunity and includes specific details and practical tips to help you understand how to incorporate it into your new lifestyle. If you don't have the time (or the desire) to read every word, you can skim the text in the shaded sidebars. They provide interesting but not essential anecdotes and additional information.

Foolish Assumptions

As we wrote this book, we made the following assumptions about you:

- ✔ You want to build your immune system to experience fewer colds, flus, and other illnesses or to manage some type of medical condition, lose weight, or fight aging, and you know that to achieve these goals, boosting your immunity makes sense.
- ✔ You understand how to eat and live healthy, and you want your loved ones to enjoy a healthy, immune-boosting lifestyle, too.
- ✔ You want to stop eating processed and unhealthy foods to feel younger, healthier, more vibrant, and happier.
- ✔ You're interested in discovering how food affects you physically and mentally and how to live a healthier lifestyle but don't want to get bogged down in too much scientific detail.
- ✔ You're open to the idea of making lifestyle changes — avoiding certain foods, making sleep a priority, and adopting healthy principles — to enhance your quality of life.

✔ You want to gain a better understanding of how the immune system works and what you can do if your immune system isn't functioning properly.

How This Book Is Organized

We've divided this book into five parts to make the different topics more manageable and easier to digest. Each part deals with certain aspects of boosting immunity and discusses the relevant topics.

Part I: Getting to Know Your Immune System

If you're interested in starting with the basics, this part is for you. The first chapter gives a broad overview of living an immune-boosting lifestyle, pointing out all the ways your decisions impact your immune system. In this part, we explain the immune system in detail, from the many organs involved to the different cells and how they interact. If you're a bit of a science geek, this is the place for you.

Part II: What Happens When Your Immune System Gets Off Track

Although most of the time the immune system functions well, other times it doesn't. If things go haywire, some disease states can develop. This part addresses the *hows* and *whys* of specific conditions, such as allergies, autoimmune conditions, and cancer, as well as immune-boosting suggestions specific to each. We also discuss immune deficiency states, both inherited and acquired, along with suggestions that help modify immune activity.

Also in this part, we discuss the impact of other medical conditions on the immune system and the immune system's impact on other medical conditions, showing you how interconnected your overall health is to your immune system.

Part III: Laying the Groundwork for Super Immunity: Nutrition, Lifestyle, and Detox

In these chapters, you find out why eating immune-boosting foods is the best choice for you and your family and how they can get you well and keep you well. Tapping into the immune properties of superfoods is one of the most amazing tools you can use to improve your health. Packed with nutrients, they provide you with the deepest nutrition. However, living an immune-boosting lifestyle goes beyond food. Lifestyle patterns also make a difference, and the chapters in this part explore the principles of living an immune-friendly lifestyle. We also show how detoxing can work its magic in people who need a cellular cleanse.

Part IV: Cooking Up Recipes for Immunity and Wellness

Getting reacquainted with your kitchen can be a gift for you and your family. We live in a busy world filled with responsibility, and this section helps you overcome the obstacle of feeling overwhelmed when you're ready to jump back into your kitchen. Chapter 13 provides tips on planning and stocking your kitchen. Chapters 14 through 19 include a collection of delicious, comforting recipes to fill every meal (and your stomach) with healthy, energizing foods. You'll find recipes for easy breakfasts, lunches, dinners, side dishes, soups, salads, desserts, teas, and smoothies that will improve your health, energize your body, and help you live longer and stronger.

Part V: The Part of Tens

Like all *For Dummies* books, this one includes the fun and exciting Part of Tens. Here, we list ten tips to avoid coming down with a cold or flu, ten ways to improve your breathing for a better immune system, ten exercises you can do anywhere, and finally ten ways to help your family adapt the immune-boosting lifestyle.

Icons Used in This Book

To make this book easier to navigate, we include the following icons to help you find key information about boosting your immunity.

This icon indicates practical information that can help you in your quest for improved health or in your progress in adopting an immune-boosting lifestyle.

When you see this icon, you know that the information that follows is important enough to read twice!

This icon highlights information that could be detrimental to your success if you ignore it. We don't use this one much, so pay attention when we do.

This icon highlights interesting but optional information that's of a more scientific nature for those who want a little deeper perspective.

Where to Go from Here

This book is organized to be read in the way that makes the most sense to you, so feel free to jump around to the information that's most relevant to you right now. You can use the table of contents to find the broad categories of subjects or use the index to look up specific information.

Do you want to know more about the foods to boost immunity? You can get started in Chapters 8 and 9. Are you ready to clean out your kitchen? Turn to Chapter 13. Want to know about the immune-boosting supplements and herbs? Check out Chapter 10, which provides an in-depth look at the nutritional underpinnings of supplementation. If you want to understand how your immune system works, jump right into Chapters 1 and 2, or if you want to understand how to deal with an overactive immune system, go to Chapter 4. If it's the recipes that interest you, Chapters 14 through 19 are for you.

And if you're not sure where to begin, read Part I. It gives you the basic information you need to understand why and how boosting your immunity can help you improve your health and quality of life.

Part I

Getting to Know Your Immune System

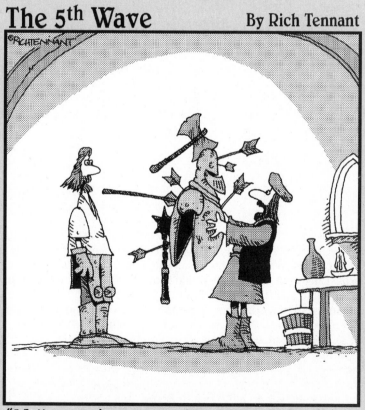

The 5th Wave — By Rich Tennant

"Well, your immune system seems to be doing its job."

In this part . . .

The pursuit of good health ultimately leads to the pursuit of a healthy immune system. This part makes clear all the ways your immune system affects your life as well as all the ways your day-to-day choices affect your immune system. The chapters in this part take you through the nitty-gritty details of the immune system and how the organs and cells interact so you understand what you can do to improve your immunity. Also, you come to understand all the ways your system can go wrong, so you can set it right again.

Chapter 1

Immunity: Your Ticket to a Stronger, Longer, and Healthier Life

. . . .

. . . .

*E*verything rises and falls on your immune system. When your immune system is strong, you avoid the pitfalls of disease, and your body expresses vitality and health. Your immune system is your shield — your most powerful protector.

Having your immune system operate at its best should be central in your life and the focus of your nutritional and lifestyle patterns. The secret to success is discovering practical tools and strategies to strengthen your immune system so it helps keep you healthy, lean, strong, and ageless.

Super Immunity 101

What does it mean to have *super immunity?* Super immunity is when your body's greatest protector — its immune system — is working to the best of its ability to get and keep you well. Having your cells express their super immunity potential can even save your life. Your immune system casts a healing shield over you, protecting you from the simplest of challenges, like the common cold, to the most threatening, like cancer.

We're passionate about bringing the concept of immune boosting to the world because we've seen tremendous value in developing tools and healthy lifestyle practices that keep people in this super immune-healing cocoon. In the following sections, we introduce you to the concept of super immunity and how it can affect nearly every area of your life.

Starting with your immune system

No matter what your goals are — whether they're to get well, stay well, lose weight, or fight aging — it all starts with creating the healthiest cells possible. Discovering the tools to help your body create these healthy cells may be one of the most important things you do for yourself.

Life can be complicated. It can be hectic, busy, and exhausting to you and your body. These things are just a few of the challenges your immune system faces. No one enjoys being stuck in bed with frequent colds, yet many adults in the United States are about two to four times per year. Simple infections can turn life threatening, and the flu can turn into a more serious and prolonged illness. People are concerned about a worldwide spread of viral illnesses, and cancers are at an all-time high (men have a 44 percent chance of getting an invasive cancer, and women, about 37 percent).

Here's the good news: Research shows that you can make a difference in protecting yourself from these illnesses. Understanding how to eat and live better helps you strengthen your body's greatest protector so it knocks out disease and keeps you well before anything serious or life threatening has a chance to take hold. Of course, you do risk some side effects of having a strong and efficient immune system — you'll look and feel amazing!

Boosting your immunity with nutritional excellence

When you start eating and living for vibrant health, it shows. You have less down time, and you enjoy life on an entirely different level. If you're suffering, take comfort in knowing that eating your way to a stronger immune system will help you a great deal, and getting well really does start with nutritional excellence. Chapters 8 and 9 explain what it means to eat foods with superior nutrition.

Nutritional excellence happens when you eat foods with *a high nutrient density,* which means foods that have a lot of nutrients in relation to the amount of calories they contain. So with each bite, you're doing something positive to your body and strengthening that healing shield.

Unfortunately, the average American takes in about 60 percent of his calories from *low nutrient density foods* — processed foods that have added flavors, colors, sweeteners, rancid oils, and are a gluten-filled, flour-filled dietary mess. When you eat these foods, every bite weakens your healing shield and opens yourself up to disease and premature aging.

Considering super immunity and modern medicine

According to former Surgeon General of the United States Dr. Richard Carmona, "Because of the increasing rates of obesity, unhealthy eating habits, and physical inactivity, we may see the first generation to be less healthy and have a shorter life expectancy than their parents." That is an unbelievable statement — that this generation will be the first to *not* outlive their parents! This means that with all the drugs, surgeries, and advancement in medicine, we're not getting any better. And now, the problem has trickled down to children.

Drugs were never designed to get you healthier. They were designed to get you out of crisis mode. Even though people have been marketed to think that more medical care means a longer, healthier life, that simply isn't the truth. If you want health, that job is up to you. No shortcut or magic pill can do this for you. It's about the lifestyle you choose to live.

Immune-boosting success story: Drew

Meet Drew, 56, horticulturist, Philadelphia, Pennsylvania:

Drew is the perfect example of someone who was a participant in his healing, which lead to astonishing results. Drew's blood sugars were creeping up to alarming levels. He and his wife decided to take action and wanted to use effective strategies that were as close to natural as possible. They transitioned their kitchen into healthy, immune-boosting foods with lean meats, low-starch carbohydrates, some fruits, and healthy fats. Much to their surprise, they really enjoyed these foods and found the transition easy with so many great recipes. Drew's blood sugars started at 350 and, in just six months' time, have plummeted to the normal range of 90 to 110. Drew and his wife were even more shocked when they found his hemoglobin A1c (average blood sugars over the previous two to three months) went from 13.8 down to an astounding 6.6! Drew feels better than ever. Every spring, he'd get sick like clockwork, but that's a thing of the past. He no longer gets sick whatsoever. Through time, he has experienced deep healing and is noticing improvements in all areas of his life.

Another problem with looking to modern medicine to get well and stay well is that taking medications does nothing to change behavior. In fact, it's your behaviors or patterns every day that may be leading to you needing the medication in the first place. Relying on medication to make you feel better allows you to continue on the path you're on, no matter how destructive it may be to your cells and overall health. Don't let modern medicine be your permission for leading a life that isn't serving you.

You have to be a *participant* in your healing to get results. Modern medicine isn't the answer. Always try to get the best results in your life; the *recipient* of healthcare has to be the *participant* as well.

Living Longer, Stronger, and Healthier

It almost sounds too good to be true, but, yes, you can live longer, stronger, and healthier when you discover how to eat and live in a way that boosts your immunity. When you stop poisoning your cells with unhealthy foods, you get rid of toxins and anything that your body can't use or eliminate. How quickly something leaves your body through your bowels says a lot about the health of that food. Certain foods cleanse you while others clog you. Eating foods that cleanse you keep you young, healthy, and beautiful, as you find out in the following sections.

When you balance your plate with lean, healthy meats, seafood, vegetables, fruits, nuts, seeds, and naturally occurring healthy fats, like the ones shown in Figure 1-1, and cut down your sugar intake, you get stronger, leaner, and healthier. We discuss the power of immune-boosting foods in Chapters 8 and 9.

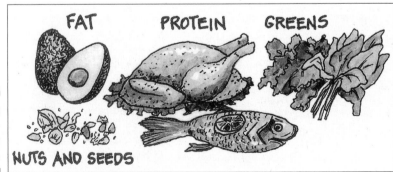

Figure 1-1: Immune-boosting foods.

Illustration by Elizabeth Kurtzman

Focusing on healthy cells

Healthy cells are different than cells under *oxidative stress* — the total burden of your cells by free radicals (unstable molecules responsible for tissue damaging and aging) in normal, everyday metabolism plus the added environmental stresses, like the toxins in air, water, or food. The biggest problem with oxidative stress is that it causes fatigue and premature aging. To turn back the hands of time and be youthful and vibrant, you have to eliminate the oxidative stress patterns placed on your body. You can do so by eating immune-boosting foods.

When you begin eating foods with nutritional excellence, your body starts to shed all its unhealthy cells. (See the discussion on cells in Chapter 2.) You begin to peel away layers of fat; you become leaner, stronger, and disease-free, and you defy your age. Immune-boosting foods do all these things and more:

- Balance blood sugar and keep your overall sugar load down
- Create a fatty-acid (omega-6 to omega-3) balance
- Balance macronutrients (protein, fats, and carbohydrates)
- Contain trace nutrient density (minerals)
- Promote and maintain acid-base balance (how acid and alkaline you are)
- Add robust amounts of fiber to your daily plate (for intestinal health)

Immune-boosting success story: Betty

Meet Betty, 83, mother, grandmother, and great-grandmother, Detroit, Michigan:

Betty is one of the most vibrant human beings on the planet. She's free of pain and, at 83, her activities aren't limited because of age. But it wasn't always that way. Betty was born premature and, as a result, was a weak, frail child. After she grew and was married, her husband suffered from heart disease, which was her catalyst for change. She became interested in finding a better way of living — a healthier lifestyle. She became intrigued with healthy foods and incorporated good nutrition into her cooking. Health became the forefront of Betty's life, and she raised her family with those food values, which are now paying off in spades. Betty lights up a room and is always on the go. Despite the fact that she endured hip replacement surgeries, she continues to exercise and maintain a positive outlook. She's 83 going on 60!

Modern-day processed and "convenient" foods won't do the trick. People are sicker and fatter than ever and are more confused about what to eat than in any other time in history. But eating immune-boosting foods cuts through the clutter and helps you become very clear about the foods that move you toward health.

Turning on your "super immunity" genes

Don't ever think that because you've had challenges in the past that you can't get healthier, look better, and live a better life. You can. You can create wellness and look amazing by giving your body the raw materials it needs and avoiding what it doesn't need.

You come into this world with your genes programmed for health. Developing bad habits and making poor choices risks your health. Remember: Your choices lead to sickness, not faulty genes or bad luck. In fact, your genes are nothing more than physical strings with a blueprint on them. Genes are either read or not read, and it's up to you how these genes are modified.

People can reprogram their genes, anytime they choose. This statement isn't fluff or soft science; it's based on a science called *epigenetics.* The fact is, every cell in your body is a programmable chip. Think of epigenetics like this: Your human gene (or genome) is like a computer. The *epigenome* found above the gene is like the software. If you're living in an environment that's congruent with how you're designed, you're all set. The software will run a healthy program. If you make choices that aren't congruent with your body's design, your outcome will be very different.

Epigenetics takes people from a place of hopelessness to a place of hope, because it doesn't matter what your situation is. Unless you're the less than 5 percent of the population with a true genetic defect, you have control of your life and your choices. You're in the driver's seat.

Nutritional excellence can make a deep impact. By eating immune-boosting foods, you're programming your genes to run a brilliant, healthy software. You're making the choice to give your body what it needs to flourish and create the healthiest cells possible. You're going to love how amazing you look and feel as a result!

Choosing health

If your body is forced to live in a way that's incongruent with a healthy, immune-boosting lifestyle, you'll continually move away from health. In fact, your body will start going through *adaptive physiology,* where your body attempts to adapt to whatever the stressor may be in your environment — smoking, drinking, eating unhealthy foods, being under constant stress, not exercising, eating lots of sugar, or even negative thinking — so you can survive. Whatever stressor your body faces, adaptive physiology will kick in to counterbalance the effects. It may even show up as some kind of chronic disease, such as high blood pressure, heart disease, or another illness. Eventually, if you don't remove the stressor from your environment, your body fatigues and stops working for you.

Think about it like this: If you're facing a threat (like running away from a wild animal), having high blood pressure and an increased heart rate is normal. You need these things to get you out of your threatening situation. On the flip side, when you're under this stress, your body doesn't need growth, so growth hormones shut down; you also don't need a working digestive system or a sex drive, so those functions shut down. So heart disease, high blood pressure, high blood sugar, or a digestive disorder may be *normal* given the environment your body is in; in fact, your body is doing exactly what it's supposed to do.

Be aware of lifestyle stressors, and work toward *choosing health*. The principles in this book and the immune-boosting recipes in Part IV are a great place to start.

Boosting Your Immunity to Look and Feel Amazing

Most people adopt an immune-boosting lifestyle because they want to create health or get some of that energy back that used to be present in their life. What they find is they get much more. Their eyes start to glisten, their skin tone evens out, their hair gets shinier, and many lose weight and have a sense of happiness.

Immune-boosting success story: Pamela

Meet Pamela, 55, registered nurse, Philadelphia, Pennsylvania:

Pamela began creating immune-boosting meals because she wanted to help her family. Her husband had high blood sugar, and even though her three children were older, she knew they needed to learn about eating real foods. What she didn't expect was what happened to her. She went from a size 8 to a size 4, and her whole body shape changed. She says, "I'm never sick, I have lots of energy, and I sleep soundly — something I haven't done in a long time. I have no wrinkles (the ones I had seem to have disappeared!), my eyes became very bright, I'm never bloated anymore, and my body feels stronger than it did when I was 25. My hair and nails now grow faster than ever before. Something good is happening inside. My kitchen is immune-boosting for life."

When your cells get the raw material they require to function at their best, magic starts to happen. If you want to boost your immunity, have perfect weight, and a youthful appearance, you have to have waste-free cells.

Clean, healthy cells keep your body in balance and are the only way to get long-term health, weight loss, or a youthful appearance.

In this section, we talk about how boosting your immunity helps you look younger, increase vitality, get a good night's sleep, clear up skin problems, and sooth digestive issues. See Chapter 11 for full details.

Looking younger

Boosting immunity foods not only keep you well but also keep you looking younger because you're ditching a lot of your sugar sources. You're no longer filling your plate or eating snacks with lots of sugar. You say goodbye to sugary carbohydrates, 100-calorie snack packs, or bottled drinks with artificial sugars.

Eating sugar causes you to have dull, wrinkled skin because of the *glycation* that occurs. The sugar in your bloodstream attaches to proteins to form harmful molecules. The more sugar you eat, the more harmful molecules are created. These molecules then damage your collagen, which is what keeps your skin firm and resilient. When this damage happens, you get saggy, dry, and wrinkled skin — definitely not a youthful look!

Also, when eating nutrient-dense foods, your cells lose waste, gain health, and make elimination easy, making your skin, eyes, and energy come alive. This kind of radiance is the cornerstone of a youthful appearance.

Increasing vitality

The body benefits immeasurably from superior nutrition. It keeps your cells clean and detoxification pathways clear; your body eliminates easily, and all your body's systems and functions begin to balance.

Just think of how many days you felt listless or sluggish and didn't have the energy to do what you wanted that day. Chances are pretty good that maybe your diet created an imbalance in one of these areas. Following are some of the properties of immune-boosting foods that keep you looking and feeling young and give you energy and vitality:

✔ Your blood sugar becomes balanced so you don't have energy swings throughout the day that make you cranky and tired.

✔ Trace nutrients (minerals) and macronutrients (fats, proteins, and carbs) become balanced, providing you with stable energy resulting from balanced, real food nutrition.

✔ Immune-boosting foods are low on the food allergy scale, so they're less likely to provoke food sensitivities that can make you fatigued.

✔ Immune-boosting foods promote a balanced pH, which promotes healing.

Immune-boosting foods give you vitality that will become the norm in your life, not the exception.

Getting a good night's sleep

One of the most priceless factors when eating and living a healthy lifestyle is improved sleep. After your body adjusts to eating cleaner, more nutrient-dense foods, you'll find that your sleep is deeper and more restful (see Chapter 11 for details).

Getting quality sleep is one of the more common frustrations of many of our patients. Maybe you have trouble falling asleep, or you wake in the middle of the night unable to drift back to sleep. No matter what the scenario, eating healthy, immune-boosting foods will completely change the quality and duration of your sleep. Here's why:

✔ You're getting foods loaded with minerals, which are grounding and calming to your body.

✔ When your blood sugars are more balanced, you don't get that blood sugar dip in the middle of the night, causing your body to release hormones to restore blood sugar, which disturbs sleep.

✔ Healthy foods contain B vitamins, which are great for calming nerves and balancing the nervous system for restful sleep.

✔ Some of the healthier foods, like eggs, turkey, nuts, fish, and some fruits, contain an essential amino acid called *tryptophan*, which helps promote sleep.

✔ When eating foods with superior nutrition, your body naturally regulates hormones and signals associated with hormones that, in turn, help you sleep better.

If you have sleep issues, eating foods with superior nutrition can be your all-natural sleep aid. It works, and there are no nasty side effects.

Clearing up skin and digestive issues

So many problems we see in our practice come down to healing the intestinal track, because an unhealthy gut is responsible for many people's problems. Your gut is filled with bacteria. Incredibly, your intestinal track is about 10,000 square feet of surface area, and within this surface area are literally trillions of cells (bacteria). Your job is to feed these cells with the right raw material and nutrients so your intestinal bacteria are plentiful and strong.

Think of all those cells as your soil. If you pot a plant that lacks nutrients or is diseased or toxic, that plant won't thrive. The same goes for you. So many people are run down or have intestinal discomforts, acne, or skin rashes because they have a deficient and toxic intestinal track.

To become vibrant and healthy and to eliminate so many of the digestive problems and skin issues, you have to first create healthy soil. The superior nutrition in immune-boosting foods begin to cultivate that healthy soil. In Chapter 7, we cover immune-related conditions, including leaky gut syndrome, acne, and other skin conditions.

You've found your nutritional blueprint. It's eating the nutritionally superior immune-boosting superfoods. When you fill your plate with these foods, your body will respond in a way it never has before. You'll literally come alive and plug back in to get healthy, stay healthy, and de-age.

Immune-boosting success story: Jennifer

Meet Jennifer, 39, business owner, Bloomfield Hills, Michigan:

Jennifer grew up eating healthy food. As she reached adulthood, she carried out the same pattern. She purchased her foods from health food stores and ate the "healthier" versions of foods, or so she thought. Even though she was eating foods from health food stores and the healthier sections of the food market, she continually battled her weight and had chronic congestion. What she came to realize was that just because foods are found in a health food store or marketed as "healthy," it doesn't always mean they're foods you should be eating. When Jennifer started eating immune-boosting foods and understood what superior food nutrition really meant, she began to look better than ever — and lost 25 pounds and 8 percent body fat to boot! She has more energy and says, "I just feel clearer and more balanced. Having this awareness has been an amazing eye opener and will be of value to me for the rest of my life."

Chapter 2

Understanding the Parts and Functions of Your Immune System

*T*o understand how the immune system works, you have to get acquainted with all the players. The immune system resides throughout the body, including organs from all over. Because the immune system's job is to protect you from the outside world, it makes sense that most of the components are found in the places where you most directly interact with the world: your skin, lungs, gut, and literally anywhere stuff that *isn't* you interacts with stuff that *is* you.

Many cell types are involved with the immune system, each with its own unique job. The pathways of communication among these cell types are long and complicated, set up in "rounds" of redundant interactions. Due to the redundant nature of the interactions, a small occurrence sends out a big message quickly. Interestingly, you're born with part of your immune system all ready to go, and another part figures out what to do based on what you're exposed to over time.

In this chapter, we explore the different organs and cell types that make up the immune system. We also discuss the functions of the immune system, how they work, and what happens when they don't work. Finally, we talk about vaccinations and whether they're really helpful to your body.

Introducing the Key Players: Your Immune Organs

Different organs in your body produce the immune system cells. The cells then move around as needed via blood vessels and lymphatics and get stored in other organs. In this section, we examine the immune system organs (see Figure 2-1) and the basics of where everyone comes from.

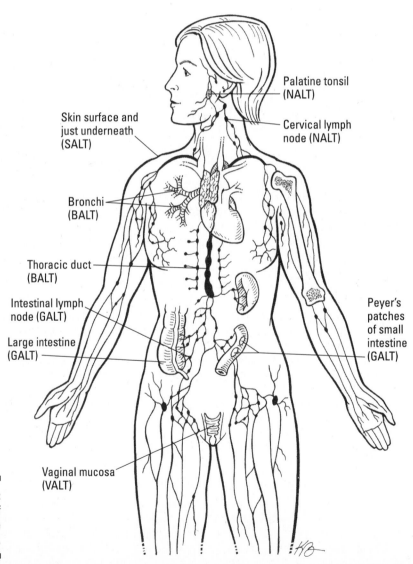

Palatine tonsil
(NALT)

Skin surface and
just underneath
(SALT)

Cervical lymph
node (NALT)

Bronchi
(BALT)

Thoracic duct
(BALT)

Intestinal lymph
node (GALT)

Large intestine
(GALT)

Peyer's
patches
of small
intestine
(GALT)

Vaginal mucosa
(VALT)

Figure 2-1:
Organs of
the immune
system.

Illustration by Kathryn Born

Bone marrow

Inside the firm outer core of bones lies the *bone marrow,* a spongy layer where blood cells are born. Most of this spongy layer is found in the flat bones, like the pelvis, skull, and sternum, as well as the end portions of the long bones of the arms and legs. In infants, most of this bone marrow is *red bone marrow,* in which lots of cell transformation takes place. As you age, some of this red bone marrow gets replaced with fat and becomes *yellow bone marrow.* In times of emergency with significant blood loss, yellow marrow can convert to red marrow to help replace lost red cells, lymphocytes, and other blood cells.

In a process called *hematopoiesis,* stem cells are converted to red cells, lymphocytes, and other blood cells. B lymphocytes (see the later section "Meeting More Players: All the Different Cell Types") undergo some maturation in the bone marrow so that they're ready to perform their job when needed; other cells leave the bone marrow still in an immature state to morph into mature cells elsewhere.

Thymus

The thymus is an organ found in the chest, directly above the heart. It's the site where thymocytes mature into T cells. In infants, the thymus is large, but it gradually shrinks with age. Immature thymocytes move from the bone marrow to the thymus, where they interact with MHC (major histocompatibility complex). Here, they're shown different *antigens,* which are compounds that may or may not be a problem for the organism. If the T cells react to antigens that are part of the organism itself, they get destroyed (otherwise, they may trigger an autoimmune reaction). If they react to only antigens that *aren't* part of the organism, then they get to hang around. However, if they fail to respond to those things that aren't part of the organism, they're also destroyed, because they're not helpful as part of the immune response. So there's active selection of both those T cells that fail to work as well as those that react to antigens that are part of self.

After this process has occurred, the mature, now immunocompetent cells go out into the bloodstream to look for invaders.

Spleen

The spleen is a smallish organ located in the upper left part of the abdomen. It acts mostly as a blood filter, gathering old red cells to destroy them, as well as recycling and processing antigens brought there by B cells, macrophages, and other cells of the immune system. It stores red cells for times of emergency and can also store platelets and lymphocytes for future use. Although it has an important function in the adult, the spleen is nonessential. If, for example, it gets damaged in an accident and has to be removed, its removal has no long-term effect on that person's immune function later in life.

Lymph nodes

Lymph nodes are small organs that are distributed throughout the body and connected by lymphatic vessels, channels through which lymph fluid flows. The lymph nodes act as filters of the lymph as well as housing for B cells, T cells, and macrophages. When an invading organism is encountered in the body, dendrites — phagocytic cells; see the section "Meeting More Players: All the Different Cell Types" — grab the organism and take it into the lymph nodes. Here, lymphocytes make antibodies that then go out into the bloodstream to fight against whatever the invader is. If there's a large infection and a lot of dendrites are bringing antigens back at once, the lymph node can become swollen, which is common in everything from colds to cancer.

Lymph nodes are scattered throughout the body but tend to be concentrated along areas where your own tissue has the most contact with organisms that aren't you. The specific types of B and T cells that congregate in specific lymph nodes are determined by the most common invaders in that part of the body. The presence of these B and T cells saves a lot of time and trouble for your immune system, because it already has the right staff to perform the job and doesn't have to wait for replacements. See the section "Barriers," later in this chapter, for further discussion.

How they work together

Structurally, the flow goes like this: Cells of the immune system get formed primarily in the bone marrow. Then they may migrate to the thymus for differentiation or to lymph nodes (or the spleen) to hang out and look for work. Due to the redundancy of the system, losing your spleen or some lymph nodes doesn't have any long-term effect on your immune function.

Meeting More Players: All the Different Cell Types

A number of cell types are involved in immune function. In the following sections, we briefly discuss each one individually and then explain how they all function together.

Phagocytes

Phagocytosis describes "eating up" substances; therefore, *phagocytes* are any cell types that act via this mechanism. The phagocytes consist of granulocytes, macrophages, and dendritic cells.

- ✔ **Granulocytes:** The granulocytes are often the first on the scene of an invasion and are programmed to directly kill invaders, often continuing until they themselves die off. Pus in a wound is largely made up of dead granulocytes. Granulocytes are also called *polymorphonuclear leukocytes* and consist of three cell types: neutrophils, eosinophils, and basophils. Their action occurs primarily via enzyme activity and is directed at parasites and bacteria. Mast cells are similar; they stay put in mucosa or connective tissue and don't have the ability to move around. What they can do, though, is let loose the secretory granules that they carry. These granules contain inflammatory chemicals, like histamine, prostaglandins, and leukotrienes, which cause inflammation to both kill invaders and send an alert message to the rest of the system. This activity is important in the allergic response and some autoimmune conditions.

- ✔ **Macrophages:** Macrophages start out as monocytes in the blood. When an invasion occurs, the monocytes transform into macrophages, which go into the tissue where the invader is and begin engulfing it. They move more slowly than granulocytes but live longer and get more done while they live. In addition to directly killing invaders, macrophages stimulate other parts of the immune system by presenting the antibodies associated with that invader, as a dendrite does.

- ✔ **Dendritic cells:** Dendritic cells (also known as *dendrites*) are also part of the phagocytes; they not only directly eat up invading organisms, but they also have the ability to stimulate the rest of the immune system. When dendrites engulf an invader, they place part of that organism's genetic material on their surface. This process is called *antigen presentation*. It's this presentation that stimulates T and B cells to join the attack.

Lymphocytes

Lymphocytes are a category of cells that include B cells and T cells. These cells are born in the bone marrow but travel to other tissues for maturation, in preparation for their work in the immune system. Each of these cells becomes specialized to recognize only one kind of antigen; the receptors on their surface will bind with only one kind of molecule.

✔ **T cells** are divided into helper T cells and killer T cells. The *helper
T cells* become activated when a macrophage or dendritic cell presents
an antigen on its surface from an organism that it just engulfed (see
Figure 2-2). If that antigen happens to be the one that the T cell is
programed to respond to, the cell becomes activated, rapidly dividing
as well as making further chemicals to stimulate other T cells and B cells
to promote the immune response. Killer T cells, however, are designed
to roam the body looking for invaders. If they run across something they
recognize as being a problem, like bacteria or cancer cells, they kill it.

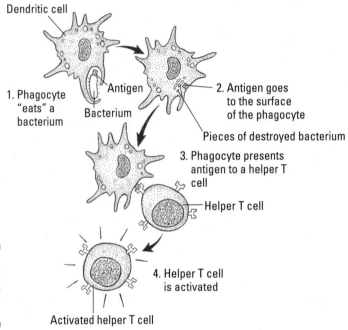

Figure 2-2:
Creation
of helper T
cells.

Illustration by Kathryn Born

✔ **B cells** roam the body looking for things that match the receptors that
are on their surface. After they run across these invaders, a triggering
signal is set off, a protein from helper T cells is added, and the B cells
begin to divide. In this process, they differentiate into plasma cells and
memory cells.

• *Plasma cells* produce a protein called an antibody that's formed
rapidly and attaches to the intruding organism. These antibodies
make it easier for the remaining immune cells to identify the
intruding organism and kill it. Antibodies can attach to more
than one organism at a time, in effect gathering the intruders into
groups for more efficient processing by the other cells.

- *Memory* cells are produced in a similar fashion (see Figure 2-3). They have the ability to make antibodies but have a much longer life span than a plasma cell. They function to respond to a similar infection much more rapidly in the future. This means that the first time one is infected by an organism, the system is often at its slowest; future infections are attended to much more rapidly due to the activity of memory cells.

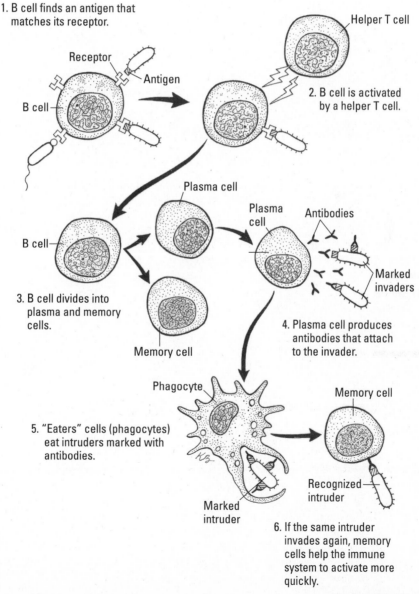

1. B cell finds an antigen that matches its receptor.

Receptor

Antigen

B cell

Helper T cell

2. B cell is activated by a helper T cell.

Plasma cell

Plasma cell

Antibodies

B cell

Marked invaders

3. B cell divides into plasma and memory cells.

Memory cell

4. Plasma cell produces antibodies that attach to the invader.

Phagocyte

Memory cell

5. "Eaters" cells (phagocytes) eat intruders marked with antibodies.

Recognized intruder

Marked intruder

6. If the same intruder invades again, memory cells help the immune system to activate more quickly.

Figure 2-3: Creation of memory cells.

Illustration by Kathryn Born

How they work together

Overall, the different cells work to activate a response and prompt the activity of all the other cells. The granulocytes and macrophages respond first, causing inflammation and damage to the invading organisms, which not only kills some of the organisms but also sends the signal that something's up. The dendrites arrive and eat some of the organisms, too. The macrophages and dendrites can then present the antigens they just ate up to the T cells, creating helper and killer T cells as well as B cell activation. After the B cells are activated, they create antibodies, which not only contribute to killing off the invading organism but also create future immunity to that organism. Figure 2-4 shows it graphically.

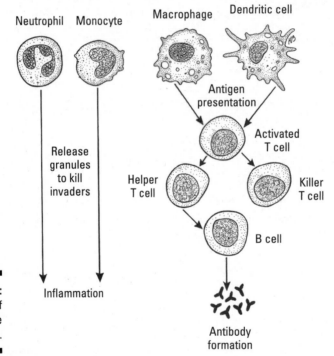

Figure 2-4:
The cells of
the immune
system.

Illustration by Kathryn Born

Tracking How the Immune System Really Works

The immune response works in phases; it's all about amplification of an initial signal and spreading that message as quickly as possible to "round up the troops" when danger is present. The response starts with nonspecific, non-induced responses but quickly switches to more broadly specific, induced responses and then to specific acquired responses, which allows for a full response, though it can take as much as five days to get to the later stages. We explain the process in detail in the following sections.

Establishing surface barriers and mucosal immunity

The first line of defense is a good barrier system. As the old saying goes, "Good fences make good neighbors"; if the virus or bacteria never make it into your body, that's a good thing. So simple barriers, such as skin, protect you. But what about all those parts of the human body that are exposed to the outside world that aren't covered by skin? Where can bugs get in? Well, you can breathe them in, or they can come in on food you eat, and women also can be exposed through vaginal contact. So at each of these places, you have a series of defenses called *lymphoid tissue,* and each one is named to reflect the area it's protecting (you can see them in Figure 2-1). Lymphoid tissue is where all the cells of the immune system hang out, waiting to go to work.

- NALT (nasopharynx associated lymphoid tissue): Tonsils and adenoids plus the upper respiratory mucosa (cells lining the airways)
- BALT (bronchi-associated lymphoid tissue): Lower respiratory mucosa and bronchial patches
- SALT (skin-associated lymphoid tissue): All the lymph tissue under and part of the skin
- GALT (gut-associated lymphoid tissue): Includes intestinal mucosa, Peyer's patches, and the appendix
- MALT (mucosa-associated lymphoid tissue): Includes all the other categories plus urogenital/vaginal lymphoid tissue (VALT)

Accepting normal flora

Ever stop to think about how many bacteria live in and on you? They're everywhere — your skin, your nose, your gut (especially your gut!). In fact, you have more individual *bacteria* in you than cells of *you* in you! Kind of makes you wonder who's in charge here, right?

However, all those normal bacteria help keep things in check. Your immune system has learned that these bacteria aren't the enemy and don't pose a threat, so it lets them hang around. In turn, they help keep things in balance, especially in the gut. If you've ever had to take antibiotics for an infection and then developed diarrhea afterward, you understand the importance of normal bacteria — the antibiotics killed off some of the good guys as well as the bad guys, and the usual balance got disturbed. The good news is that it can fix itself pretty quickly. (In Chapter 10, we discuss how to use this to good advantage).

Making sure the body has plenty of normal bacteria is important to healthy function of the immune system. Studies show that exposure early on makes a difference; infants born by Cesarean section develop different normal bacteria than those born vaginally, because they get exposed to different bacteria. Kids raised in households that are *too* clean (yes, there is such a thing!) tend to develop more cases of asthma and allergies because their immune systems don't get exposed to enough normal bacteria. To make sure your normal bacteria are in place, consider taking a supplement, eating naturally fermented foods, and avoiding antibacterial soaps or unnecessary antibiotics.

Complement system

The complement system is also important in the immune response. It consists of various proteins produced by the liver that flow through the bloodstream in inactive form. When the proteins encounter an infection, they become activated and cause an inflammatory response. These proteins have the ability to launch a rapid cascade of reactions to stimulate other complement molecules, hastening the inflammatory response rapidly. The activity of these proteins not only kills invaders but also marks them for easier recognition by other cells in the immune system.

Relying on innate immune response

The innate immune response refers to the stuff you're born with. The innate system kicks in first, during the first 96 hours or so after infection by a virus or bacteria. Initially, structural issues respond in a nonspecific, non-induced way, such as by trying to flush out the invader in saliva or respiratory mucus. The innate system also includes all those cilia that line the respiratory tract;

the little hair-like organs that move particles back out if you breathed them in. Also part of this structural system is your reflex to cough things back out, and if something you ate is particularly a problem, you'll vomit it back up.

After this first nonspecific response comes a broadly specific, induced response from your immune cells. When a pathogen is encountered, dendritic cells and macrophages move in to eat it up. Polymorphonuclear leukocytes also can move in and engulf the invader, breaking it down into pieces. If a virus or cancer cell is encountered, usually the killer T cells do the job. All these cell responses are general and "reflex" in nature.

The innate immune response manages to recruit immune cells to the site of an infection, activate the complement cascade, and produce a controlled inflammatory state to repel the invader. No previous exposure to this invader is required for it to get in motion. What is required is exposure to pathogen-associated molecular patterns (PAMPs) and damage-associated molecular patterns (DAMPs). Both are specific types of chemicals that tell the body that a stranger's here (PAMPs) and that the stranger is a problem (DAMPs). PAMPs are chemicals found only in viruses and bacteria, so they're pretty easy to recognize. DAMPs are chemicals that occur through injury or necrosis of the cell but not after usual *apoptosis* (planned cell death, which we discuss further in Chapter 6). If a stranger is present that isn't a problem (like one of the normal gut bacteria that you live with every day), no DAMPs are created, so the response isn't triggered. It takes both stranger and danger.

The amazing thing is how fast these signals get amplified and sent to the rest of the immune system; it takes only a day or so! This happens so fast because the immune system triggers NF-kB (nuclear factor kappa-light-chain-enhancer of activated B cells — whew!) and other transcription factors. NF-kB is a protein that stimulates the production of some of the proteins that make up antibodies. It plays an important role in regulating the immune response; when it goes haywire, the body gets weird messages so that cancer and autoimmune conditions may develop. When the transcription factors are activated, they cause production of inflammatory cytokines, free radicals, and eicosanoids, all of which produce a controlled inflammatory condition.

Inflammation is part of the normal response and is important when things go wrong.

Acquired immune response

After the innate immune response kicks in (as described in the previous section), the acquired response begins. These two responses function together, though through different pathways (see Figure 2-5). The acquired immune response varies from person to person because it depends on the invaders each individual is exposed to. Although the process is the same, the actual antibodies vary. After the dendrites and macrophages have eaten up the invader, they take parts of that invader and present them on the surface of the dendrite. This action, called *antigen presentation,* shows the rest of the immune system what the invader looks like.

This antigen presentation stimulates helper T cells and cytolytic T cells to come into the area to help fight off the invader. It also stimulates B cells to make antibodies. These antibodies help mark the invader so other cells find it more easily; they also bind particles of the invader together to "corral" them and make them easier to fight. This whole process takes a while, usually four to five days. That explains why the typical viral infection takes nearly a week to resolve — when your immune system is working as well as you want it to.

The acquired immune response involves specialized T and B cells; each T cell has structurally unique antigen receptors that were randomly generated during maturation. When they interact with the appropriate antigen and get the correct stimulating signal from the innate immune system cells, these T cells rapidly regenerate themselves, making thousands of copies to fight against this specific invader.

T cells randomly make as many receptors as they can to be ready for anything. Sometimes, that means they make receptors for something that's actually "self." These cells get deleted either by "supervisor" cells in the thymus, or by regulatory T cells out in the peripheral blood. If they somehow escape this deletion process and happen to replicate, it can cause an autoimmune response.

Cell mediated immunity, humoral immunity, and cytokines

Cytokines are proteins that are part of cellular communication; in this case, we're specifically referring to immunomodulating agents that are part of proliferating the immune response. Helper T cells create two categories of cytokines: Th1 cytokines are involved in cell mediated immunity and delayed sensitivity, and Th2 cytokines are part of humoral immunity and the allergic response. Th2 cytokines promote cell growth and recruit mast cells, basophils, eosinophils, and B cells to the area. See Table 2-1 for a comparison of the two types.

The body needs to have a balance of these two categories of cytokines. Otherwise, you run the risk of either having too much inflammation or too little inflammation (the whole system isn't working), or you start creating a response to yourself, which is an autoimmune disease. Different specific cytokine chemicals are associated with specific Th1 and Th2 responses;

some are inflammatory and some are anti-inflammatory. These cytokines can be measured in the bloodstream, so healthcare providers can try to figure out what exactly your immune system is doing when it's acting up. For example, TNF-alpha and IL-17 (tumor necrosis factor alpha and interleukin 17) are both specific markers of inflammation. The levels of these two markers start to rise long before most of the symptoms of an inflammatory condition really get started. A smart practitioner who sees signs of impending trouble or notices a genetic predisposition to an inflammatory state can measure these levels and then, if they're elevated, take steps to normalize them before they cause damage.

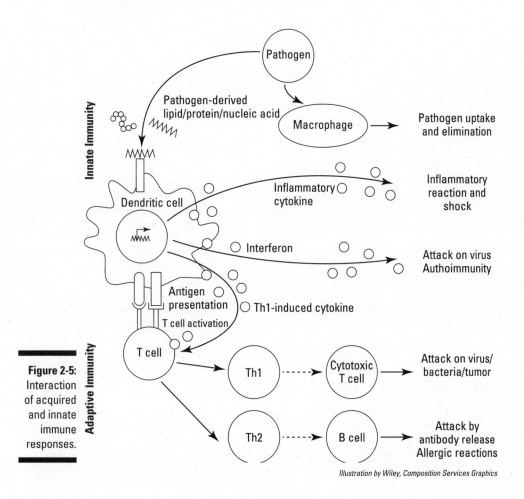

Figure 2-5:
Interaction of acquired and innate immune responses.

Illustration by Wiley, Composition Services Graphics

Table 2-1		Comparison of Th1 and Th2 Systems	
T Cell System	*Cytokines Produced*	*Activation*	*Predominant Diseases*
Th1	IFN gamma, TNFB, IL-1, IL-2, IL-12	T cell mediated activation of macrophages, neutrophils	Rheumatoid arthritis, MS, thyroiditis (Graves' and Hashimoto's), Crohn's, Lyme arthritis, Type I diabetes mellitus
Th2	IL-4, IL-5, IL-6, IL-10, IL-13	B cell mediated activation of mast cells, eosinophils, basophils Leads to increases in IgE and IgG4 antibodies	Allergic diseases, asthma, Scleroderma, ulcerative colitis, lupus, pregnancy

Regulatory T cells

One of the main ways you achieve balance between Th1 and Th2 systems is by regulatory T (Treg) cells. These specific T cells are produced as a response to a dendrite showing up with a specific antigen on its surface. After Tregs are stimulated, they produce chemical signals to impact both the Th1 and Th2 systems. They can suppress autoimmunity as well as modulate the changes in immune function produced by UV radiation. In the gut, they function to maintain normal tolerance by dampening the response you make to ingested food antigens. They also function to keep you from rejecting tissue grafts. If too much Treg activity occurs, however, it can be immunosuppressive and lead to cancer formation. Recently, Treg activity is shown to improve with Tai Chi Chuan, the Asian movement/energy exercise.

Considering Vaccinations and How They Work

The usual time for the body to mount an immune response to a viral or bacterial infection is somewhere between four and seven days. During that time, you get symptoms of the infection. Usually these infections are simply troublesome, but they can also be severe, even fatal. Prior to the advent of vaccinations, contracting a disease was the only way to gain immunity to it: When you survived the first infection, your body had the ability to fight off the next infection, thanks to the activity of memory cells and antibodies.

In the following sections, we explore the ways your immune system fights infections, from being exposed to the infection before to taking vaccinations. We also touch on the common flu shot vaccination. At www.dummies.com/ extras/boostingyourimmunity, you can find additional coverage of the common HPV vaccination Gardasil.

Teaching your immune system to remember and fight

Vaccines were discovered by accident. A vaccine allows for the intentional introduction of a pathogen (or part of one) into a healthy individual to prompt an immune response. After that response is generated, if that individual encounters that same pathogen in the future, the body recognizes it and fights it off right away. Time saved and symptoms avoided!

When a vaccine is given, macrophages and dendrites notice the antigens from the pathogen involved and go into action. They engulf the pathogen and then present the antigens on their surface so the lymphocytes are activated. T cells go into action by either killing the pathogen (killer T cells) or alerting the B cells (helper T cells), just as we discuss in the earlier section "Lymphocytes." The B cells create antibodies to this pathogen, as usual, and ultimately, memory cells are created. The ultimate goal of the vaccination is to form memory cells so you don't contract the disease in the future, because the immune response is rapid if the pathogen is encountered again.

The reason folks usually don't get very sick after a vaccination is that the particle used to make the vaccine is changed and isn't as potent as usual. Some vaccines, called *live attenuated vaccines,* use microbes that have been changed in the lab and weakened in such a way that they can't cause the full-blown illness. These vaccines are easiest to make for viruses, because their smaller number of genes are easier to manipulate; bacteria are more difficult to control due to their larger number of genes. The downside of live attenuated vaccines is that these damaged pathogens could theoretically revert to their normal potency and cause illness; for this reason, these vaccines shouldn't be used in individuals with compromised immune systems (very young infants, individuals who have recently undergone chemo, or those with HIV). These vaccinations also need to be refrigerated, so they're less helpful for use in developing countries where proper refrigeration can't be assured.

Inactivated vaccines contain microbes that have been killed either with chemicals or by heat changes. The good news is that no chance exists of reverting to a virulent form, so anyone can receive the vaccine. Inactivated vaccines also don't require refrigeration. The bad news is that the immune response tends to be weaker than to the live attenuated microbes, requiring booster shots in most instances. The lesser response to the vaccine likely is due to changes in the pathogen from killing it in the first place.

Weighing pros and cons of vaccination

Although a lot is to be said for vaccination, it isn't all just one big happy picture. However, preventing a disease, which is often cheaper and easier, makes more sense than treating one. Also, a phenomenon called *herd immunity* suggests that if a lot of folks all in the same place have been vaccinated against the same disease, then even those who aren't vaccinated have a lesser chance of contracting it, because fewer people will be susceptible to it. Some illnesses don't seem to even exist anymore in parts of the world because so many folks were vaccinated against it.

On the other hand, as we explain in the previous section, some vaccines can revert to active forms and actually make you sick. Also, some vaccines work with the immune system in an odd way to increase the chance of problems as well as cause immunity. And last, some vaccines are made each year against specific viruses, with the assumption that those particular strains will be the ones we see — and it doesn't always work out that way. So folks end up taking vaccinations that aren't specific for the virus they're exposed to, and they get sick anyway.

Some people worry about the way kids currently receive vaccines. Years ago, fewer vaccines were available, so people got only one or a few at a time, and they were spread out over a number of years. This gave the immune system time to adjust and do its job. Nowadays, many more vaccines are available, and infants and young kids are receiving a lot over a short period of time, sometimes many all at once. Some people worry that this amount may cause problems and, in effect, short circuit the immune system, overwhelming it and causing a confused response. Although no direct evidence suggests this reaction, there's concern that the increase in asthma and atopic diseases in kids comes from a malfunction of the immune system by overexposure in a short time.

There's also some concern about the actual processing of the vaccine itself. Many vaccines contain *adjuvants,* which are chemicals added to make the vaccine work better. Some people worry that the adjuvants may cause problems, though no data truly links these chemicals with potential problems.

Making an informed decision about flu shots

Influenza (better known just as the flu) is a viral illness that causes fever, sniffles, cough, and can even lead to pneumonia and death. For the average person, it's an uncomfortable inconvenience that costs a lot in doctor visits and lost work. For some, however, it can be much more severe.

Annual flu vaccinations have been available for a number of years. Unlike other viruses, the influenza virus has a high mutation rate, meaning it changes often, so making a vaccine that will still recognize the flu virus that ends up infecting a given area is difficult. The World Health Organization has a collaboration each year — sites all over the world collect samples of viruses that are then used to create the vaccine. The vaccine contains three different strains, and it's hoped that the specific versions of these strains will be the actual virus to infect the targeted area. Some years, this collaboration works well; some years, not so much. In the worst-case scenario, people are given a vaccine that gives them protection to the wrong flu virus, and they get sick anyway. Also, sometimes people wait too long to get the shot; it can take up to two weeks to gain immunity, so if they get infected in the mean-time (even to the correct strain), they still get sick. In some years, the vaccine causes a not-so-mild reaction, and a large portion of people actually get nearly as sick as they would have had they contracted the virus.

The overall usefulness of the flu vaccine has been studied for years, and the research has had mixed results. Studies in normal adults show that although good immunity is built, there's little impact on illness and hospitalizations overall, which is likely due to immunity against the wrong strain. Studies in infants show essentially the same thing — good immunity but no real change in illness. However, in the elderly, most studies have actually shown a difference in illness, as do studies in immune-compromised individuals, such as with people who have HIV/AIDS.

So the flu vaccine can be helpful or it can be a waste of time. It really depends on the year, who you are, and when you get the shot. Makes you wonder whether boosting your natural immunity and assuming your body will take care of things for you may be easier.

Part II

What Happens When Your Immune System Gets Off Track

The 5th Wave   By Rich Tennant

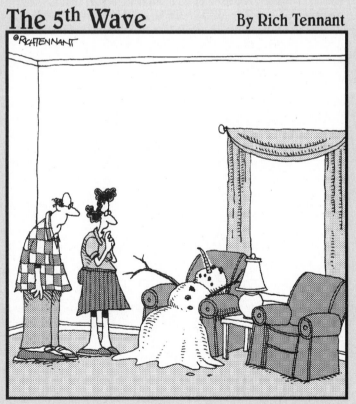

"He gets like this every summer."

In this part . . .

The immune system can sometimes go wrong; it can't tell the difference between "you" and "not you," or it fails to stop a growing cancer, or it overreacts to everything in an allergic reaction. This part goes into detail of how those things occur; if you're having symptoms, you'll find yourself in these pages. The chapters in this part also explain the hows and whys of treatment to minimize symptoms. Even if you're born with an immune system that doesn't work as well as it should, this part explains why, the implications of the defects, and how best to optimize function. This is where you find out that you can always do something to increase function and stay healthy.

Chapter 3

Strengthening Your Allergy Defense System

In This Chapter

▶ Understanding what allergic rhinitis is and how to manage it

▶ Clearing the air and treating asthma

▶ Recognizing eczema and soothing your skin

▶ Knowing the difference between food allergies and food sensitivities

*I*n some people, the usual response of the immune system when it meets certain antigens is to get a bit overexcited, and the response triggers physical symptoms that can be irritating, alarming, and downright disturbing — sometimes even fatal. After some of these responses get hard-wired into your response system, they can't really be changed, but they can be modified and managed to reduce symptoms and to keep you safer.

Allergies and asthma are becoming more prevalent in society in part due to the increasingly artificial environment in which people live. Natural environments are less bothersome to your immune system, but human-made fabrics, highly processed foods, recirculated air, and other things surprise and confuse your natural defenses. This chapter looks at ways you can modify your environment and minimize allergy and asthma triggers to reduce your overactive responses. We also guide you through common diagnosis and treatment methods.

Of course, eating the immune-boosting diet we suggest throughout this book is an essential part of keeping your immune system ready to help you out when needed.

Battling Sneezes, Sniffles, and Itchy Eyes

Hay fever actually doesn't involve either hay or a fever, so the more accurate term is *allergic rhinitis*. Allergic rhinitis has a genetic component and occurs as an IgE-mediated response. Because IgE antibodies (long-lasting antibodies that cause a histamine-based reaction) last forever, when a person develops this allergic reaction, he'll likely have this allergy for life. (See Chapter 2 for details about different kinds of antibodies and how they act.)

Typical allergic rhinitis symptoms include sneezes, sniffles, runny nose, and itchy, watery eyes, and perhaps a cough. These symptoms can be irritating and disruptive, but if you look at what's really happening, it makes perfect sense. Your body is simply trying to get rid of the allergen. Because the allergen is inhaled, it gets trapped in the lining of the nasal passage, so the body tries desperately to flush it out. What better way to do that than to increase fluid production and cause sneezing (so you blow it out)?

In the following sections, we dig deeper into what allergic rhinitis is, what causes it, how to diagnosis it, and how to treat it.

Getting to the root of the allergic reaction

Why some people are prone to allergic rhinitis and others aren't is unclear, but we know that genetics come into play because it tends to run in families. Exposure to certain substances in utero or early in life can possibly put someone at increased risk of allergic rhinitis. Some chemicals in the environment, like ragweed and mold, are just inherently more prone to trigger a reaction, so if you live near these things, your body is more likely to respond.

In susceptible individuals, a specific IgE to a specific allergen gets produced and coats the surface of mast cells that live in the mucosal lining of the nose. When that individual is exposed to the allergen again, it triggers the mast cells to initially produce histamine, kinins, heparin, and other chemicals. Secondarily, the mast cells produce inflammatory products, such as prostaglandins and leukotrienes. These chemicals cause dilation of blood vessels, production of mucus, and stimulation of sensory nerves — hence the typical symptoms of swollen eyes, sneezing, runny nose, postnasal drip, itchy eyes, and scratchy throat. All these symptoms are referred to as the *early phase response*.

Over several hours, the immune system calls other cells to action, including eosinophils, lymphocytes, and macrophages. The actions of these cells lead to what are called *late phase reactions,* which are also inflammatory in nature.

They look a lot like the early phase but are more about congestion and swelling and less about itchiness and sneezing (because no histamine is involved).

The local reaction in the nasal passages and sinuses can lead to more systemic reactions, such as fatigue, malaise, and sleepiness. The lack of fever is one of the main ways to distinguish the allergic response from an infectious rhinitis found in colds and flu.

Pinpointing causes of allergic rhinitis

What causes allergic rhinitis? The answer comes from one of two categories: seasonal allergens and year-round allergens. As we explore further in the next sections, *seasonal allergens* primarily include pollen from trees, weeds, and grasses, while *year-round allergens* include dust mites, mold, and other allergens found in the home or workplace. Pets are also a pretty common cause of year-round allergic rhinitis. Of course, some people are affected by both seasonal and year-round allergens, so they should consider that possibility when searching for causes of allergic rhinitis.

Seasonal allergens

The presence of pollen from trees, weeds, and grasses varies both seasonally and geographically. Unfortunately, you can't simply move and get away from all allergens, because virtually every place on earth contains some form of common allergen; for example, ragweed is found in all 50 states of the United States, including Alaska and Hawaii. You can, however, check a few resources, such as the following, to find out what grows in your area and when to expect it:

✔ www.pollen.com/allergy-weather-forecast.asp

✔ www.webmd.com/allergies/healthtool-pollen-counter-calculator

Year-round allergens

Year-round allergens can be difficult to determine and even harder to avoid. The most common indoor source of problems is dust mites. They feed on organic matter, such as dead skin cells from both humans and pets. They're commonly found in carpets, bedding, curtains, upholstered furniture, and stuffed toys around the house. Pet dander is also a common cause of year-round symptoms, although it may be a source of only intermittent symptoms if you're exposed to an animal that you're not usually around. Cockroach infestation is a very common source of allergens, leading to both asthma symptoms and allergic rhinitis. Mold in the house, which may not even be apparent to the eye, can cause symptoms and should be searched for and remediated if found.

Diagnosing allergic rhinitis

The presence of allergic rhinitis isn't hard to determine — the clinical symptoms are pretty self-explanatory. However, knowing what the triggers of those symptoms are, which you can determine by various testing methods, may be important. Here are a few common tests that your care provider can administer:

- **Skin testing:** For this test, your doctor places an extract of a common allergen on your skin and then scratches or pricks under the skin with a needle, exposing the skin mast cells to the allergen, and a wheal-and-flare reaction occurs. The central area becomes infiltrated with cells and fluid, causing swelling, and the surrounding area becomes red from vasodilation. The size of the wheal roughly correlates with your sensitivity to the allergen.

- **In vitro testing, such as RAST:** RAST testing uses a blood sample to look for the amount of specific IgEs floating in the bloodstream. With this test, you're able to look for multiple allergens with one blood sample.

- **Total IgE:** Total IgE can be drawn as a blood test as well. The total IgE is higher in people who have allergic rhinitis, but this number doesn't really tell you much. Your total IgE can't tell you what you're specifically sensitive to or how much of a problem it is, so the test isn't very helpful.

- **Blood eosinophil count:** Blood eosinophil count is a measurement routinely done during a CBC (complete blood count). It's elevated in people who have allergic rhinitis, especially during the time of year they have the most symptoms, but again, it isn't specific. Sometimes, it can help determine whether rhinitis symptoms are from allergies or something else (such as infectious causes), but otherwise, it isn't of much value.

- **ELISA/act testing:** ELISA/act testing looks for activated lymphocytes in the bloodstream. This testing looks for delayed sensitivity rather than just the immediate sensitivity markers found in RAST testing. Although it's somewhat controversial and often not used in conventional medical offices, ELISA/act testing can be helpful in determining causes of immune response when they aren't obvious.

Testing isn't completely without incident. Rarely, people develop a severe reaction to skin testing. Some practitioners prefer introducing the allergen deeper into the dermis. Although this technique is more sensitive than prick testing, it should be done only by trained specialists. It also can have high false positive and false negative results, meaning it can look like you're sensitive when you're not, or it can miss things you really are sensitive to. This is also an issue with RAST testing.

Allergy-friendly dogs

If you're a pet lover, don't worry: Plenty of dogs are low allergen. Here's a partial list:

- ✔ Airedale terrier
- ✔ American hairless terrier
- ✔ Basenji
- ✔ Bedlington terrier
- ✔ Bichon frisé
- ✔ Cairn terrier
- ✔ Chinese crested
- ✔ Fox terrier (wire)
- ✔ Havanese
- ✔ Irish water spaniel
- ✔ Kerry blue terrier
- ✔ Lhasa apso
- ✔ Maltese
- ✔ Poodles and poodle hybrids
- ✔ Portuguese water dogs
- ✔ Schnauzers
- ✔ Shih Tzu
- ✔ Soft-coated wheaten terrier
- ✔ Yorkshire terrier

Using conventional medicine treatment for allergies

Avoidance is actually a pretty smart way to start treatment for allergic rhinitis — if you're not around an allergen, you won't react to it. For seasonal allergies, this means staying indoors when possible during high pollen days (usually hot, dry, and windy days). For year-round allergies, this could mean using air filters and purifiers in the home, especially in the bedroom because you spend more time there. Wash bed linens in hot water to kill dust mites, and consider purchasing impermeable mattress and pillow covers to reduce exposure. Either replace carpets with hard flooring or vacuum them frequently, and use blinds instead of drapes or at least clean fabric drapes as often as possible. Of course, to avoid pet dander, you have to either not keep pets or have pets with low or no dander production (see the nearby sidebar "Allergy-friendly dogs").

Typical medications given for allergies include the following:

- ✔ **Antihistamines:** These meds stop histamine production and its symptoms. Over-the-counter options include older meds such as Benadryl and Tavist, which can cause drowsiness, and newer options like Claritin, Zyrtec, and others, which are less sedating. Prescription options tend to last longer and include drugs like Clarinex.

✔ **Decongestants:** These options treat the swelling and include Sudafed, Actifed, and others. Use these meds for only a few days at a time; otherwise, they can cause rebound swelling and make matters worse. Also, some contain pseudoephedrine, which can raise blood pressure.

✔ **Nasal corticosteroids:** Sprays such as these stop the inflammation, so they reduce symptoms, such as itchy eyes, runny nose, and sneezing. Common examples are Flonase, Nasonex, and Nasocort.

✔ **Leukotriene modifiers:** Because leukotrienes are inflammatory mediators, blocking their production also decreases itchy eyes, runny nose, and sneezing. Leukotriene modifiers don't cause drowsiness, and you need to use them only once a day. Options include Singulair and Accolate.

✔ **Cromolyn sodium:** This older, over-the-counter medication prevents the release of histamine. It's best to take this med before symptoms even start (even if you've just been exposed or expect to be exposed to something you know you're allergic to).

✔ **Nasal atropine:** Atropine causes constriction of blood vessels, so it's useful in stopping severe runny noses. Contraindications include glaucoma or an enlarged prostate.

Also known as *desensitization* or *allergy shots,* immunotherapy treatment consists of injection of high-dose allergens to block the allergic response. Although it's been shown to be about 80 to 90 percent successful for some allergens, it requires up to three to five years of treatment to get relief. Immunotherapy can be associated with severe systemic reactions in some cases and should, therefore, be considered only if medical treatment is ineffective.

Choosing natural medicine treatment for allergies

Sometimes avoiding allergens simply isn't possible. So one way to physically remove allergens from the system without using medication is to do nasal irrigation, best done via a neti pot. This ancient practice consists of using a small vessel the shape of a watering can (without the handle) to instill a mild salt solution — using filtered water only, not tap water — into one nostril, letting it flow back through the nasal passage and through the sinuses and then drain out the other nostril. Although this process can feel pretty strange the first time you do it, it's very effective. We think it's more effective than some of the more recent squeeze syringe devices that require you to blow all the fluid back out — which is much less efficient and can leave fluid trapped in pockets of your sinus cavity, increasing the chance of infection.

Allergic to this? Avoid that!

Many common sources of pollen have cross-reactivity with specific foods. So if you know you need to avoid a certain kind of pollen, you should also be careful about the corresponding food item. Here are a few that go together:

✔ Ragweed: Melon, cucumber, banana, apple

✔ Birch trees: Apple, stone fruit (peach, plum, cherry, apricot)

✔ Mugwort: Celery, carrot

✔ Grasses: Potato, tomato

Many natural substances have the same activity as some of the pharmaceutical agents we mention in the previous section. They include the following:

✔ **Antihistamines:** Butterbur *(Petasites hybridus)* has been shown to both stop histamine production and modulate leukotriene production. Butterbur contains chemicals called pyrrolizidine alkaloids that can be toxic to the liver and kidneys; these chemicals are removed from the extract and should be marked as *free of pyrrolizidine alkaloids* on the bottle. If it doesn't have this phrase, don't use that particular product.

Interestingly, butterbur is from the ragweed family, so if you know you're allergic to ragweed, don't use this remedy. Stinging Nettle also has antihistamine activity and can be taken as an herb or harvested and eaten as a green, like spinach.

✔ **Leukotriene modulators:** Quercitin, a flavonoid found in brightly colored produce as well as onions and garlic, has been shown to slow leukotriene production as well as prevent production of histamine. It's fairly short acting, and some products require use several times a day.

✔ **Anti-inflammatories:** Omega-3 fatty acids are essential fatty acids, meaning you must get them in your food; among other activities, they stop inflammation by halting prostaglandin and leukotriene production. The active forms of omega-3s are EPA and DHA, which are found only in animals (best source is cold-water fish). Plant sources of omega-3s include flax, walnuts, and others. Unfortunately, humans don't do a very good job of converting plant omega-3s to the active form, so consider taking fish oil even if you eat a lot of flax and walnuts. Carotenoids, the pigments that turn foods bright colors, are also anti-inflammatory, so if you're prone to allergic rhinitis, the brighter your diet, the better.

Catching Your Breath Again: Asthma

Asthma is a common condition that causes wheezing, coughing, and shortness of breath; it's inflammatory in nature and is primarily caused by allergic triggers. Although asthma usually consists of a genetic component, environment also plays a big role.

The hygiene hypothesis of asthma suggests that the increased incidence in recent years is from not enough exposure to different allergens early on; kids in large families or going to day care as infants tend to have a lower incidence of asthma. Early use of antibiotics is also correlated with development of asthma, likely from changes in gut flora (see Chapter 2 for details). Likewise, infants born by Cesarean section are also at risk for asthma, due to changes in gut flora development (they don't pick up the same bacteria from their mother that children born vaginally do). A strong correlation also exists with maternal smoking during pregnancy and continued exposure to smoke after birth, even if no one smokes in the house directly. Individuals with allergies and atopic conditions have a much stronger chance of developing asthma.

Common triggers for asthma are similar to the triggers for allergic rhinitis — animal dander, cockroaches, and dust mites. Asthma is also commonly triggered by exercise and emotionally stressful situations. Environmental pollutants, such as volatile organic compounds (VOCs) and phthalates, have also been linked to increased asthma risk.

In the following sections, we discuss how doctors diagnose asthma and the different methods for treating it.

Diagnosing asthma

Practitioners diagnose asthma based primarily on clinical symptoms of characteristic breath sounds heard on auscultation of the lungs (when they listen with a stethoscope) as well as spirometry, which measures air flow, lung capacity, and airway resistance. The diagnosis can be confirmed when someone responds well to treatment.

Using conventional medical treatment for asthma

Obviously, one way to treat asthma is to stay away from triggers, which can usually be easily avoided after you've identified them. However, conventional healthcare practitioners also rely on two forms of medication: control drugs, such as corticosteroids, beta-agonists, and leukotriene inhibitors, and "rescue" drugs, such as bronchodilators and oral corticosteroids. Most of these medications are given as inhalers.

Choosing natural medicine treatments for asthma

A more natural way to head off an impending attack is to use lobelia, or Indian tobacco *(Lobelia inflate),* mixed with capsicum (cayenne pepper) in a three-to-one ratio. Take 20 drops of the mixture in water at the beginning of an attack and repeat every 30 minutes as needed up to three to four total doses.

For long-term control of symptoms, a high enough intake of essential fatty acids is, well, essential! Omega-3 fatty acids found in cold-water fish and fish oil capsules have been shown to lower the incidence of asthma attacks in chronic disease. Gamma linoleic acid (GLA), found in borage oil and evening primrose oil, is also helpful. (If you're taking large doses of fish oil, more than 3 to 4 grams daily, you must also take additional GLA to keep the anti-inflammatory profile of the oils in the appropriate ratio.)

One other herb has also been shown to be beneficial: butterbur (sold in the United States usually under the name Petadolex). As we mention in the earlier section "Choosing natural medicine treatment for allergies," butterbur isn't only an anti-inflammatory but also a smooth muscle relaxer. Routine use of the herb has been shown to decrease asthma attack frequency and severity.

Another smooth muscle relaxer is magnesium. Although it's a common mineral, many people are deficient. The usual daily dosage is 200 to 400 mg.

Soothing Scaly, Itchy Skin: Eczema

Eczema (also known as *atopic dermatitis*) is a common skin condition caused by an allergic hypersensitivity reaction. Basically, the immune system thinks there's an invader, so it revs up activity, but it only serves to cause inflammation and irritation for no good reason! It occurs most often in individuals who have other allergic sensitivity, but it isn't the same as *contact dermatitis* (where you get an allergic reaction only when your skin comes in direct contact with something). Various things make it worse: a flare of allergic rhinitis, cold and dry weather in the winter, strong emotions, and overexposure to water, to name a few.

The rash that occurs tends to happen most often in children, even as young as 2 to 6 months. It tends to appear on the neck, hands, and feet, often preceded by severe itching. Other related symptoms include blisters; dry skin with bumps on the backs of the arms and thighs; ear itching, discharge, and bleeding; skin color change; and thickened, scaly patches of skin.

In the following sections, we explain how eczema is diagnosed and the best forms of treatment.

Diagnosing eczema

No true test exists for diagnosing eczema other than physical exam and history. In cases where some question remains as to whether it's eczema or something else, doctors may choose to do a skin biopsy. The main point is to keep it in mind, especially if other issues with allergic reactions are present.

Using conventional medical treatment for eczema

Conventional practitioners usually focus on keeping the skin moist and treating the itching. Therefore, they prescribe either topical corticosteroid creams or emollient creams to prevent dryness. Long-term use of corticosteroid creams can lead to thinning (atrophy) of the skin, as well as bacterial or fungal skin infections. If needed on the face, be sure to use only mild steroids for brief periods of time, because scarring can occur from atrophy.

Another option is topical immunosuppressants, such as pimecrolimus (Eladil and Douglin) and tacrolimus (Protopic). Although these drugs can be effective, they can lead to increased risk of cancer because they "squash" immune function rather than simply modulate it.

In cases that don't respond to other treatments, you can use oral immuno-suppressant drugs, such as cyclosporine and methotrexate; however, they carry quite a few risks as well and should be used only if absolutely necessary.

Choosing natural medical treatment for eczema

Prevention of eczema may be possible with the use of probiotics. When pregnant women whose infants are at risk of developing eczema take probiotics and then those infants continue to receive the same probiotics after birth, the incidence of eczema is much less than otherwise expected. People who've already developed eczema can also use probiotics, but they really only help individuals with food allergies (see the section "Treating food sensitivities," later in this chapter).

The most commonly used probiotic is *Lactobacillus GG.* Other strains include *Lactobacillus fermentum VRI-033 PCC, Lactobacillus rhamnosus, Lactobacillus reuteri,* and *Bifidobacteria lactis.* The prebiotic *galacto-oligosaccharides* have also been used. These compounds are found in human milk and some vegetables, which serve to help beneficial bacteria thrive. It also helps explain why breastfeeding can be so beneficial to the development of a healthy immune system in a newborn.

Here are a few other natural remedies for eczema:

- ✔ *Gamma linoleic acid,* an essential fatty acid, can help prevent eczema outbreaks. This fatty acid helps modulate inflammation and has a nourishing effect on skin, hair, and nails. It's found in borage oil, evening primrose oil, and black currant seed oil. It works slowly and may take several months to really make a difference, so be patient!

- ✔ Topical use of licorice root gel has been shown to help reduce inflammation and itching; in some studies, it performed better than hydrocortisone cream. A 2 percent gel is more effective than a 1 percent gel; essentially no side effects occur (though if there's a great deal of absorption systemically, it can raise blood pressure, so be sure to watch for that). Licorice is known to affect stress hormone levels, which is likely the mode of action on eczema.

- ✔ Chlorine can aggravate eczema, so using a chlorine filter for the shower is a good idea. Also avoiding highly chlorinated pools or at least rinsing off right away can help.

- ✔ Because food allergies are often — though not always — associated with eczema, newly diagnosed individuals should be tested for food allergies. If any issues are discovered, avoiding those foods appropriately can lead to limited eczema flares. And eating immune-boosting foods, such as the ones we discuss in Chapters 8 and 9, will help.

Distinguishing between Food Allergies and Food Sensitivities

Two forms of food allergies exist: immediate/acute and delayed. Then you have the issue of food intolerance (or sensitivity), which isn't really a true allergy at all. Determining whether you have an immediate food allergy is pretty easy, but the delayed type of reaction is much sneakier. We explain both types, as well as the difference between a food allergy and sensitivity, and effective methods of treatment in the following sections.

Immediate/Acute food allergies

The immediate/acute allergy is the "classic" food allergy, where you experience a rash, swelling, hives, or trouble breathing after eating a food. In these cases, your body has responded to a protein in the food, creating an IgE antibody to it. After you eat the food, your body reacts to the IgE-coated particle by creating histamine, which causes the typical rash, hives, itching, swelling, and difficulty breathing. (See Chapter 2 for details on how this reaction works.)

Some foods have proteins that don't break down completely with digestion. These foods are the most likely to trigger allergic reactions. And, just as with all other allergies and atopic conditions, your genetics affect whether you have a food allergy. Also, because IgE antibodies last forever, after your body has created them, you never get rid of them. So when you've developed a true hypersensitivity reaction to a food, you'll always have a problem with it. Having food allergies is much more common if you also have other immune-related conditions, such as asthma and allergic rhinitis (see related sections earlier in this chapter for more info).

The signs and symptoms of an IgE-mediated food allergy include hives, itching of the mouth, eyes, nose, and swelling of those areas. You can also have difficulty swallowing, a hoarse voice, and wheezing. All these symptoms develop in less than an hour or so of eating the food. Nausea and vomiting can also occur within about two hours.

We dig deeper into diagnosing and treating food allergies in the following sections.

Diagnosing food allergies

Just as with allergic rhinitis, skin testing and blood testing can determine IgE food allergies. (See the section "Diagnosing allergic rhinitis," earlier in this chapter, for details about these types of tests.) Usually people already know what foods give them rashes, but sometimes the testing can help them know in advance what foods may cause a problem so they can avoid them.

Treating food allergies the conventional way

Prevention is always the easiest thing to do here — simply avoid the foods that cause trouble! Because the immune system will always respond with a histamine reaction, eating these foods isn't safe.

Sometimes, though, you're surprised — you never expected your food allergen to be in what you just ate. Under those circumstances, epinephrine (in the form of a self-administered dose called an EpiPen) can block the allergic reaction most of the time. Because using epinephrine causes significant short-term side effects, such as heart racing, sweating, and anxiety, some people try to avoid using an EpiPen if possible. You can sometimes use oral antihistamines, such as Benadryl, to block smaller reactions. In severe reactions, you may need to use oral corticosteroids after epinephrine initially begins to work.

Taking the natural approach to treatment

You can follow all the natural approaches we mention in the "Choosing natural medicine treatment for allergies" section, earlier in this chapter, to treat food allergies. Of note is that if a family history of food allergies exists, breastfeeding an infant for at least four months drastically lowers the incidence of food allergies. Another treatment is the homeopathic remedy *Apis,* which almost always helps with the rash and hives.

Delayed food-allergy reactions and food sensitivities

Delayed food allergies are much harder to diagnose than the IgE-mediated (immediate/acute) ones. The problem here is that the reaction is slower and lasts longer, mediated by IgG antibodies. These antibodies may not show up for several days, and the allergic reaction can last for several days. The symptoms can vary from fatigue to diarrhea and bloating, from foggy headedness to muscle pain. Also, these reactions tend to occur to just about anything you eat, and because the symptons take a while to show up and last a long time, putting your finger on the culprit is difficult.

Unlike the immediate/acute allergies, delayed allergies aren't necessarily for life. IgG antibodies last for only about three months. However, if the IgG is made in response to a food you eat frequently, your body makes more antibodies each day, so the symptoms never get a chance to resolve on their own.

Leaky gut syndrome commonly describes these delayed allergies, or food sensitivities. If inflammation, chronic use of antibiotics or steroids, or high levels of stress hormones damage the lining of the gut wall, food particles can pass between cells rather than through them on the way to the bloodstream. Then, because the gut is lined with pockets of immune complexes that notice that a three amino acid chain, for instance, is going by rather than a single amino acid, in response, it sounds the alarm by creating IgG antibodies to that food. The resulting condition leads to bloating and pain after eating, constipation or diarrhea, or intermittent urge to defecate followed by mashed-potato consistency stools.

In the following sections, we describe the process of diagnosing food sensitivities and how to go about treating them.

Diagnosing food sensitivities

If the symptoms fit, only two good ways exist for diagnosing this condition: a food elimination diet or testing for IgG antibodies in the blood:

- ✔ A food elimination diet consists of avoiding the most common allergens (cow's milk, gluten, eggs, peanuts, soy, and so on) for several weeks. When all the symptoms have resolved, you add each food into your diet one by one, waiting several days between each food to see whether symptoms return. If they do, that food is a problem and you should avoid it for at least four to six months to give the IgG antibodies time to die off.

- ✔ Testing for IgG antibodies in the blood can be especially helpful when you have multiple foods that are a potential problem (or when the elimination diet results are difficult to interpret). However, a good deal of cross-reactivity occurs on these tests, so false positives and false negatives are fairly common.

Treating food sensitivities

After you've discovered and eliminated the offending foods, you can use anti-inflammatory supplements (such as fish oils, turmeric, and rosemary) and healing nutrients (like glutamine) to help the gut heal from all the inflammation, allowing the tight connections between cells to get reestablished. Vitamins A and D are essential to the appropriate function of the immune system at this level, so adequate intake of these vitamins is important. Zinc and magnesium are also important in this healing response. Probiotics are necessary to reestablish the normal gut flora, which is usually compromised in light of significant inflammation. Olive leaf extract is a good healing herb for the gut wall, as is oregano. Use these until the gut is healed and symptoms resolved.

Because high-stress hormone levels are commonly associated with gut wall damage, leading to IgG-mediated food sensitivities, some form of stress management, as we discuss in Chapter 11, is essential to truly heal the gut wall. To help support efforts of stress management, you can use herbal adaptogens, such as holy basil, rhodiola, and ashwaganda. These herbs have the ability to help normalize the stress response and modulate the amount of inflammation produced by stressful situations.

Chapter 4

Autoimmune Disorders: Dealing with an Overactive Immune System

....

....

*M*ost of the time, the immune system does a pretty good job recognizing what is you and what isn't. However, because your T cells are constantly making different antibodies as quickly as they can, sometimes they make antibodies to you, not an invader. These antibodies and the T cells that made them are supposed to be destroyed, but sometimes that doesn't happen. When the antibodies persist, they can cause disease.

Autoimmune disorders can manifest anywhere in the body. More than 80 conditions are thought to be caused by autoantibodies; they may look dissimilar on the surface, but the same inflammatory process occurs in each. How to modify that process to avoid further damage to normal tissue is the key to managing an autoimmune condition.

In this chapter, we explore different autoimmune disorders, how they occur, why certain people develop them and others don't, and how to treat them.

Getting to the Root of a Confused Immune System

Why some people develop autoimmune disorders and others don't isn't entirely clear. It's been shown that most people have some degree of autoimmunity — that is, their body *occasionally* makes antibodies to stuff that is actually them and not an invader. However, in most people, that never gets out of control and actually causes disease. In the following sections, we look at contributing factors, such as genetic predisposition, gender, the environment, and immune dysregulation, to understand why some people develop autoimmune conditions.

Uncovering a genetic predisposition

Finding clusters of different autoimmune diseases within a family is common; one person may have rheumatoid arthritis while another family member has Hashimoto's thyroiditis and yet another develops lupus. Although they have separate diseases, they all stem from the same confused autoimmune system dysfunction.

A classification system of genes called HLA (human leukocyte antigen) is a gene type that only humans have. Different versions of these HLA genes exist, and people with a predisposition to developing autoimmune disorders tend to have certain ones. If you're concerned about your own risk, you can ask your care provider to test you for these HLA markers. Having that HLA type doesn't mean you necessarily *will* develop the condition, but it shows you have increased risk. Doctors can use this information, for example, to help family members of an individual with celiac disease determine their own risk prior to ever developing symptoms.

If you have increased risk based on HLA typing, you can use nutritional and supplemental interventions to modify the immune response to avoid damage to organs. HLA typing can also help make a diagnosis, if needed, as well as inform you of other conditions you may be prone to, once a diagnosis of a particular disease has been made.

Weighing the impact of gender

Most autoimmune disorders occur much more often in women than in men. The range can be from 2:1 to as much as 10:1 (see the female to male ratios of autoimmune diseases in Table 4-1). Studies show that although women are diagnosed more frequently, the disease progression is usually worse in men with the same disease. The reason is unclear, though women tend to have a more robust immune system than men in general. See the later section "Estrogen: A Hormone, a Helper, and a Potential Time Bomb" to understand the impact of estrogen and its metabolism.

Table 4-1   Female to Male Ratios in Autoimmune Diseases

Autoimmune Disease	Female to Male Ratio
Hashimoto's thyroiditis	10:1
Systemic lupus erythematosus	9:1
Sjögren's syndrome	9:1
Secondary antiphospholipid syndrome	9:1
Primary biliary cirrhosis	9:1
Autoimmune hepatitis	8:1
Graves' disease	7:1
Scleroderma	3:1
Rheumatoid arthritis	2.5:1
Primary antiphospholipid syndrome	2:1
Autoimmune thrombocytopenic purpura (ITP)	2:1
Multiple sclerosis	2:1
Myasthenia gravis	2:1

Factoring in the environment

Although the underlying cause of autoimmune diseases isn't entirely clear, evidence suggests that any change to the DNA in the cells can cause that cell to look foreign, triggering the immune system to respond. Many environmental toxins are known to damage DNA, and studies show that regular exposure to these toxins is associated with a higher incidence of autoimmunity. Chapter 5 has more information about environmental toxins, such as mercury and PCBs. Some medications also damage DNA; several drugs, such as procainamide and hydralazine, are known to both damage DNA and induce a lupus-like illness in some people, even those with no genetic predisposition!

Specific viruses, bacteria, and even parasites are also associated with stimulation of the immune system to produce autoantibodies. Studies have shown increased autoantibodies (not causing any damage; just present in the system) in spouses and pets of individuals with lupus, which implies that people may be exposed to a common exposure or infectious agent, but only one person gets the disease.

Blaming immune dysregulation: Imbalance of Th1 and Th2

As we discuss in Chapter 2, the interaction between the Th1 and Th2 mucosal immune systems controls the balance between the innate and acquired immune functions. It's generally believed that a Th1 dominant state leads to *systemic* inflammatory diseases, such as lupus, and a Th2 dominant state leads to a *tissue specific* disorder, such as Hashimoto's thyroiditis. In the long run, though, knowing which of the two is out of balance may be less important than simply knowing how the imbalance impacts the body and how to resolve the imbalance. The balance can vary over time, leading to small flares of symptoms of a different autoimmune disease in someone with a known condition. For example, in someone with Hashimoto's, although the majority of autoantibodies are to the thyroid, if a fluctuation occurs in Th1/Th2 balance, that person may feel neurologic symptoms consistent with multiple sclerosis or some other autoimmune disorder for a short period of time.

When the immune system is turned on to make autoantibodies, the process also causes inflammatory cytokines to be produced, as we discuss in Chapter 2. These cytokines can cause damage to skeletal muscle, leading to significant changes in body composition in people with autoimmune disorders. With less skeletal muscle, more fat tends to exist; this fat is also inflammatory, which leads to continuation of the inflammatory processes started by the immune system.

Contributing Factors Essential to the Autoimmune System

In an autoimmune disorder, the body gets a signal that the immune system recognizes as foreign, resulting in the release of chemicals triggering a cascade of inflammation. The details of this pathway are important to know so you can take steps to prevent progression all along the way. We outline these details in the following sections.

NF-kB

NF-kB stands for *nuclear factor kappa beta,* which is a protein that acts as a transcription factor. In other words, its job is to make your DNA produce specific proteins. NF-kB usually floats around in the cell attached to another protein that keeps it from being active; a Th1/Th2 imbalance causes the NF-kB to detach from this protein, replicate, and move into the nucleus of the cell. In the nucleus, it binds to specific places on the chromosomes and causes them to produce inflammatory mediators, such as prostaglandins and leukotrienes. The activation of these inflammatory mediators leads to a release of catabolic cytokines, inflammatory chemicals that lead to the loss of skeletal muscle. Because this whole pathway is dependent on activation of NF-kB, slowing that activation down is one way to decrease damage to tissue in those with autoimmune disorders.

Inflammatory cytokines

Inflammatory cytokines are produced as part of the pathway described in the previous section. They include TNF-alpha and the many interleukins. Their job is to cause inflammation and damage to the cell that they believe to be foreign. As part of the normal immune response to bacteria or other invaders, the inflammation takes on the form of fevers, aches, and pains, even that moodiness and whininess that some people show when they're sick (caused by inflammation in the brain, changing how they feel!). This response shows that the cytokines can cross into the brain, where they cause inflammation. If this inflammatory response is part of the autoimmune process, that inflammation can actually cause damage to brain cells. In fact, some studies question whether Alzheimer's and other dementias are actually autoimmune in nature.

Free radicals

Free radicals are molecules that have been oxidized, causing them to become unstable and react with other chemicals nearby. In the body, free radicals cause damage to tissue. During the autoimmune process, when T cells attack cells that they think are damaged, free radicals are produced from the inflammatory cytokines mentioned in the previous section. These free radicals then damage more cells nearby, causing change to the DNA of both the cell itself and the mitochondria in it. This damage leads to more cells looking foreign, which perpetuates the inflammatory cycle.

So a cycle is set up as follows: The immune system reacts to damaged cells that no longer are identified as you, causing NF-kB to be produced, which causes inflammatory cytokines to be produced, which induce free radicals, which cause more cells to have damaged DNA. These cells are recognized as not you and the process continues. In the usual immune response to a viral or bacterial infection, a limited amount of foreign matter is present, so the process eventually comes to a close. Here, because your own cells are being damaged, the process can continue for a long time, because there isn't really a limit to the amount of damaged cells.

Cortisol and the stress response

Cortisol is the main stress hormone produced as part of the fight or flight response. Its job is to send blood to the brain and to muscles to think fast and either stand and fight or run away. *Stress* is a non-specific response of the body to any demand. Small amounts of stress can be a good thing; they're what keep you motivated to improve performance at work or with sports. However, large amounts of unrelenting stress can overwhelm the system. Studies show that prolonged cortisol elevation has a negative effect on the immune system and contributes to production of inflammatory cytokines. Control of this response leads to improvement of autoimmune conditions and lessening of cellular damage. See Chapter 3 for more information on stress and how it contributes to immune function.

5-MTHF

5-MTHF stands for *5-methyltetrahydrofolic acid,* which is folic acid (a B vitamin) with a methyl group attached. *Methyl groups* are chemicals that attach to DNA to protect areas of the protein from damage. If cells don't have enough methyl groups, areas of the DNA become under-methylated. If cells have under-methylated DNA areas, they'll appear to be abnormal and not you, which can trigger an immune response. Under-methylation can occur as a response to specific drugs and environmental toxins. It also can occur when individuals don't have the genetic ability to attach methyl groups correctly (true of a whopping 30 percent of the population!). Not all people who are poor methylators develop an autoimmune condition, but it's probably a contributing factor for disease development in a lot of individuals.

High dose folic acid or 5-MTHF can increase methylation in the cells. If methylation isn't occurring correctly, it shows up in the blood as an elevated homocysteine level. To check your own status requires a simple test. If the homocysteine is high, taking a supplement of folic acid or 5-MTHF can lower damage to the DNA of the cells.

Pinpointing Dietary Influences on Autoimmune Conditions

What you eat changes how your immune system works. We go into detail in Chapters 8 and 9 about specifically what to eat, but in terms of keeping the immune system from creating autoantibodies, some specific nutrients are important to keep in mind.

In the following sections, we cover how specific dietary components impact the autoimmune system, from the amount of animal protein you eat to the amount of omega-3 fatty acids you consume.

Lower arachidonic acid

Arachidonic acid is a fatty acid found primarily in animal sources, like fish, eggs, beef, and other meats. As part of a chain of fatty acids, it leads to the production of inflammatory prostacyclins and prostaglandins. Studies have shown that lowering the amount of arachidonic acid in the diet improves clinical signs of inflammation in those with rheumatoid arthritis and augments the beneficial effect of fish oil in these individuals. We're not saying that everyone needs to be a vegan, but watching your total intake of this fatty acid is important. Small amounts of meat at any one time is fine; large amounts, especially if you have a deficit of other fatty acids, leads to increased inflammation and continuation of the autoimmune cascade. Think of it this way: Eating a serving of 3 to 4 ounces of steak at one time is fine, but eating a 28-ounce steak all by yourself in one sitting is a recipe for inflammation!

Higher omega-3 intake

Omega-3 fatty acids are fats that make up your cell membranes; you can't make them yourself, so getting them from your diet is essential. Omega-3 fatty acids are a type of polyunsaturated fatty acid and come from fish, flax, walnuts, and almonds, among other foods.

Omega-6 fatty acids are more common in the diet and compete with the omega-3s, moving into place in cell membranes and chemical reactions where the fats act. Omega-6s are found in corn, safflower, sunflower, and soybean oils. Optimal ratio of omega-3 to omega-6 fatty acids is 1:1, but in North America, the ratio most commonly is skewed far in favor of omega-6s.

Omega-3s, especially the long chain EPA and DHA found in fish, have been shown to be anti-inflammatory and specifically modify the immune system. They appear to suppress cell-mediated immunity and specifically block the proinflammatory cytokine IL-1, which is responsible for the inflammation associated with several autoimmune conditions, including rheumatoid arthritis, lupus, and Crohn's, among others. You can get EPA and DHA from plant foods as well, but that source is inefficient, so we suggest that you not rely on them and get your omega-3s from either eating fish or taking a supplement.

Vitamin D

Vitamin D is actually misnamed. It has such broad effects that it should really have been named a hormone, not a vitamin. Among many other places in the body that it effects, it directly impacts the immune system. Vitamin D has been shown to lower production of select inflammatory cytokines, it decreases B cell proliferation, and it improves regulatory T cell production and activity, all which help blunt the autoimmune response.

In North America, vitamin D deficiency is common. Vitamin D has to either come from food or get produced in the body by sun exposure and its effect of acting on a precursor molecule in the skin. People don't commonly get vitamin D from food sources (fish and sea vegetables, primarily), and production in the skin from sun exposure is limited due to not going outside without sunscreen very often. Some data shows that in more northern latitudes, the rays of sun hit the skin in an angle that doesn't create optimal vitamin D amounts, so even if you're outside, the skin conversion is really inefficient.

Gluten

Gluten is a protein found in some grains, including wheat, barley, spelt, and kamut. Over the past 50 to 60 years, wheat has been hybridized to make it a more efficient food source; unfortunately, in making these changes to the plant, the gluten proteins changed significantly. (For example, did you know that wheat isn't 8 feet tall anymore? Through the hybridization process, it's now only 2 feet tall! So much for "amber waves of grain.") Now, it's common for individuals to become sensitive to the gluten proteins and develop inflammatory responses. See the next section on gut inflammation for more details.

Gluten has been shown to cause inflammatory reactions in the gut wall, which can trigger specific inflammatory cytokines and lead to cell damage. Many studies have shown that removing gluten from the diet of those with autoimmune disorders leads to reduced symptoms of disease and damage. Although you can be tested for celiac disease — an autoimmune gut condition responsive to gluten — the testing can be deceiving. You can also be tested for the genetic HLA markers associated with celiac disease, which can be helpful, but those same HLA markers are also found in many individuals who haven't developed celiac disease.

Our suggestion: If in doubt, get gluten out of your diet!

What Do You Mean My Gut Is Involved?

Most of your immune system is in the gut wall, because that is where the body most often encounters something that isn't you. The GALT (*gut associated lymphatic tissue;* see Chapter 2 for details) is the primary responder among all the different major parts of your immune system. It's also the place where many mistakes can be made in terms of confusing you and not you. In the next sections, we tell you how to increase gut permeability and antibody formation as well as how to fix your gut to improve your immune system.

Developing increased gut permeability and antibody formation

The gut is basically just a big tube that runs through you and is where your immune system has to figure out which abnormal bacteria to fight and which helpful bacteria to leave alone. The lining of the gut wall has tiny, fingerlike projections called *villi,* which is where absorption of nutrients takes place. If these villi get damaged, nutrients aren't taken in correctly; some larger, not yet fully broken down molecules can slip between cells and into your bloodstream. All along the gut wall is the GALT, patches of lymphoid tissue that watch what nutrients are coming through. If anything abnormal gets in, an immune response and inflammation occurs. This inflammation, though essential to fighting off the invader, also can increase the damage to the villi themselves, which can actually lead to more abnormal absorption of molecules. This process leads to what is commonly referred to as *leaky gut syndrome* or *irritable bowel syndrome.*

Gut wall villi can be damaged in a number of ways, including long-term use of steroids, multiple rounds of antibiotics (due to loss of normal bacteria from the antibiotics), and long-term use of nonsteroidal anti-inflammatory agents or aspirin, among other drugs. Improper nutrition can also lead to abnormal bacterial population of the gut, which increases the chance of villous damage. When this process of increased gut permeability begins, the immune system produces IgG antibodies to the molecules it sees, which means that pretty much any food eaten can become the cause of antibody production. If that food continues to be eaten, more and more antibodies will be produced, causing not only continued inflammation in the gut and loss of normal function (leading to gas, bloating, diarrhea, or constipation) but also continued stimulation of the immune system in general and autoantibody production specifically.

A good example of this cycle is the correlation of celiac disease and the development of autoimmune conditions. *Celiac disease* is a genetic condition in which individuals can't tolerate the protein gluten found in wheat, barley, and other grains. Continued exposure to gluten in these individuals increases the incidence of autoimmune diseases; if they stop eating wheat early after their diagnosis, they tend to not make autoantibodies and, therefore, don't develop any other illness or damage to their tissues.

It has also been shown that when abnormal bacteria develop in the gut of individuals with rheumatoid arthritis, another autoimmune condition, they tend to have a flare up of inflammation and a worsening of their illness. Normalization of the gut bacteria leads to improvement in symptoms.

The good news is that the antibodies that the gut makes tend to be IgG antibodies. As we discuss in Chapter 3, these antibodies don't live forever. They tend to die off after about three months, unlike IgE and IgA antibodies. So eliminating foods that are causing the reaction stops further antibody production, and after a time, the immune system calms down and further exacerbation of the autoimmune process also stops.

Fixing your gut to fix your immune system

When the gut is inflamed, the immune system gets the wrong signals and furthers the autoimmune process. Healing the gut wall and reducing inflammation leads to decreased autoimmune response and fewer symptoms of disease. You can take a few fairly easy steps to heal the gut, but do them in the right order for best effectiveness: removal, replacement, reinnoculation, and repair.

Remove

Of course, no process can stop easily if the reason it got started is still present! So first order of business is to remove offending agents that triggered the inflammation. These agents may be pathogenic (abnormal) bacteria, antigens from food, or toxic agents. Rarely, abnormal bacteria require antibiotics for full removal, although herbal remedies can also be used. Consult with a professional herbalist or holistic physician for suggestions on which herbs to try.

To determine which foods need to be taken out of the diet, you can either get IgG food allergy testing done (a blood test that's helpful but not foolproof), or you can do an elimination diet.

An *elimination diet* is a carefully constructed way to figure out what food may be causing an immune response. You can do this process in many ways, but the idea is to limit the types of foods eaten for several weeks, waiting for symptoms to normalize. (Usual symptoms of food intolerance are gas, bloating, diarrhea, constipation, and urgency to defecate.) When these symptoms have been gone for at least a week, you add back each restricted food one at a time, waiting several days to see whether symptoms return. If they do, this food was one of the reasons for the immune response, and it's again restricted from the diet for at least six months. You then carefully add each food back one at a time, looking for return of symptoms. In this way, the offending agents become clear.

Foods to restrict vary, but the most common offenders to focus on include gluten, corn, soy, dairy, most nuts, oranges, and all processed foods (to avoid food colorings, additives, thickening agents, and such, because they are common offenders as well).

During the reintroduction phase, sometimes GI symptoms return. If this happens, plan on restricting these foods indefinitely. This occurrence is fairly uncommon, unless the gut wall hasn't been properly healed with proper herbs, vitamins, and nutritional counseling administered by a knowledgeable healthcare practitioner.

Replace

After offending agents have been removed, it may be necessary to replace either a normal stomach pH (by simply drinking water with lemon) or pancreatic enzymes (common nutritional supplements) to achieve adequate digestion of food. This step is important because either of these processes can be disrupted by the inflammation of the immune process; without appropriate stomach pH and enzyme activity, large food particles make it out of the stomach, and the small intestine won't be able to process such big particles correctly. The result is abnormal bacterial overgrowth, which is one of the things that caused a problem in the first place!

Reinnoculate

During the course of gut inflammation, normal bowel bacterial flora becomes disrupted, which you can restore with prebiotics and probiotics. *Prebiotics* are foods and nutrients that normal bacteria use as fuel. The compounds involved, fructans, arabinogalactans, and fructooligosaccharides, are found in many kinds of produce, including greens, legumes, and some fruits. *Probiotics* (helpful bacteria) are found in fermented foods, including yogurt, kefir, and natural (unpasteurized) fermented vegetables, such as sauerkraut. See Chapter 19 for how to make your own kefir and kombucha, a fermented tea. You can also take probiotics in the form of supplement capsules or powders.

Repair

After you've removed the offending agents, supplemented the digestive process as needed, and restored the normal bacterial balance, the gut wall inflammation needs to be healed. Many nutrient supplements have the capacity to stimulate this healing. Most commonly used include L-glutamine, L-arginine, omega-3 fatty acids EPA and DHA, zinc, vitamin E, and aloe vera. These agents have all been shown to stimulate healing of the gut mucosa or act as anti-inflammatory agents, or both.

64 **Part II: What Happens When Your Immune System Gets Off Track**

Curcumin, ginger, rosemary, peppermint, plantain, and fish oils also have been shown to specifically affect the activity of GALT in a positive way. See details in the section "Nutrigenomics: Using Food Nutrients to Modify Autoimmunity Specifically," later in this chapter.

Estrogen: A Hormone, a Helper, and a Potential Time Bomb

Most autoimmune disorders occur in women more often than men (refer to Table 4-1). Sex hormones play an important role as modulators of auto-immunity. Estrogens enhance humoral immunity. Androgens (testosterone, DHEA, androstendione), progesterone, and cortisol act as immunosuppressors. Many autoimmune disorders have their onset at a time of hormonal change — puberty, pregnancy, and perimenopause — so an imbalance in these hormones likely helps trigger the immune change. In the following sections, we focus on estrogen and its effect on autoimmune disorders.

Influencing estrogen breakdown products

After estrogen has done its activity in the body, it goes to the liver for processing. Estrogens are broken down in the liver in two phases to make them water-soluble and able to be eliminated in either urine or feces. The same processes that break down estrogen also break down toxic chemicals. (We've always found it fascinating that our bodies handle toxins and estrogen the same way, as though the body thinks estrogen is toxic. Wonder why?)

The elimination happens in two stages: First, estrogens become either 2-hydroxyestrone, or 16-hydroxyestrone, or 4-hydroxyestrone, which simply means that a chemical group called a *hydroxyl compound* gets to put on the number 2 or 16 or 4 carbon. All these chemicals are still active, and the 16- and 4-hydroxyestrones are fairly inflammatory. They specifically increase the production of NF-kB-mediated production of inflammatory cytokines (see discussion in Chapter 2). In studies of patients with lupus and rheumatoid arthritis, the activity of 16- and 4-hydroxyestrone was much greater than controls, in both men and women, regardless of the overall estrogen level.

To some extent, which of these breakdown products you make the most is genetically predetermined, but the pathways can be influenced by nutrient intake. In animal studies, agents that block the effects of estrogen and its breakdown products have been shown to decrease symptoms of autoimmune diseases. It's also clear from studies that estrogen-to-androgen hormone ratios tend to be out of balance when there's the most autoimmune activity.

Processing chemicals and estrogens in the liver

The liver is the biggest processor of chemicals in your body. Situated on the upper right-hand side of the abdomen, tucked under the ribs, the liver has a large blood supply that feeds it blood from all over the body. Carried in this blood are all the chemicals your body has made or absorbed; many of them are detoxified by chemical reactions in the liver cells. The plan is to turn these chemicals into benign, water-soluble chemicals that can be passed into the stool or urine for elimination.

The detoxification process occurs via two main steps. The first group of chemical reactions produce metabolites that are still generally pretty active and only partially water-soluble; the second group of reactions finishes the job. Both sets of processes need to be working optimally to get the job done. See Chapter 12 for further information on this process and how to expand and enhance it in general.

When it comes to estrogens, the liver's ability to process them can greatly change how the body expresses autoimmunity. As we mention earlier in this chapter, several chemicals and drugs have the potential to trigger a lupus-like illness. This doesn't happen in everyone who takes the drugs but is likely related to how well the individuals process the drug and get it out of their bodies. If they do a quick, clean job, no illness — otherwise, it can trigger inflammation and illness.

Many people with autoimmune conditions need to take pain medication and anti-inflammatory drugs. All of these are processed by the same liver enzymes. So if a perimenopausal woman with unbalanced estrogen and progesterone happens to also have lupus and needs to take ibuprofen for pain, imagine all the work the poor liver is asked to take care of! No wonder it doesn't always work so well.

Modifying liver activity and the amount of estrogen to process

To help the liver do its job correctly and efficiently, a number of simple dietary interventions work. First, getting enough B vitamins, vitamin A, flavonoids, and appropriate phospholipids help the first step in liver detoxification. The second step of the pathway is spurred along with glutamine, methionine, and specific amino acids. See Chapter 12 for details about what foods contain these chemicals and what exactly they do.

You can also take pretty simple steps to modify estrogen production and breakdown. Indole-3-carbinole (found in broccoli, cauliflower, and their relatives), along with flax, help direct estrogen breakdown toward safer breakdown products. Magnesium helps the final pathway in estrogen breakdown, as does stress management. With better stress management, fewer methyl groups are being syphoned off to make stress hormones and more are available to finish breaking down the estrogen. See Chapters 11 and 21 for more information.

You can also work toward avoiding an estrogen imbalance in the first place so that less is needed to break down. Eating a high glycemic index diet (and therefore letting your blood sugar go too high) leads to the production of more insulin to keep the glucose in check. Insulin stimulates the enzyme that makes estrogen and also decreases the protein in the blood that binds up and regulates the activity of estrogen. So eating sugars and starches raises the blood sugar level, which causes more insulin production. This high insulin level leads to more estrogen production directly and also due to less of it being bound on the regulator protein.

On top of this, excess body fat produces more estrogen (it can convert other hormones into estrogen within the fat cells themselves). Excess insulin causes more body fat, which leads to more estrogen. So maintaining an appropriate weight (and appropriate fat-to-muscle ratio, which doesn't always mean the same thing!) is important for those with autoimmune conditions. Appropriate movement and exercise maintains muscle mass, so the fat-to-muscle ratio will stay normal. Stress management is also helpful here; long-term stress leads to increased inflammation that directly breaks down muscle.

Mercury and How It Wreaks Havoc on the Immune System

Mercury is a metal that used to be in thermometers; now, exposure is primarily through eating certain fish contaminated with mercury as well as through old dental amalgams containing mercury. Studies in both animals and humans have shown significant changes in the immune system from chronic, low-level exposure to mercury. Primarily, lymphocytes get stimulated to produce antibodies. In human studies of women with mercury exposure, the higher levels of mercury were correlated with the highest levels of thyroglobulin antibody, found in autoimmune thyroiditis. In a study of Brazilian miners exposed to mercury, a significant amount of autoimmunity existed compared to the general population.

So higher levels of mercury lead to increased levels of antinuclear, antithyroid, and other autoimmune antibodies by stimulating T cells inappropriately, especially in folks with a genetic predisposition to autoimmune disease.

You can handle your exposure to mercury by cutting back on mercury-heavy fish, having dental work redone to remove mercury, and getting your mercury levels tested, all of which we discuss in the following sections.

Scaling back on mercury-heavy fish

The most common exposure to mercury is through eating certain kinds of fish. Large, bottom-feeding fish, such as tile fish, shark, swordfish, and tuna, have the most mercury. You should limit these in your diet. Smaller fish and those from unpolluted fresh water, such as anchovies, sardines, haddock, and salmon, have much less mercury and can be enjoyed without much concern. Pregnant women and small children need to be especially careful about the type and amount of fish they consume, because the effect of mercury on the fetus and small children is much more powerful than in adults.

Dealing with mercury in dental work

The other main exposure to mercury many of us have is via dental amalgams, the combination of metals including mercury that were put into cavities in the past. If you have fillings that once looked shiny and now look gray or black, that's an amalgam. Whether the simple presence of an amalgam is problematic is controversial. If it's not that old (less than 15 years or so) and the tooth containing it doesn't appear loose or cracked, the amalgam may not need to be removed. However, if the tooth has a crack in it or if it's loose and you've just been diagnosed with an autoimmune disorder, it may be time to have the amalgam removed.

Almost every dentist is knowledgeable about the issues around mercury toxicity. That, unfortunately, doesn't mean that all dentists know how to remove it carefully. Here are appropriate ways dentists should deal with mercury toxicity from an amalgam:

- ✔ Use a dental dam, which traps the mercury as it's removed.
- ✔ Use suction because mercury is a vapor at room temperature, and the rate of vaporization increases as the amalgam is drilled out.

✔ Talk to you ahead of time about using a chelating agent to remove any mercury that does escape into the bloodstream. Chelating agents can include something as simple as cilantro or chlorella extracts, which escort the mercury out of the body when they encounter it in the blood.

✔ Replace the filling with porcelain or composites that don't contain metal.

✔ Don't suggest removing all your fillings at once, just in case (don't want to overwhelm the system, after all!).

Ask dentists specific questions about training in mercury removal. Being listed on a website doesn't necessarily prove they know anything; some websites are more about marketing than they are about expertise. Also, be sure they follow the guidelines in this section.

Testing for mercury toxicity

If there's concern for mercury toxicity, you can get testing done. Blood testing for mercury isn't helpful because it tells you only what you've been exposed to recently. The body tries to move mercury out of the bloodstream as quickly as possible, putting it into fat, nails, hair, and other organs where it causes less trouble than in the bloodstream. Hair analysis is often used to evaluate mercury levels; it's really only helpful in diagnosing long-term exposure and may give confusing results because hair can get contaminated from chemicals found in shampoos and personal care products.

Urine testing done after provocation with a small dose of a chelating agent gives the best results. A chelating agent, such as DMSA, is a chemical that binds to heavy metals, allowing them to be excreted by the urine along with the DMSA. If you take a small dose of this chemical and a urine test reveals a higher than normal amount of mercury, it's clear that the tissues are contaminated. At this point, you can undergo full chelation with the same or a similar chelating agent. Be sure to seek guidance of a qualified holistic care provider.

Nutrigenomics: Using Food Nutrients to Modify Autoimmunity Specifically

Nutrigenomics is the study of how foods and nutrients interact with gene expression. A wide range of gene expression exists in humans, with varying predisposition to diseases and other conditions. Having a gene doesn't mean that the gene necessarily gets expressed. Nutrigenomics looks to see how different foods modify that expression. It's possible to create diets appropriate for each person, aimed at modifying genes such that diseases are avoided or ameliorated with food, not drugs.

Throughout this book, we talk about ways you can boost immune system function with food and nutrients. We'd much rather have you use food than take a handful of pills every day, even if those pills are supplements and not pharmaceuticals. In this section, though, we refer specifically to what works if autoimmunity is a problem. Some overlap occurs with overall immune-boosting efforts, so you can explore chapters in Part III for specific foods and Part IV for recipes that help bring the whole picture together.

Caffeine

Specific chemicals called *protein kinases* modulate how the autoimmune process proceeds in any individual. These protein kinases are found in excess during an inflammatory flare up of an autoimmune disease. Caffeine and theophylline, both found in coffee and tea (black, green, or white), have been shown to be weak inhibitors of one of the most common protein kinases associated with autoimmunity. So feel free to drink a cup or so a day to help keep things in check.

Hops-derived compounds

Hops, the grain from which beer is made, contains chemicals called *reduced iso-alpha acids,* which have been shown to calm down the kinase pathway and slow down inflammation. They appear to specifically block the activity of NF-kB. In this instance, taking the compound as a supplement is best; just drinking a beer hasn't been shown to work (and the alcohol in it is known to be inflammatory anyway!).

Omega-3 fatty acids

We talk about fish oil in various places throughout this book. If you want a healthy immune system, you need to get adequate omega-3s. Eating fish several times a week is a good idea, as long as it's low in mercury; supplementing as well gives you good insurance that your intake is enough.

Omega-3 fatty acids have been shown to modulate the inflammatory process by blocking COX 2, a proinflammatory precursor to prostaglandins that is itself inflammatory. Omega-3s also promote production of anti-inflammatory prostaglandins. Studies have shown specific symptom reduction in a number of autoimmune conditions, including lupus and rheumatoid arthritis, when folks are given omega-3 supplementation.

Curcumin and rosemary

The herbs curcumin and rosemary are generally helpful as anti-inflammatories and immune boosters. They also block the production of COX 2 and help modify protein kinase production. The recipe chapters in Part IV offer several ways to add these herbs into your diet with ease.

Selenium and zinc

Adequate selenium and zinc work together to modify the kinase pathway and calm the inflammatory response. Lack of selenium is associated with increased activity of NF-kB and increased levels of COX 2. Zinc works together with selenium, modulating its activity and improving its performance. In studies, those with the highest selenium levels had the least amount of autoimmune symptoms.

Selenium is fairly easy to get in the diet. Three Brazil nuts a day will get you all the selenium you need. Taking excess amounts hasn't been shown to improve autoimmunity, so no need to take a supplement if you have adequate nut and seed intake.

Vitamin D

Food sources of vitamin D are a bit limited: primarily some fish, eggs (the whole thing, because it's in the yolk!), beef liver, and some cheeses. Other foods that are available have been fortified with vitamin D, but we recommend that you eat whole, unprocessed foods whenever possible. Sea vegetables also contain small amounts of vitamin D, so seaweeds are a good addition to the diet as well (think sushi and seaweed salad). See the prior discussion of vitamin D in the section "Pinpointing Dietary Influences on Autoimmune Conditions," earlier in this chapter.

Considering Specific Autoimmune Conditions

There are many autoimmune conditions, too many to go into in depth individually. In this chapter, we discuss these conditions as a whole, laying out what they have in common. This section focuses on two specific autoimmune disorders — rheumatoid arthritis and autoimmune thyroiditis — because they're the most common, and they often appear in conjunction with other disorders.

Rheumatoid arthritis

Rheumatoid arthritis (RA) is a chronic, systemic, autoimmune condition that generally causes inflammation of the *synovium,* the lining of joint capsules. The synovial cells overgrow and create excess fluid in the joint causing swelling and pain. Ultimately, fibrotic tissue forms in the joint, which can cause distortion of the joint by tying down tendons attached to the joint and resulting in twisted, knobby fingers.

In addition to joint disease, the lung can become inflamed, as can the lining around the heart and the white of the eye. Nodules can also form under the skin, generally over an affected joint.

Diagnosis

Because more than one kind of arthritis exists, determining whether the arthritis is autoimmune in nature or simply from overuse is important. Generally speaking, the joints in RA are stiff in the morning and get better with use, the opposite to what is seen in osteoarthritis (OA). Most often, the joints affected by RA are symmetric, meaning it occurs on both sides of the body. Like most autoimmune conditions, RA occurs more often in women than men and is often diagnosed around the time of hormone change (puberty, after pregnancy, menopause).

Often, a good clinical history is all a healthcare provider needs to make a diagnosis, but lab testing can also be helpful. Here are some tests that can shed light on the situation:

- **ANA (antinuclear antibody):** Not specific to RA, ANA can be positive with other autoimmune conditions, such as lupus, scleroderma, or polymyositis. Some folks with RA won't have a positive test.

- **Rheumatoid factor:** Tests the amount of specific antibody to gamma globulin most often seen in RA.

- **HLA typing:** These genetic factors are often seen in those with autoimmune conditions. HLA B27 is often found in Reiter's syndrome, a version of RA that causes inflammation of the joints, eyes, and urethra.

- **Sed rate (ESR, or erythrocyte sedimentation rate):** A marker of inflammation. Can be used both for diagnosis and to mark progression of the disease/improvement from treatment. It's not specific to RA but will be positive in most autoimmune disorders.

- **Joint fluid testing:** Various tests can be done on fluid taken from the painful joint; they can help look for bacterial causes for the inflammation as well.

- **X-rays:** Doctors may order X-rays to determine the extent of tissue and joint damage. Usually, plain X-rays are enough; CT or MRI aren't needed, because the bones are what's important, not the soft tissue around them.

Treatment

Whether a care provider is coming from a conventional medicine mindset or a holistic one, everyone agrees that consistent movement or exercise and an anti-inflammatory diet are essential to managing symptoms. See Chapters 8, 11, and 22 for more information about these lifestyle issues.

- ✔ **Conventional medical treatment:** Generally two categories of pharmaceutical agents are used to treat RA: Disease-modifying antirheumatic drugs (DMARDs) and anti-inflammatory drugs.

    - The DMARDs include methotrexate and leflunomide, which are cytolytic, and remicade, humera, and others, which are TNF blockers. All these drugs can cause serious side effects and require close monitoring. Each of them actively changes how the immune system works, which means they can also lead to increased infections and other immune-related problems.

    - The anti-inflammatory drugs include celebrex, aspirin, and nonsteroidal anti-inflammatories, such as ibuprofen. NSAIDS and aspirin, although not associated with strong side effects, can lead to gastrointestinal bleeding and ulcers as well as potential heart problems. Celebrex, a COX 2 inhibitor, can lead to stroke and heart attack in some people.

    Another type of medication often used for RA patients is an antimalarial called Plaquenil. When used for autoimmune conditions, it interrupts communication within the immune pathways. It's slow acting; results may not be seen for up to six months. Unfortunately, it's also associated with *retinitis* (inflammation of the retina, leading to loss of vision), which isn't always reversed once the drug is stopped.

- ✔ **Holistic medical treatment:** In addition to lifestyle changes, including diet and exercise modification, anti-inflammatory supplements, such as fish, oil, ginger, curcumin, rosemary, and hops extracts, are usually suggested. Vitamin D, vitamin A, and selenium are also used. You can find discussion of these supplements in the "Nutrigenomics: Using Food Nutrients to Modify Autoimmunity Specifically" section, earlier in this chapter.

    Tai Chi, yoga, meditation, and other mind-body practices lead both to symptom control and lowered inflammatory markers in those with RA, likely from the effects these practices have on cortisol levels and other stress hormones.

    Long term, RA can lead to issues with fatigue, insomnia, and malaise. General treatment with acupuncture, hypnotherapy, and aquatic therapy can all be helpful.

Autoimmune thyroiditis

Notice that we haven't labeled this section *Graves' disease* or *Hashimoto's thyroiditis*. Although both are included in this section, it's appropriate to discuss them together because they come from the same disease pathway and often either coexist or the body moves between the two over time. However, most healthcare providers have been taught that the two diseases are separate. But because we know that the autoimmune function is the underlying problem here, fixing that imbalance can fix either or both thyroid conditions.

Graves' disease is the autoimmune condition that leads to hyperthyroidism, or overactive thyroid. *Hashimoto's thyroiditis* is the opposite; it leads to hypothyroidism or underactive thyroid. So how can they occur together or move back and forth?

The underlying problem in autoimmune thyroiditis is with the immune system, not the thyroid. The specific immune problem can be any of the following:

✔ Thyroid stimulating immunoglobulin (TSI) may be formed, which causes overproduction of thyroid hormone.

✔ Thyroid peroxidase antibodies may be produced, which halts the activity of an enzyme needed to make thyroid hormone.

✔ Antithyroglobulin antibodies may be formed, leading to underproduction of thyroid hormone directly.

Symptoms

Many symptoms of either overactive or underactive thyroid are the same: fatigue, insomnia, menstrual irregularity, moodiness, night sweats/hot flashes, muscle pain, difficulty thinking or concentrating, and hair loss. Specific to underactive thyroiditis: weight gain and constipation. Specific to overactive thyroiditis: eye issues, such as irritation and double vision, diarrhea, and tremors. If the two conditions are coexisting, the person can feel symptoms that fit into both categories at the same time.

The immune system can be making antibodies for both Graves' and Hashimoto's at the same time, so don't assume that the diagnosis of one excludes the diagnosis of the other.

Diagnosis

Often, the early symptoms of autoimmune thyroiditis can go unrecognized for years because they're so non-descript. Imagine that you're a typical midlife woman. You feel tired, you aren't sleeping well, you're irritable and moody, your periods aren't as regular as before, and you've gained a little weight. These could easily feel like symptoms of aging or being stressed or being too busy. Many women wait for a long time before seeking help, or even when they do, they're told nothing's wrong.

Specific blood tests can tell you what's going on, but be sure your care provider is drawing the right tests! The full panel measures TSH, free T4, free T3, and the three antibodies (TPO antibodies, TSI, and antithyroglobulin antibodies). Avoid tests such as free thyroxine index, T3 uptake, and the like because they're less accurate. Years ago, no one knew how to measure the levels of the thyroid hormones directly. Once upon a time, we relied just on TSH (thyroid stimulating hormone), which is actually a brain hormone that tells your thyroid what to do. If the thyroid is slacking off, the TSH goes up (basically it yells louder at the thyroid to get to work). If the thyroid is already working overtime, the TSH goes down. The problem with using this test alone is that it isn't always accurate. Just because the TSH is okay doesn't mean the body is actually getting enough thyroid hormone. And, if the TSH is high, it may be just that there's interference from the adrenal (stress) hormones or some other issue.

Treatment

After the diagnosis has been made, treatment of autoimmune thyroiditis from a holistic vantage point is quite different from conventional treatment. Many patients benefit from initially using conventional treatment to stop immediate symptoms, but the reason for antibody production is the focus of holistic therapy. If the antibody production can be slowed or stopped, you may not need medication; it also helps to avoid production of unrelated antibodies and other autoimmune disorders by the revved up immune system.

> ✔ **Conventional medical treatment:** The conventional medical treatment of Hashimoto's aims at restoring appropriate thyroid hormone levels to relieve symptoms. So after testing has been done to rule out thyroid cancer (if nodules are present), a prescription for thyroid hormone is given. This would most commonly be only T4 (levothyroxine, Synthroid); it's given with the assumption that the body will be able to convert it to T3. T4 is also easier to prescribe, because it's slower acting and more predictable than T3.
>
> The conventional treatment for Graves' disease aims at calming down the thyroid hormone production to reduce symptoms and avoid long-term complications from overproduction (heart disease, liver disease, and exophthalmos or "bulging eyeballs"). Options include the following:

- A prescription of a drug that blocks thyroid hormone production, such as propylthiouracil (PTU) or methymazole (Tapazole). The prescriptions may take months to reach peak activity; symptoms will continue until that time.

- Destruction of the thyroid gland with radioactive iodine. The radioactive iodine usually damages the thyroid so much that one becomes underactive and requires thyroid hormone replacement, just like with Hashimoto's.

- Surgery to remove a portion of the thyroid so the remaining portion will be left making just enough hormone and not too much.

Generally, during conventional treatment, measurement of the antibodies involved is no longer done, because it's believed that once the antibody levels have risen, they'll always remain high. Although antibody levels may drop some with treatment, this isn't a treatment goal of the conventional practitioner.

✔ **Holistic medical treatment:** The foundation of holistic treatment is removing inflammation and boosting appropriate immune response. The basics here are simple: stress management, removal of inflammatory foods from the diet, and thyroid-specific nutrient supplementation as well as overall immune modulation.

- **Stress management:** The stress hormones produced by the adrenal glands tend to overstimulate the immune system and, in those with a genetic predisposition, increase the chance of autoantibody production. Therefore, any form of stress management that appeals to the individual should be pursued, be it meditation, yoga, HeartMath techniques, or breathwork; we cover these methods in Chapter 11.

  The adrenal glands tend to respond to emotional states — fear, anger, worry, anxiety — all tell the adrenals they need to stay on. Joy, happiness, appreciation, and gratitude tell the adrenals they're safe, and they can stop hormone production. Calm and peaceful, although better than angry or worried, are likely seen by the adrenals as neutral — not good, not bad, not safe, and not really a problem. Therefore, those emotions aren't usually tied in with normalizing of adrenal function. So shoot for joy and happiness, not just calm and peaceful.

- **Elimination of inflammatory foods:** Inflammatory foods are pretty simple: sugar and sugar substitutes, starches and grains that turn into sugar, food additives, and *excess* animal products. We obviously are okay with eating animal products, but having too much at one time, especially if it's not well balanced with nutrients from plants, is actually just as inflammatory as a lot of sugary junk.

Gluten is especially inflammatory for those with autoimmune thyroiditis. A direct correlation exists between the amount of inflammation produced from gluten in most sensitive individuals and the amount of antibodies and symptoms in those with thyroiditis. So if you have either of these diagnoses, avoid gluten indefinitely.

- **Nutritional supplementation:** Supplements helpful for autoimmune thyroiditis are many of those we've already discussed as being helpful for the immune system in general. Optimization of vitamin D levels (at least 50 to 80 on a blood test) has been associated with fewer autoimmune flares of any kind and thyroiditis in particular. Selenium is important in thyroid hormone production, so either supplementation with selenium at 200 mcg daily or eating three Brazil nuts (they contain this much selenium) will do the trick. Direct supplementation of iodine is controversial; although it's important in thyroid hormone production, direct supplementation can actually lead to severe imbalances. Perhaps a safer way to supplement is seaweed extracts, which include iodine and other minerals helpful in thyroid hormone production.

  Basic anti-inflammatory supplements are also helpful in these situations. Fish oil, curcumin, rosemary, and hops extracts all have a place. The adrenal herbal supplement ashwaganda has been shown to be specifically helpful in those with autoimmune thyroiditis as well. See Chapter 10 for more about herbs for immune balancing.

If caught early enough, it's possible to avoid damage to the thyroid and the need for either suppressive treatment or supplemental thyroid treatment. Management of the disease requires a dance of stress management, appropriate diet, and immune-boosting supplementation. Management of the autoimmune processes can help avoid the development of further autoimmune conditions and the organ damage associated with them, so we feel that focusing on the activity of the *immune system,* not just what the thyroid is doing, is important.

Choosing gluten-free options carefully

If you're going gluten-free, be careful: It's easy to just substitute gluten-free pasta, bread, and muffins for those containing wheat. Not a good idea. All the non-gluten grains have more calories and less fiber than gluten-containing grains, so substituting gluten-free items is a great way to gain weight and actually increase inflammation, and that's what you most definitely don't want to do.

Chapter 5

Cancer: When the Immune System Takes a Vacation

*F*or most people, the word *cancer* is incredibly frightening. When someone hears the words "you have cancer," the healthcare provider may as well stop talking, because that person isn't going to hear anything else for a while. However, the process of cells changing and becoming cancerous is common, and it's something your body can fight off. Most of the time, your immune system weeds out these problematic cells and keeps them from being an issue. But if your system checks out and lets things get out of hand, cancer may be the result.

In this chapter, we explain the process that leads to cancer and what different things slow it down, modify it, or stop it. We also tell you what you can do to help prevent it from happening again. There's always something you can do!

Understanding the Changes in Cells that Lead to Cancer

Ever wonder what cancer actually is and how it got that way? A cancerous tumor occurs when a cell loses the usual control mechanisms regulating cell division and planned cell death. Typically, there's tight control over these two processes; otherwise, your organs wouldn't be able to stay the same size and shape. Most mutations simply change what that cell is capable of doing; only specific mutations within a cell's genes can transform it into a cancer cell.

In the following sections, we break down how cancer develops in your body and how your immune system fights to ward off those cancer cells.

Tracking dangerous cell mutations

Each cell contains tumor suppressor genes and some contain oncogenes. The tumor suppressor genes code for proteins that do just what the name says — suppress tumors. If these genes aren't working, cancer can keep growing unchecked. *Oncogene* refers to genes that, when altered, express proteins that allow cancer to grow.

It usually takes multiple mutations (and a long time) for this whole process to occur. For example, the tumor suppressor gene in one cell may become inactivated, which allows cells to proliferate. Then a DNA repair gene mutates and becomes inactivated, leading to further growth of the abnormal cells. Then another mutation can cause an oncogene to be turned on, which may lead to suppression of even more tumor suppressor genes. So, ultimately, multiple levels of control have gone awry, and a tumor has formed.

So why wouldn't your immune system notice that all this mutation is going on? Well, think of it this way: Macrophages and other immune cells are designed to notice things that aren't you. Bacteria, viruses, and the like look a lot different than your own cells, so immune cells notice them and sound the alarm. Cancer cells, however, don't always look all that different from normal cells in terms of the proteins on the surface, so nothing gets the attention of your macrophages. Think of bacteria and viruses as invading armies from a foreign land, easy to spot because they look different, and think of cancer cells as spies coming to infiltrate the ranks, not easy to spot.

Another control system that the body has is a specific gene in most cells called *P53*. This gene is the "proofreader" in that it proofreads the genetic code of your cells as they grow and divide, helping to weed out those cells that didn't do it right and developed mutations. Often, as a cell becomes cancerous, it's able to suppress this gene. Low vitamin D is also associated with poorly functioning P53 genes. If P53 is working poorly, any mistakes in the genetic code of the cell will get replicated as the cell divides, potentially leading to the growth of a cancer.

Skipping apoptosis: Planned cell death and how it relates to cancer

Your cells aren't supposed to live forever. They wear out and need to be replaced via a process called *apoptosis,* or planned cell death. Triggers from either inside or outside the cell can start the process. External triggers include toxins, hormones, and inflammatory cytokines. Internal triggers tend to occur in the face of a stressor, such as nutrient deficiency, excess heat, viral infection, stress hormones, and lack of oxygen.

When apoptosis is triggered, a huge cascade of reactions occurs in the cell, ultimately leading to degradation of the filaments that hold the cell in its usual shape. The cell membrane breaks down and the cell is divided into small globules that are engulfed by phagocytes. The cellular components are then digested and recycled to make new cells.

If apoptosis is disturbed and doesn't occur, cells become immortal and fail to die. Certain strains of cancers have achieved this state, such as the HeLa strain of cervical cancers, which is used in research. Inhibition of apoptosis also occurs in autoimmune disorders and other inflammatory illnesses; reduced cell death can lead to a cell passing on mistakes in its genetic makeup to its daughter cells (which is how a changed cell can mistakenly be seen as not you by the immune system and trigger an autoimmune response).

Weeding out cancer cells

Normally, the immune system follows several fairly simple steps to weed out cancer cells that it notices. First, when a cancer cell is recognized, natural killer cells, dendritic cells, and macrophages surge into the area and produce IFN gamma, which causes some damage to the cells and initiates the production of *chemokines*. These chemicals have the ability to stop the production of blood vessels, which in a sense smothers the cancer cells by cutting off their oxygen and nutrient supply. At this point, the dendrites engulf the dead tumor cells and other debris and moves them into the lymphatic system for disposal, triggering the differentiation of Th1 cells and the production of CD8 T cells, which are specific tumor-killing cells.

Meanwhile, natural killer cells and macrophages are stimulating each other to get to work by producing IFN gamma and IL-12. These compounds speed up the process of apoptosis and cause damage-producing reactive oxygen species *(free radicals)*. Finally, tumor-specific CD4 and CD8 T cells kill off any cancer cells that they recognize by attaching to them and destroying their cell membranes.

Sometimes, cancer cells survive this process and enter what can be called an *equilibrium phase*. T lymphocytes and IFN gamma continue to work against the cancer cells, but the process of destroying them and the process of their growth pretty much balances out; growth is slowed and kept in check but not completely destroyed. Of course, sometimes the equilibrium phase is short lived and the cancer continues to grow. Other times, the cancer remains in the body in low levels and becomes a chronic condition for people to live with and manage, not something that kills them.

Realizing that even a good immune system can't always keep up

Most people who develop cancer don't have any obvious problem with their immune system. So how does the cancer get started and take over? People are exposed to damaging conditions every day: viruses, ionizing radiation from a medical test, flying in a plane, bacteria in the environment — you name it. Every day, these factors change some cells, which then undergo several mutations. If the immune system notices the changes in time, it disposes of the cell prior to its transformation into a cancer cell.

Unfortunately, sometimes the immune system doesn't have everything it needs to function correctly, so the situation gets out of hand. Occasionally, a genetic problem is to blame; for example, a person with a genetic predisposition to a certain cancer may need even more support for the immune system than average, because their cells tend to mutate more often and faster than usual. The good news is that you can modify much of what triggers the pathways toward cancer by what you eat, what you drink, where you live, and how you handle stress.

Reducing Your Chances of Recurrence after Chemotherapy or Radiation

If you've developed cancer and have been treated successfully, a prime goal may now be to keep your immune system working even better than before. Treatment for cancer in and of itself has the ability to initially worsen the immune response. Most chemotherapy drugs target rapidly dividing cells, which is why they kill cancer cells. Unfortunately, they also kill other rapidly dividing cells, such as those in the bone marrow, leading to decreased numbers of neutrophils. During chemotherapy, people are at higher risk of developing infections; usually between treatments, the bone marrow is able to replenish the stock of neutrophils. Long term, the immune system tends to go back to its baseline ability to function.

Radiation therapy kills cancer cells by damaging their DNA past the point of repair. Unfortunately, normal cells nearby or overlying the area are also exposed and damaged. No long-term damage appears to affect the immune response in people who were treated with radiation, but an increased incidence of secondary cancer can occur from damage to normal cells in the area of treatment; for example, risk of breast cancer increases in someone who was treated for Hodgkin's disease with chest irradiation.

In the following sections, we explain how modifications to diet, stress levels, and your environment can boost your immunity and decrease your chances of recurrence of cancer.

Making dietary interventions specific to cancer

Because each individual is unique, each person gets slightly different nutrients from various foods. One person may not be able to break down and assimilate particular foods as well as the next. Because what nutrients your body takes in from foods is unpredictable, we suggest that you try to focus on whole groups of foods, even entire recipes, instead of homing in on individual foods and specific nutrients themselves. That way, your body will likely absorb more individual nutrients, which will benefit the immune system.

Having said that, knowing what each individual food is good for is important. Use the following list to boost your immune system both during treatment for cancer and afterward to prevent recurrence. This list isn't all inclusive but does highlight those foods that can help the most. Also, see Chapters 8 and 9 for foods that boost immunity in general.

- **Asparagus:** Asparagus is anti-inflammatory, with action similar to a COX-2 inhibitor. It contains lots of vitamins A and K and folic acid, which have all been shown to improve immune function.

- **Basil:** This herb has antimicrobial and antibacterial properties to help fight infections during the time your immune system is weak from treatment. It also has flavonoids that have been shown to help protect normal cells from radiation treatment.

- **Beets:** The red color comes from an antioxidant that fights off free radical damage. The fiber in beets also increases the level of glutathione in cells, which helps produce energy and remove toxins.

- **Bell peppers:** Filled with lycopene, vitamin C, and lots of fiber, peppers have been shown to offer protection against colon, cervical, bladder, prostate, and pancreatic cancers.

- **Cruciferous vegetables:** These vegetables include broccoli, cauliflower, cabbage, and all their relatives. They contain lots of chemicals to help out: *Sulforaphane* slows the growth of leukemia and melanoma, *glucosinolate* inhibits breast cancer growth, and *indole-3-carbinole* helps metabolize estrogen so it doesn't cause trouble.

- **Cranberries:** Cranberries inhibit the growth of liver cancer cells as well as lung, cervical, prostate, and breast cancers.

- **Green tea:** The polyphenols in greet tea inactivate many carcinogens.

  Green tea may block the action of the anticancer drug Velcade, used for multiple myeloma treatment.

- **Lemons (and other citrus):** Filled with vitamin C, citrus also contains compounds, such as limonene, that promote apoptosis and other compounds that likely stop cell division of cancer cells. It's also antimicrobial.

- **Mushrooms:** Any are good, but focus on shiitake, maitake, and reishi in particular. The polysaccharides and lectin help stop cancer cell division. They also appear to boost production of interferon.

- **Onions, leeks, and other alliums:** All the foods in this category, including shallots and garlic, are anti-inflammatory and antibacterial; some help usher carcinogens out of the body quickly.

- **Swiss chard:** This green has it all: fiber, vitamins A and C, and carotenoids, such as beta carotene.

- **Tomatoes:** Tomatoes contains lycopene, which has been shown to reduce risk for pancreas, prostate, breast, and colon cancers. Studies show that eating tomatoes with broccoli has a synergistic effect (and tastes good!).

We could list many other foods here, but we wanted to show that some foods are specifically important for cancer prevention and have actually been shown in clinical trials to be beneficial. Other foods listed in this book are equally important but may not have been studied in cancer specifically.

Managing stress: Cortisol and cancer prevention

Cortisol is the body's main stress hormone. In small amounts, it's a good thing: It helps you get away from the tiger that's chasing you by increasing blood flow to your muscles, it makes you smarter (improves blood flow to the brain), and it gives you a small boost in immune function. It also promotes vasoconstriction, which helps you from bleeding if you get hurt in the supposed battle that cortisol is preparing you for.

However, prolonged, inappropriate levels of cortisol lead to all the wrong responses. In terms of immune function, changes occur on a few levels: Cortisol directly lowers T cell proliferation but doesn't affect natural killer cells. Negative emotional states, which are correlated with elevated cortisol levels, are directly related to a decrease in IgA levels in saliva, which is actually a profound effect: Only five minutes of anger and frustration lead to a blunting of IgA production for up to six hours! Can you imagine what happens to your immune system when you spend eight hours a day at a job you hate or have to live with someone who causes you continued frustration and irritation?

This immunosuppressive effect of cortisol is fairly easy to overcome. You can't eliminate all the stresses in your life, but you can learn to react to them differently. Cortisol goes up with negative emotions; DHEA (which is immunoprotective) goes up with positive emotions. Your emotions are something you can easily control.

You can achieve normalization of cortisol and DHEA levels by practicing techniques created by the Institute of HeartMath (see Chapter 11), an organization that has been looking at the effect of stress and emotional management on human physiology for decades. These techniques vary somewhat among each other, but they have one thing in common: The basis of the techniques is to focus on your heart, breathing as though you're breathing through your heart and feeling some positive emotion by remembering a time when you felt happy, joyous, grateful, or successful. The Institute of HeartMath has a body of research that shows the efficacy of the techniques in lowering cortisol and raising DHEA as well as the physiological consequences of that. Positive emotional states, like care and appreciation, boost the immune system directly, while negative emotional states, like anger, suppress immune function for hours, as Figure 5-1 illustrates.

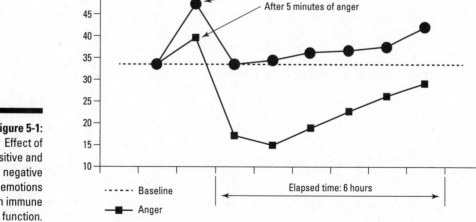

Figure 5-1:
Effect of positive and negative emotions on immune function.

Illustration by Wiley, Composition Services Graphics

Various forms of meditation and breathwork are also valuable in boosting immune function, though they're mostly less studied as to the detailed physiology involved. See Chapter 21 for details.

Cleaning up your environment

A number of environmental issues impact your immune system and its ability to prevent cancer cells from growing. Once you've had cancer, look into cleaning up the stuff around you that may be causing problems! A number of contaminants, such as the ones in the following sections, can potentially cause trouble: protecting yourself from absolutely everything is nearly impossible, so don't go crazy trying. Attend to the most obvious problems in your area and do the best you can.

Heavy metals

Heavy metals, such as lead and mercury, have been shown to change how T lymphocytes do their work. Lead inhibits antigen presentation, thus leading to decreased antibody production. It also switches B lymphocytes from producing IgM and IgG toward production of IgE instead, so the body is more geared toward allergic reaction than cell damage control.

Mercury induces inflammatory cytokines, which can alter the usual cascade of repair mechanisms and lead to cellular damage. It also reduces production of glutathione, which is a necessary component of the cell's detoxification processes. In disturbing these and other pathways in the cell, mercury promotes cell damage that can lead to cancer.

Removing these metals from your environment isn't really all that hard. Lead is mostly found in old paint and outdated plumbing, so simply remove and replace when possible. Mercury is found in fish (essentially all fish have some level of contamination), so be careful how much you eat. Also, avoid eating big fish that are bottom feeders because the mercury gets more concentrated the higher up the food chain you go. Some debate exists as to whether people should remove old mercury amalgams in teeth. If a tooth is cracked around an old filling, definitely repair that, but going in and removing stable amalgams may actually stir up trouble. Definitely discuss this option with a qualified biological dentist, and don't consider it during cancer treatment at all.

PCBs

Polychlorinated biphenyls (PCBs) have been in the news a lot. They make plastics softer and more pliable and were once used in other industrial applications. PCBs have been shown to impact the growth of the thymus in infants exposed either in utero or early in life. They've also shown varying impact on both B cell and T cell function. Although their use is less prevalent now, they unfortunately persist in the environment. Current exposure tends to come from river water, so avoid it (and the fish that grow there). Some plastic water bottles still have PCBs in them as well, so avoid them and never reuse or drink from them after they've had a chance to warm up (like after leaving them in the car on a hot day!).

PAHs

Polycystic aromatic hydrocarbons (PAHs) are found in cigarette smoke, asphalt roads, and vehicle exhaust. They appear to alter antigen receptor signaling pathways, which blunt the usual immune response. They also can lead to increased apoptosis of lymphocytes, making it difficult for the body to maintain adequate forces to avoid cancer overgrowth.

Avoiding these compounds is actually not hard: Don't smoke and avoid those who do. Have someone else change the oil in your car, and don't hang out where you'll be exposed to a lot of exhaust fumes. Make sure your garage is well ventilated, and don't leave the car running inside the garage. Consider using an air purifier if you live or work near a busy street.

Taking Supplements Post-Treatment: Possible Drug Interactions

If you've had cancer, you may still need to take prescription medication long term. Some of these medicines are for long-term treatment or modulation of a cancer that you'll continue to live with, and some are for prevention of recurrence in the future. This section addresses what you need to know about specific nutrients and supplements and how they interact with these drugs, in both good ways and bad. Check with a qualified holistic practitioner about specific dosing for your situation.

Omega-3 fatty acids

These fatty acids interact in a good way! Fish oil has been shown to improve appetite and slow or stop weight loss from chemo and cancer. No change occurs in the efficacy of the chemo drugs, and the proven benefit is lower proinflammatory cytokines and oxidative damage.

Probiotics

Although not a lot of specific studies of probiotics and cancer treatment agents exist, there's no obvious cause for concern of negative interaction. Because antibiotics are often needed for treatment of infections when the immune system is compromised from treatment, using a broad spectrum probiotic both during treatment and long term makes sense. These probiotics help normalize the bowel flora after prolonged antibiotic use.

Vitamin D3

Taking this supplement is a no-brainer. Vitamin D has been shown to boost immune function. People with cancer or a strong family history of cancer need supplementation. Although you should always strive to get adequate nutrients from food when you can, in this case, it's not possible. Get your blood levels drawn and strive for a blood level of 60 to 80 mg/dl, which will likely require daily intake of 5000 IU for quite a while. Just keep checking and adjust as needed.

Vitamin C

Okay, this one is tough. Yes, vitamin C is helpful, but you need to be careful, and be sure to consult your care provider. Usually, vitamin C helps during chemo, but it should be avoided during radiation therapy due to its interaction with free radicals — the substances produced by radiation that make it work! Vitamin C can interact with some chemo drugs, however, so consult with someone experienced in integrative/holistic medicine about your specific situation. IV vitamin C has shown benefit in some situations, but high dose oral vitamin C can also be harmful, especially when not supervised by a knowledgeable care provider. Generalized recommendations really can't be made, because they're so dependent on the individual, the type of cancer, and the chemo or radiation dose involved.

Calcium and magnesium

Not a lot of research exists on the relationship between calcium and chemo drugs or radiation. If you're taking cyclosporine or cisplatin, be careful with magnesium — they can make you lose magnesium quickly and become deficient, so you may need to increase your supplementation levels. Signs of low magnesium include muscle weakness, fatigue, cramps, and constipation. Ask your care provider to check an RBC magnesium level, not a serum magnesium level, because it's far more accurate!

Zinc and selenium

Zinc and radiation — one of those "oh good!" interactions! Zinc helps prevent that horrible taste in your mouth that radiation often produces. Even if your treatment is over, it's not too late to reap the benefits of zinc, so try some now. Be careful to balance it with copper, however, and ask your care provider to check your levels to be sure you're staying balanced between the two.

Selenium is another good thing. It's been shown to help chemo do its job when treating ovarian cancer, probably due to reducing oxidative stress and improving the function of glutathione peroxidase. Food tip: Two to three Brazil nuts each day get you a days' worth of selenium.

Aloe vera

Another good thing to have around during treatment is aloe vera! Aloe is good for healing the mouth and throat ulcers caused by many chemo agents. Use as much as you like of oral aloe in a liquid form; it likely won't interfere with any chemo or radiation. (Aloe is also helpful if you simply get reflux from a change in your gut flora after treatment.)

Astragalus

This herb has traditionally been used in Asia as part of a protocol for cancer treatment. It boosts the production of immune cells from bone marrow, specifically platelets and white blood cells of all forms. Everyone taking chemotherapy and radiation should be taking this herb because these treatments are notorious for dropping counts of these cells. It's also really helpful in chronic viral infections like Hepatitis C or HPV.

Cat's-claw

Cat's-claw is another helpful herb for those undergoing treatment of cancer. Although it's generally thought of as an anti-inflammatory, for use with arthritis and other conditions, cat's-claw has also been shown to repair damaged DNA. Take this herb after chemo or radiation. It's also okay to use during treatment, because it doesn't interfere with the mode of action of these treatments.

Echinacea

Echinacea is a somewhat confusing herb: Although studies show that it works when used correctly (soon after infections begin and in high doses), it has varying results when combined with chemo agents. Use this herb under the supervision of a skilled integrative care provider; it can help potentiate some chemo agents, but it may need long-term administration to improve dampening of bone marrow activity.

Ginseng

Ginseng is a superstar when it comes to chemotherapy. It may decrease drug toxicity and improve efficacy through a variety of pathways. It also has the ability to build up stamina and endurance after treatment as well as avoid the weight loss often seen after treatment. You should definitely use ginseng as pretreatment and along with both chemotherapy and radiation, under appropriate supervision by a trained professional.

Nettle

Traditionally, herbalists use nettle to improve hair growth after the alopecia caused by chemo or radiation. As far as the immune system is concerned, no good studies show that it's beneficial during cancer treatment, but no studies indicate negative effects, either.

St John's wort

St John's wort has a wonderful effect on mood, so taking the supplement when you're dealing with the news that you have cancer may seem logical. Unfortunately, because it has a significant and well-studied effect on liver enzymes that are important to detoxification and metabolism, St John's wort is *very* contraindicated with most chemotherapy agents and even anesthesia, so you shouldn't consider taking it at all during treatment.

After treatment, you may want to take St John's wort to help your immune system and boost your mood.

Viewing Cancer Treatments from around the World

Conventional Western medicine sees cancer in the terms used throughout this chapter: uncontrolled growth of cells caused by changes in DNA structure and the loss of usual control mechanisms. Other healing traditions see cancer differently and view immunity and how to resolve disease from different vantage points. We explore their methods of cancer treatment in the following sections. If you want to use these healing methods, consult a qualified provider who uses quality herbs; some herbs from overseas may be contaminated with heavy metals and drugs.

Traditional Chinese medicine

Traditional Chinese medicine (TCM) sees health as an appropriate balance of opposites: *yin* and *yang, blood* and *qi,* and *jing* and *shen.* All these terms are for energies and fluids in the body, which should flow freely and not be stagnant or deficient. When an imbalance occurs or stagnation happens, a tumor can grow. Interestingly, although Chinese medicine has a concept of tumor, or growth, no concept of cancer per se exists. Also, Chinese medicine doesn't have the concept of immune system as we know it in Western medicine.

Chinese medicine dates back over 3,000 years; the idea of treating tumors is as old as that. During the intervening years, people used Chinese medicine to treat the swelling and inflammation of a mass, improve host defense, potentiate conventional Western cancer therapies, and prevent or control symptoms and side effects of conventional Western treatments.

Many factors can lead to impedance of the flow of *qi* or *blood;* Chinese medicine even sees prolonged emotional states, such as sadness or anger, as potential causes. Traditionally, emotional or physical events are equally important as potential instigating events for disease.

The overall pathway to a tumor growth may look something like this: Stagnation and depletion of *qi, blood,* and *moisture* occurs from some pathologic event, be it physical or emotional. The persistence of deficiency and stasis leads to poor coordination of function within the system of organs, which leads to further weakness, obstruction, and depletion of *essence* (the original source of *qi* and *blood*). Malignancy is seen as highly disordered function. If this process continues, the depletion of *qi, essence,* and *blood* begins to disrupt the balance of *yin* and *yang,* leading to separation of *yin-yang* and chaos. Disorganization of cellular function is the manifestation of this chaos, leading to loss of control over proliferation and differentiation of cells.

In this view, different cancer cell types are caused by varying patterns of phlegm, toxins, deficient *qi* and *blood,* and stagnation of blood. The same kind of cancer Western medicine would diagnose could be caused by several patterns as viewed by a TCM practitioner. Therefore, treatment is tailored to the individual and the patterns expressed instead of using an overall treatment "protocol" for breast cancer, for example. Patterns of acupuncture needle placement as well as herbal formulas are specific to each individual and may even vary slightly among different practitioners based on their own interpretation of the imbalances and stagnation expressed in the patient.

Traditional Chinese medicine sees chemotherapy and radiation as worsening the very underlying cause of the tumor growth in the first place: stagnation and depletion. Chemotherapy is seen as an extreme form of *yin,* a poison that damages the *yang* energy and the ability of *qi* to move *blood* and *moisture.* Radiation is seen as extreme *yang,* heating the body to excess and drying up *yin, blood,* and *moisture.* Just when the body needs the most support in providing *qi* and blood, chemotherapy and radiation undermine that ability. Traditional practitioners focus on restoring balance within the body, allowing for improvement in flow. This focus on restoration of balance can be helpful in enabling patients to tolerate and bounce back from conventional therapies. The following sections cover a couple of specific treatments associated with Chinese medicine.

Acupuncture

Acupuncture has not only been used for pain control and anesthesia but also been well studied for control of nausea and vomiting caused by conventional chemotherapy and surgery. The use of acupuncture has also been shown to improve the suppression of immune cells caused by chemotherapy; white blood cell counts, macrophage activity, and natural killer cells have all shown improvement. Studies in women with hyperplastic nodules in their breast tissue have shown either complete resolution or significant reduction in more than 50 percent of cases. Acupuncture is also very effective in reducing menopause symptoms in women who have been thrown into that hormonal state by chemotherapy or who are experiencing those side effects from tamoxifen, a drug used to prevent recurrence of breast cancer.

Herbs

Herbs aren't traditionally used separately in Chinese medicine but as formulas that may include as many as 20 herbs. These formulas were designed hundreds of years ago and haven't varied much over time. Modern Chinese medicine has a huge number of studies looking at how herbal formulas can be used to help either potentiate conventional Western cancer treatment or help relieve the side effects it produces. Many of these studies are dramatic, showing a doubling of survival rate in those individuals combining the two approaches. The severity of side effects, including bone marrow suppression and nausea, can be greatly reduced with the addition of herbal formulas or medicinal mushrooms, such as maitake. Obviously, this would need to be coordinated by an appropriately trained healthcare provider but can be considered quite safe with essentially no adverse interactions with conventional chemotherapy or radiation protocols.

Ayurveda

Ayurveda is the traditional healing system of India and likely predates even traditional Chinese medicine. Like TCM, ayurveda focuses on promoting good health and long life instead of treatment of disease. It's practiced by both physicians and surgeons and has two ancient main texts, one describing medical management of disease and one describing surgical instruments and procedures.

In this healing system, different stages of tumor development are categorized as

- Chronic inflammatory and intractable diseases with the potential of malignancy
- Precancerous growth/probable malignancy *(granthi)*
- *Arbuda* or definite malignancy

According to ayurveda, cancers arise from lifestyle errors, such as improper choice of food, poor hygiene, or poor behavior, and trauma. These errors lead to imbalances in the three main energies *(doshas)* of the body, *vata, pitta,* and *kapha.* The imbalance then causes disruption in one of six levels of skin as well as the formation of abnormal branches of blood vessels. This physical change then produces either *granthi* or *arbuda.* Both types of swelling can be inflammatory or non-inflammatory, based on the doshas that are disrupted.

The four main foci of treatment of cancer from the ayurvedic approach include

- Health maintenance
- Restoration to normal
- The spiritual approach
- Disease cure

Treatment includes surgical removal of the tumor, herbal remedies, dietary changes, and spiritual treatment (which can include such diverse practices as detoxification, prayer, music therapy, gem therapy, sound therapy, yoga, meditation, and astrology).

The medical management of cancer starts with strong purification techniques, including both internal and external purification, known collectively as *panchakarma chikitsa.* Treatments include oil massage, purgatives, and enemas; modern treatment includes chemotherapy, radiation, and surgery as well. Because one focus is on maintaining the strength of the patient during treatment, practitioners use a milder approach for weaker patients. After completing the purification procedures, practitioners use balancing treatments to rejuvenate the body prior to focusing on treatments aimed at the specific dosha imbalance.

As early as the seventh century, surgery was seen as the first choice for treatment of *arbuda,* because practitioners recognized that herbal treatment was only helpful in the earliest stages of disease. The ancient texts describe multiple surgical techniques as well as postop care for wound healing.

Although specific oncogenes, suppressor genes, and components, such as nuclear factor kappa beta, were obviously not yet recognized, many herbs traditionally used in ayurveda have been shown to target these molecules. For example, *Vinca rosea* is described in ancient texts; it's the plant from which modern vincristine is derived, a common chemotherapy agent. A main difference between conventional Western cancer therapies and ayurvedic herbal medicine is that whole plant extracts are used in ayurveda rather than single chemical entities, which may explain the observation of lesser side effects of ayurvedic treatments, because other compounds in the plant may blunt any unwanted actions of the herbs.

As with traditional Chinese medicine, many ayurvedic herbs have been shown to improve outcomes when used in conjunction with both conventional chemotherapy and radiation. This appears to be primarily from the plant's ability to enhance immune function. Other herbs can minimize side effects of treatment, such as nausea or vomiting and weight loss. The strong focus on rejuvenating therapies, such as yoga postures, breathwork, and sound therapy, have been shown in clinical trials to improve outcomes of conventional Western treatments as well. As is often mentioned, ayurveda is one of the original holistic medicines developed by humankind.

Chapter 6

Immunodeficiency Disorders: When the Immune System Slows Down

• •

In This Chapter

▶ Investigating inherited defects of the immune system

▶ Accounting for acquired defects of the immune system and where they come from

▶ Determining what you can do to treat or modify immunodeficiency conditions

• •

As we discuss throughout this book, the immune system generally works well, kicks into gear when it should, and performs automatically. However, sometimes people are born with a faulty system that never works as it should. Also, some situations can overwhelm the system to the point where it never regains its usual ability to fight for health. We discuss both types of immune system defects in this chapter and explain the best forms of treatment. Most of these conditions are rare, but they can be devastating and require modification to daily living to remain healthy. Chronically impaired or absent immune response leads to frequent, severe infections from otherwise benign bacteria, viruses, or fungi.

Uncovering Inherited Immunodeficiency Disorders

Inherited disorders are present from birth. More than 200 known conditions fit into this category, all of which are fairly rare. The disorders are categorized based on whether they produce impairment of B cells, T cells, complement proteins, or some combination of these.

Many of the inherited immunodeficiency disorders are *X-linked,* meaning the abnormality is found on the X chromosome. Because the disease is manifested with just one abnormal chromosome (and no normal one to function in its place), these conditions occur in men and boys. That explains why more than 60 percent of individuals with inherited immunodeficiency disorders are male.

Problems with B cell production and function are the most common types of inherited immunodeficiency disorder. We explore several congenital immunodeficiency disorders, including how they're diagnosed and treated, in the following sections.

Symptoms of inherited immunodeficiency disorders generally arise in infancy. The most common is severe, recurrent, or hard-to-treat infections. Many of these infants exhibit "failure to thrive," where they grow slowly, have difficulty maintaining appropriate weight, and fail to meet developmental milestones in a timely fashion. Other symptoms of concern are chronically enlarged lymph nodes or spleen as well as recurrent deep abscesses of internal organs. A family history of such immunodeficiency syndromes can help reach a diagnosis.

B cell immunodeficiency syndromes

In some immunodeficiency conditions, only the B cell production or activity is compromised. Some of these conditions are noted at birth; others may not be diagnosed until people are in their 20s or 30s. The following are B cell immunodeficiency syndromes:

- ✔ **Common variable immunodeficiency:** Even though this immunodeficiency is one of the most common conditions, the exact genetic inheritance is still unclear. It affects both males and females and leads to an inability to fight against bacterial and viral infections. Commonly affected areas include lungs, sinuses, ears, and the gastrointestinal system.

- ✔ **Specific Ig deficiency:** Any of the specific antibodies can be affected, such that the body doesn't produce that particular antibody but has normal levels of all the other antibodies. The most common is IgA deficiency. Because IgA is related to mucous membrane infections, these individuals tend to have infections of the mouth, airways, and digestive tract. They may lead fairly healthy lives other than requiring more frequent or longer courses of antibiotics for infections. IgA deficiency is commonly associated with autoimmune conditions, so when an individual is diagnosed with autoimmunity, he'll be screened for IgA deficiency if he has a history of multiple infections.

- ✔ **X-linked agammaglobulinemia:** Individuals with this immunodeficiency are unable to produce a specific protein called *Bruton's tyrosine kinase,* which is needed for B cells to develop properly. Therefore, affected individuals have insufficient B cells to make antibodies of any kind.

✔ **Transient hypogammaglobulinemia of infancy (THI):** All infants are born with antibodies from their mother that function for the first several months of life, while the baby's own system is developing. Usually, these maternal antibodies are gone between 3 and 4 months of life; the baby's own antibody formation may not be completely up-to-speed until 6 months of age. If antibody formation is low beyond 6 months of age and severe infections occur, THI is diagnosed. THI is a self-limiting condition and generally resolves by 2 to 4 years of age. Up until then, the child may need additional antibiotics for infections, though many children do well without a lot of assistance.

T cell immunodeficiency syndromes

In some conditions, the immunodeficiency is limited to T cell production or function, meaning that response to fungal infections are primarily affected. The following are T cell immunodeficiency syndromes:

✔ **Chronic mucocutaneous candidiasis:** In this condition, T cells function poorly or not at all, though the remainder of the immune system functions normally. Yeast infections commonly start in infancy with thrush or chronic diaper rash. Other commonly affected areas include the mouth, nails, skin, or vagina, involving a thick, crusty rash that can ooze and be painful.

✔ **DiGeorge syndrome:** This T cell deficiency occurs due to absence or underdevelopment of the thymus gland. It's a genetic condition associated with abnormalities of other organ systems, such as congenital heart defects, absent or underdeveloped parathyroid glands, and facial abnormalities. Symptoms include low calcium and muscle spasm from the parathyroid abnormality, severe infections due to the immune function issues, and cardiac conditions.

The overall presentation and progression of this disease can vary because T cell function may be severe or simply reduced. Often, the heart defect or facial defects are a larger concern.

Combined B and T cell deficiency

As the name of this section implies, the following conditions affect both B and T cell function or production:

✔ **Ataxia-telangiectasia:** This condition affects several parts of the body, including the immune system. The primary immune dysfunction is poorly functioning B and T cells as well as low levels of IgA and IgE, leading to chronic infections primarily of the respiratory tract and sinuses. Also associated with this condition is an increased risk of certain cancers, including leukemia, lung cancer, and stomach cancer.

Ataxia refers to incoordination, which occurs from an abnormality of the brain's cerebellum. Dilated capillaries, or *telangiectasia,* also develop on ears and eyeballs. The muscle weakness and mental retardation common to this condition steadily progresses with age; the average lifespan of these individuals is only 30 years.

✔ **Severe combined immunodeficiency:** This condition can be caused by several genetic changes; they all lead to absence of T cells and, therefore, the inability of B cells to make antibodies. In essence, no functioning immune system exists. In the past, the best form of preventative treatment was to keep these children in protective, isolated plastic environments, leading to the common term *bubble boy syndrome.*

Common early symptoms are pneumonia, thrush, and diarrhea prior to 6 months of age. The thymus is underdeveloped, and serious infections can develop. If untreated, most infants with this condition die by age 1. Current treatment is bone marrow stem cell transplants; if done by age 3, most children live and do well.

✔ **Wiskott-Aldrich syndrome:** This condition affects only boys. The genetic defect leads to a defective protein that both B and T cells need to function; thus, low antibody levels and poor T cell function occur. In addition, platelets are defective because the spleen destroys them, leading to low platelet counts and bleeding issues.

Infections of the respiratory tract are common, as is eczema. Lymphomas and leukemia are also common in these individuals.

Problems with phagocytosis

If immune cells can't "eat" invaders as usual, the immune response can't move forward the way it normally would. The most common condition arising from this process is *chronic granulomatous disease.* In this condition, the cells can ingest the invading organism but are unable to produce the hydrogen peroxide and superoxide needed to actually kill the invader. Thus, severe infections can occur. Many but not all forms of this disorder are X-linked, so more boys are affected than girls. Lymph nodes become massively enlarged as they fill with white blood cells containing the not-yet-killed organisms; the nodes often drain spontaneously. Over time, granulomas occurs, which is a chronic inflammatory condition that creates firm nodules on the skin. Pneumonia is also common with this condition, especially with the unusual fungus aspergillus.

Problems with complement proteins

Complement proteins are an essential part of the immune system's ability to respond rapidly to an invader. If these proteins aren't made in appropriate amounts or if they function poorly, the overall immune function suffers.

✓ **Hereditary angioedema:** This condition arises from a defect in the gene that codes for C1-inhibitor, resulting in either inadequate amounts of normal protein or normal amounts of nonfunctioning protein. This C1-inhibitor protein regulates a complex interaction of the immune system, blood clotting system, and inflammatory response. Without its action, the imbalance produces peptides that stimulate the capillaries of the vasculature to allow fluid to leak into the space between cells, causing edema (swelling) of the tissue.

When this happens in the throat, airways can be compromised, and it can be fatal. The swelling also commonly occurs in hands, face, and feet; when it occurs in the walls of the intestines, it leads to severe abdominal pain, nausea, and vomiting. Undiagnosed individuals with this condition commonly undergo surgery during an attack because the abdominal pain mimics a "surgical abdomen" and appears to be an emergency, such as appendicitis.

✓ **Specific C protein deficiencies:** Many complement proteins are in the cascade, and a deficiency of any of them affects the immune system response. However, a wide range of responses can occur, depending on the complement protein involved. Most common is an increased incidence of infections, the type depending on which complement protein is missing. Other individuals primarily show rheumatic illnesses similar to lupus, and still others may be completely asymptomatic.

Testing for inherited deficiencies

First, you need an accurate diagnosis. Each condition varies slightly, but overall, the symptoms lead a care provider to look for the answer. If a family history of these illnesses exists, the care provider can search for a carrier. If you're found to be a carrier, a genetic counselor can help you understand your risk with each given pregnancy. When you're pregnant, some of these conditions can be evaluated in either blood, amniotic fluid, or cells from a pregnancy to determine whether that pregnancy is affected. Otherwise, when a baby starts to show signs, blood testing can determine whether the baby has one of these deficiencies.

Many of these conditions can be shown in either direct genetic testing or inferred by levels of immune components in the blood. If a T cell deficiency is suspected, you can also have a skin test done; when the skin is pricked with specific antigens, a reaction should occur — when it doesn't, T cell function is compromised.

Exposing Acquired Immunodeficiency Disorders

Not all immunodeficiency conditions are genetic; some occur as a reaction to certain drugs, infections, or cancers. Acquired conditions can often be temporary or at least more easily treated than genetic conditions. In the following sections, we give you the lowdown on many acquired immunodeficiencies and share different methods of treatment.

Identifying the main culprits leading to deficiency

Acquired immune conditions can be broken down into those arising from drug exposure, infections, and lifestyle issues. Here are the details:

- **Drugs:** Several medications can lead to short- or long-term issues with immune compromise. Some medications, like Imuran, are given specifically to lower immune response in those individuals who have received an organ transplant, in an attempt to avoid rejection of the transplant. These medications are necessary for success of the transplant, but they put these individuals at risk for developing certain infections over time. Corticosteroids, such as prednisone, are used fairly routinely in treatment of infections and allergic reactions. Although they can be lifesaving in situations like acute asthma attacks, corticosteroids suppress immune function over time; avoid long-term use or use when not specifically needed. These drugs are used entirely too often to treat otherwise minor infections, and this use will ultimately lead to poor immune function in these individuals.

  Biologic drugs designed for treatment of autoimmune conditions, such as Remicade and Humira, are successful in treating the autoimmune issues. However, they've been shown to double the chance of long-term immune deficiency and triple the chance of developing certain cancers, such as breast, lung, gastrointestinal, and skin cancers. The manufacturers suggest that the risk/benefit ratio justifies their use, but some patients aren't really aware of the true risk they may be incurring and, at times, these drugs are started earlier than really necessary.

✔ **Infections:** Infection with different organisms can lead to short- or long-term immune deficiency. One of the simplest (and usually only temporary) compromises of the immune system occurs after infection with the Ebstein Barr virus. This virus causes mononucleosis; it infects B cells, which then are attacked by T cells geared toward that virus. Because these B cells are destroyed, a temporary drop in antibody production can lead to impaired immune function. Clinically, this is only a problem if the infection lasts for a prolonged period of time, which isn't often the case.

Worldwide, the most common infectious cause for immune compromise is infection with the human immunodeficiency virus, or HIV. This virus attacks the immune system, leading to permanent compromise of the system in most infected individuals. Once almost uniformly fatal, this disease is now manageable if treated early with an array of immune-modulating drugs. Unfortunately, these drugs are expensive and not always available worldwide.

✔ **Cancer treatment:** During cancer treatment, most patients experience an enormous drop in their immune capacity. Surgery, radiation, and chemotherapy all tend to cause myelosuppression, or a "squashing" of red and white cell production from the bone marrow. This, of course, is a problem both from an overall health standpoint as well as from the standpoint of actually killing the cancer! Medications called *myeloid growth factors* are used to counteract this. They include Neupogen, Neulasta (a longer-acting version of Neupogen), and Leukine. Although they can be helpful in raising immune function, they can also cause significant nausea, vomiting, and fatigue. Once cancer treatment is over, most patients resume normal immune function over time.

✔ **Splenectomy:** Occasionally, the spleen needs to be either partially or completely removed, either as treatment for a disease (such as ITP — idiopathic thrombocytopenic purpura, an autoimmune platelet disorder) or when it's ruptured in an accident or enlarged as a reaction to another condition. Although the spleen isn't a vital organ, removing it does lower the body's ability to fight certain kinds of bacteria and viruses. Therefore, when performing a splenectomy is necessary, the person is usually first given vaccinations against pneumonia and the flu; these vaccinations are also recommended yearly thereafter. Prophylactic antibiotics are also routinely given if any question of exposure to bacteria is present. Most individuals without a spleen do well with just a few precautions, though it's a long-term management issue for them.

✔ **Chronic stress/poor sleep:** Although not technically thought of as a medical condition, chronic stress and poor sleep are perhaps the most common causes of altered immune function in our society, along with poor nutrition. Prolonged, unremitting stress leads to a decrease in antibody production and altered immune function via abnormal cortisol and DHEA levels. Poor sleep, whether hours of insomnia each night or fitful interrupted sleep throughout the night, also leads to lowered antibody production and slow immune response. Sleep is often interrupted due to chronic stress, but it also may be insufficient due to lifestyle choices. Many people think they're "too busy" to get enough sleep at night, or they fall asleep with the TV on, which leads to fitful sleep. Drinking alcohol or taking drugs can also interfere with restful sleep. All these situations are well within an individual's ability to change; see Chapter 11 for details.

✔ **Undernutrition:** We specifically use the term *undernutrition* rather than *malnutrition* because it refers to a broader range of problems with diet. *Malnutrition* refers to more severe nutrient deficiencies, such as may be seen in developing countries during a time of environmental or weather-related disaster. *Undernutrition* refers to those individuals in developed societies who, though they may be adequately fed or even overfed, still lack appropriate nutrition due to poor food choices. This condition is startlingly common, especially in this country. Because junk food is usually less expensive than nutrient-dense foods and because many major cities lack appropriate access to healthy food in poorer neighborhoods, many people keep themselves full with foods lacking appropriate nutrients, like sugary drinks and chips. The lack of vitamins C, A, D, and the B vitamins directly affect immune function. Lack of minerals, such as magnesium, obtained from leafy green vegetables also contributes to immune disruption.

Unfortunately, undernutrition usually leads to insulin resistance and diabetes due to the high sugar content of the foods chosen. Poorly controlled insulin leads to poor wound healing, increased incidence of fungal infections, and more severe bacterial and viral infections. The good news is that it's not only preventable but also easily reversed, given the right lifestyle changes!

Diagnosing acquired deficiencies

Care providers are likely already on the lookout for immune deficiency in some of these situations because they're such a common problem. For instance, white blood cell counts are routinely checked during the course of chemotherapy because low counts are so common and can affect the course of treatment. Any time someone becomes severely ill from a normally minor infection or when someone has repeated infections or requires multiple rounds of antibiotics to clear an infection, the provider becomes suspicious of an immune dysfunction. Also, if certain unusual cancers develop, they can trigger investigation for immune deficiency, as in the case of Kaposi's sarcoma in patients with HIV/AIDS.

Care providers can do laboratory testing in most circumstances to confirm the dysfunction. These tests can range from a simple CBC (complete blood count) to check white blood cell counts to checking complement protein levels and amounts of specific immunoglobulins. Some states push to routinely screen newborns for inherited immunodeficiency with simple blood counts.

Treating Inherited and Acquired Immunodeficiency Conditions

So it's all fine and good to know that a condition exists, but can you do anything about it? Because the inherited conditions are genetic, making them simply "go away" isn't possible, but you can modify their impact on your life.

You can do many things to help lessen the impact of all these deficiencies. For example, avoiding people who are ill and sticking to good personal hygiene (hand washing, keeping your hands away from your face, practicing good dental care) help prevent infections from occurring. Avoiding exposure can also mean drinking only filtered water and never eating uncooked, undercooked, or poorly washed food.

The other strategies we discuss throughout this book are, of course, helpful here as well. Eating well, getting adequate sleep, and exercising are all good ideas to keep the immune system functioning as well as it can. The herbs and supplements we discuss in Chapter 10 are also helpful. However, if someone is incapable of making antibodies on her own or her white cells can't move into the area of an infection, she'll likely need antibiotics, antifungals, and antiviral medications.

We discuss specific treatments for both inherited and acquired immunodeficiency disorders in the following sections.

Nutrition and stress management

No matter which type of immunodeficiency we're talking about, the best way to optimize immune function is to start with good nutrition and stress management. This is just common sense. As we discuss in the "Identifying the main culprits leading to deficiency" section, earlier in this chapter, without healthy food, good sleep, and appropriate response to stress (more balanced adrenal stress hormones), even a *normal* immune system can't function correctly! Logically, if someone is faced with a challenged or compromised immune system, it's even more important to focus on these basics. In the case of an inherited immunodeficiency, the best food in the world won't be able to make B cells work when they simply can't, but the good food *will* be able to help T cells function optimally. It's still worth the trouble!

If poor nutrition is the culprit to start with, cleaning up the diet is essential. Many studies show how improved eating leads to improved insulin control and, therefore, better wound healing, fewer hospital days, and reduced complications of diabetes. Studies done by the Institute of HeartMath and others show how essential stress management can be in improving immune function. Again, even though genetic conditions are causing a portion of the immune system to be nonfunctional, these techniques can improve the function of the immune system that's still operating.

Antibiotics, antifungals, antivirals

As alluded to earlier in the chapter, if portions of the immune system are simply "off line" and unable to work, severe infections can occur. For those individuals, it's imperative to use antibiotics, antifungals, and antivirals as needed to either treat a current condition or prevent a potential infection. Prescription medications can be lifesaving for these folks. Currently, natural medicine approaches don't exist for either treatment or prophylaxis in those with inherited immune deficiencies. In fact, because many natural medicines work to improve your own immune function rather than directly affect the infecting organism, there's a limited number of even potential candidates to study. However, people with many acquired conditions, such as during cancer treatment, can use some herbs and supplements in place of prescriptions. For instance, astragalus, a Chinese herb, is well known to boost killer T cells, prevent low white blood cell counts due to chemotherapy, and decrease infections in people undergoing cancer treatment. See Chapter 5 for what's available and what works.

Interferon

Interferons are naturally occurring substances that fight viruses and stimulate the immune system. Human-made interferon is available for injection and is used as treatment for some of the inherited immune disorders as well as conditions like hepatitis in patients with AIDS. It does have side effects, such as flu-like symptoms, abdominal pain, fatigue, depression, irritability, hair loss, nausea, and vomiting. Individuals must balance the chance of these side effects occurring and their severity with the benefit of the treatment.

Immunoglobulin infusions

Intravenous immunoglobulin infusion (IVIG) is a blood product that contains IgG from more than 1,000 individuals. None of the other immunoglobulins are present. The injection confers passive immunity to the recipient as it increases the amount of antibodies present in the blood. Because IgGs have a fairly short life span, you need this injection every three to four weeks to maintain immunity.

IVIG is primarily used for those with primary immune deficiencies and is safest for those with XLA (X-linked agammaglobulinemia), because they lack antibodies. In other individuals, the antibodies they do have may react with the IVIG and cause anaphylaxis or other immune reactions. IVIG won't protect tissues defended by IgA antibodies (eyes, lungs, gut, and urinary tract) because it doesn't contain IgAs.

Common side effects include headache, peeling skin, and other allergic reactions, including anaphylaxis. The infusions are also sometimes used for treatment of autoimmune conditions; the actual mechanism of action in these cases is unclear. Although IVIG can be lifesaving for some individuals, it's enormously expensive: thousands of dollars per infusion for each individual!

Bone marrow transplant

Because the bone marrow is the site of production of most of the immune cell function in the body, bone marrow transplantation has been done for patients with primary immunodeficiency since the 1960s. The theory is that transplanted bone marrow would "graft" into the recipient's marrow and allow that individual to produce blood products, including immune cells, giving them normal immune response. If a closely matched donor is available (usually a sibling), the success rate is fairly high; less well-matched donors, such as a parent or unrelated donor, can lead to more frequent graft versus host reaction and failure of the transplant.

Typically, prior to bone marrow transplantation for cancer treatment, the recipient's own bone marrow must be destroyed to make room for the donor marrow. During that time, the individual is at high risk of life-threatening infections. In individuals with primary immunodeficiency disorders, some transplantations skip this step, because the recipient has so little functioning bone marrow already. Avoiding the pretreatment destruction of bone marrow increases the success rate of the transplant and helps avoid long-term side effects of that pretreatment (autoimmunity, later cancers, and so on). In some immunodeficiency conditions, pretreatment must be done because the person does have some bone marrow, even though it doesn't function well.

Side effects and long-term issues with bone marrow transplantation include failure of the transplant (the cells don't "take"), failure of a portion of the graft (obtaining T cell function but not B cell function), graft versus host disease, and side effects from pretreatment, including nausea, vomiting, hair loss, and fatigue. The issues in bone marrow transplantation are complex and vary widely with the specific disease, the type of donor available, and the choice of pretreatment used. We don't have the space in this book to go into all the details involved; we encourage you to discuss your own specific condition with an expert in transplantation.

Chapter 7

Uncovering the Influence of Immunity in Other Conditions

In This Chapter

▶ Exploring illnesses associated with chronic inflammation

▶ Looking at what causes IBS, or leaky gut syndrome

▶ Getting to the root of skin conditions

Many of the ways the immune system influences the body don't appear on the surface to have anything to do with the immune cells and systems. In this chapter, we briefly cover a few disease processes to show you how interconnected the immune system really is with the rest of the body. When you understand these connections, it's easier to see how other processes are involved as well.

Chronic Inflammation: From Achy Joints to Alzheimer's

You've heard it before: Most chronic illness is based on chronic inflammation. But what does *chronic inflammation* really mean? And how can achy joints, way out in the periphery of the body, have anything in common with a scary dementia state like Alzheimer's? Or heart disease? Or high cholesterol and high blood pressure? All these conditions share one thing in common: inflammation. Getting to the root of that leads to a better understanding of each disease. We explain these connections and the common causes for chronic inflammation in the following sections.

In other chapters, we discuss common inflammatory pathways in the body: NF-kB, histamine release, prostacyclins and prostaglandins, and cytokines. All of them have connections to the immune system, mostly as either the inciting event or the mediating process. So modifying the immune system's activity to influence the progression of these diseases makes sense.

The inflammatory process

The inflammatory process can start in many ways: activation of macrophages, exposure to antigens, the presence of oxidized LDL (that bad cholesterol) or glycosylated end products, which are proteins with extra glucose molecules attached (from diabetes). No matter what the trigger, a set of common pathways get started, all of which end up producing proinflammatory cytokines.

These molecules end up activating a lot of other cells types, including leukocytes, platelets, and fibroblasts. Activation of the platelets and fibroblasts leads to increased arachidonic acid, which gets converted into prostaglandins, thromboxanes, and leukotrienes. Mast cells and basophils release histamine. The complement system is activated as well. (See Chapter 2 for details of these processes.)

So how does all of this show up in the body? Sensory nerves get overstimulated and create pain. Redness shows up, as does swelling of the area. Leukocytes roll along the surface of the area in question and end up getting stuck in place. All these things lead to increased blood flow to get debris and pathogens out of there. Fluid moving into the space between cells helps dilute toxins and pathogens. The chemicals produced lead to a walling off of the area to limit the spread of the inflammation, and the creation of pain helps activate a withdrawal response in some situations to limit further exposure.

Normally, there's a balance in the immune/inflammatory response; any reaction has limitations so it doesn't cause damage along with whatever good it produces. In states of chronic inflammation, the regulating systems have stopped, and nothing stops the pathway from becoming harmful.

Achy joints

Joint pain can result from rheumatoid arthritis (RA), an autoimmune condition that we discuss in Chapter 4; osteoarthritis (OA), an overuse condition; or an inflammation of the tendons and ligaments attached to the joint (tendonitis, bursitis). A different phenomenon starts each condition: In RA, it's an autoantibody; in OA, it's chronic overuse; in tendonitis or bursitis, it's also overuse. However, each process is the same, regardless of what starts it: The production of cytokines and prostaglandins lead to heat, pain, and swelling, as discussed in the previous section.

Heart disease

Heart disease is an inflammatory process? Really? Despite the obvious link to cholesterol and lifestyle, the actual process of plaque formation in your arteries involves the immune system.

If a lot of inflammation courses through blood vessels (usually from starches and sugars in your diet, along with the high insulin levels they create or high levels of stress hormones like cortisol), then the body responds by producing LDL and HDL cholesterol. The LDL is the patch material to repair damage to the wall of the vessel from the inflammation. LDL becomes *oxidized* (gets oxygen molecules added to it), and the body responds by sending macrophages out to grab this oxidized LDL in the lining of the blood vessel and pull it into the wall of the vessel. There, it mixes with fibrin, other oxidized lipid, and cell debris to form a plaque. If the inflammation continues, the amount of plaque progresses, the cap over the area becomes thin, and eventually the whole thing ruptures, sending plaque, oxidized lipid, and cell debris into the blood vessel, where it mixes with blood and forms a clot. This clot goes downstream and occludes the vessel, stopping blood flow and causing a heart attack.

Without the action of the immune system, none of this plaque formation could progress. The good news about the macrophage ingestion of oxidized LDL is that it removes it from the blood vessel lumen. The bad news is that if lifestyle factors lead to continued production of LDL, the process has a chance to progress and cause trouble. You can interrupt the process fairly easily by managing stress, changing unhealthy eating patterns, and exercising/ moving your body. Also, taking probiotics can improve the bacteria present in the body, modulating how much you react to LDL. Other anti-inflammatory substances, such as fish oil, turmeric, vitamin D, and resveratrol, lead to improvement in heart disease by decreasing the amount of inflammation, which stabilizes the plaque and keeps it from rupturing.

Diabetes

Diabetes is a condition where blood glucose levels are poorly regulated, going too high and leading to cellular damage from the excess glucose. The two types of diabetes are caused by two different events, but each one leads to the same inflammatory processes.

✔ **Type 1 diabetes (insulin-dependent; autoimmune)** creates inflammation via all the usual autoimmune pathways we discuss in Chapter 4. Therefore, modulating the autoimmune segment improves the outcome of the diabetes, with better glucose control and fewer long-term consequences of the disease.

✔ **Type 2 diabetes (from excess insulin resistance)** also causes inflammation. As insulin resistance worsens and glucose levels become chronically elevated, inflammatory markers, such as prostaglandins and leukotrienes, are triggered. Over time, excess glucose gets attached to proteins to form AGEs, *advanced glycosylation end products,* which get carried through the blood vessels, inciting inflammation and ultimately causing damage to tissues when they become stuck in small capillaries of the kidneys, eyes, fingers, and toes. The damage to blood vessels eventually causes compromise of the body's ability to heal itself, because the immune system response relies on appropriate blood flow to get different components into place. Research also points to a change in gut bacteria in many individuals with Type 2 diabetes, ultimately leading to a change in the immune system response, as we discuss in Chapter 2.

Alzheimer's disease

Although most people think that getting Alzheimer's disease is inevitable if it's part of their family history, it's actually a preventable disorder. The underlying processes in the brain that lead to the typical dementia seen with this disorder are the same inflammatory processes we've been discussing throughout this chapter. TNF-alpha, NF-kB, and cytokines are all part of the disease process. Yes, a genetic predisposition is present in many people who develop the disease, but in recent decades, many folks with no family history have experienced a great deal of inflammation as a causative agent.

Some research even suggests that the herpes virus may be a contributing factor in the development of Alzheimer's. The immune reaction to the herpes in the brain tissue, and the subsequent inflammation, triggers the production of neurofibrillary "tangles" and amyloid plaques that are characteristic of the disease. Once considered the cause of the disease, all treatments aimed at removing the plaque cause a worsening of symptoms. This implies that the tangles may be an effect of the body's attempts to wall off the herpes virus, not a cause of the illness at all!

You can prevent or modulate the Alzheimer's disease process by using many of the anti-inflammatory substances we discuss in this and other chapters. The eating plan we present in Part IV is also appropriate for prevention and treatment of Alzheimer's.

For further discussion of Alzheimer's and inflammation, we recommend holistic neurologist Dr. David Perlmutter's *The Better Brain Book* (Riverhead Trade), with coauthor Carol Coman, and *Power Up Your Brain* (Hay House), with coauthor Dr. Alberto Villoldo.

Irritable Bowel Syndrome (IBS), or Leaky Gut Syndrome

When people who experience chronic constipation or diarrhea are evaluated by a conventional gastroenterologist, they're often told that "Everything is all right; you just have IBS." This diagnosis actually describes only a set of symptoms, not a disease process. Conventional medical treatment is, therefore, aimed at alleviating the symptoms, not at changing the underlying process, which requires slowing down the inflammation and effect on the immune system.

Leaky gut syndrome is a term found in the lay press but isn't really used in medical circles. It also describes a condition of chronic constipation and diarrhea, often worse with stress. Ultimately, irritable bowel syndrome (IBS) and leaky gut syndrome are the same condition. Here, we discuss both, using the terms interchangeably.

The GI tract is one long tube from mouth to anus; it's one of the places in the body where you have the most exposure to things that aren't you. There-fore, not surprisingly, a huge amount of immune complexes, collectively known as the GALT, line the gut wall. The job of the GALT, is to monitor what comes into the body, sounding the alarm if there's an intruder. At the same time, it has to become familiar with normal, friendly bacteria and leave them alone.

Generally, the cells that line the gut wall are uniform and connected tightly to each other. They form a barrier for chemicals to penetrate on the way to the bloodstream. Usually, as food is digested, it's broken down into the smallest possible components; for example, protein is broken down into the individual amino acids of which it's made. These amino acids travel through the cells that line the wall, pass by the GALT, and go into the bloodstream for trans-port elsewhere in the body. If this is done in the usual fashion, the GALT is on the alert but able to remain quiet.

This process is easy to disrupt. When the gut is exposed to long-term use of nonsteroidal anti-inflammatory agents (like motrin and Tylenol) or aspi-rin, steroids, and long-term or frequent antibiotic use, the cells lining the gut become damaged. They develop *gap junctions,* which are minute areas at the cellular level where a gap exists between the cells. These gaps allow the influx of not-yet-fully-digested food particles between cells and into the bloodstream (see Figure 7-1). As they pass by the GALT, the unfamiliar particles are recognized as foreign, and they trigger an immune reaction. IgG antibodies are formed to the foods just eaten and lead to inflammation in the gut wall and subsequent change in gut function. Generally, this presents clinically as chronic diarrhea, loose stools, urge to defecate with unformed stools, or constipation. The anatomy is still perfectly normal, so a colonoscopy would at most show some mild inflammation of the gut wall. Sometimes, individuals with this condition are told "nothing's wrong."

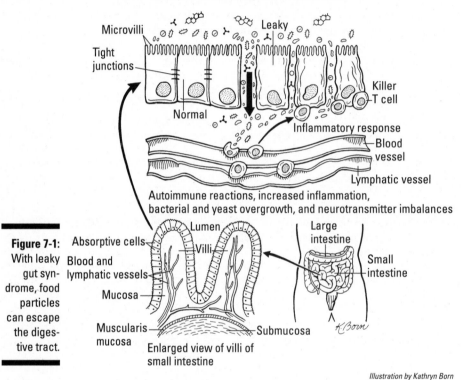

Figure 7-1: With leaky gut syndrome, food particles can escape the digestive tract.

Enlarged view of villi of small intestine

Illustration by Kathryn Born

In Chapter 3, we tell you that IgG antibodies aren't long lived; generally each individual antibody survives about 120 days. You'd think that IBS would be a self-limiting disease then, right? Wrong. The problem here is that the body is reacting to whatever you're eating; some foods have a tendency to trigger more or less IgG production. Because you're reacting to foods you eat nearly every day, putting your finger on which food is causing it is almost impossible. IgG antibodies are being made each day, so the level rarely falls low enough to stop the inflammation and other symptoms.

In the following sections, we describe how IBS (or leaky gut) is diagnosed and different methods for treating it.

Diagnosing IBS

To determine a diagnosis of IBS, a care provider needs to ask specific questions about bowel habits. In our culture, bowel habits are generally not discussed, so few people know what *normal* bowel function is. People tend to assume that whatever is normal for *them* is normal, which is why someone with a bowel movement every three days and someone with one five times a day may each assume that's okay and never mention it.

Here's what a normal bowel movement is: A formed but not hard stool produced one to three times daily, often stimulated by eating. There should be minimal gas, never putrid smelling. (Okay, no one has gas that smells good, but if it literally smells like something died, seek help.) There should be no bloating and no pain. After a bowel movement, you should have a feeling of being emptied.

If symptoms fit the diagnosis of IBS, the easiest way to confirm it is to do an elimination diet and restrict certain foods from your diet for several weeks; if one or more of the foods are the reason for the symptoms, the symptoms will dissipate as fewer antibodies are being produced. After all symptoms are gone, the eliminated foods are reintroduced into the diet one by one; if any of them cause the symptoms to return, they're one of the causes of the reaction.

At this point, you leave the offending foods out of your diet for three to six months and use anti-inflammatory supplements and probiotics to normalize the gut wall and stop the inflammation. See the discussion of this process in Chapter 4, where we point out the role of leaky gut syndrome and the autoimmune process.

Elimination diet

You can do an elimination diet in many ways, but one of the less complex and least time-consuming ways goes as follows. You eliminate

✔ Soy, beef, eggs, shellfish, and processed meats

✔ All dairy

✔ Gluten-containing grains (wheat, spelt, farrow, kamut, and barley) as well as corn

✔ Most nuts and seeds other than pine nuts and flax seeds

✔ Most fats and oils other than olive oil and ghee

✔ Essentially all processed foods

This list contains the statistically most likely foods to cause inflammation and the immune response. Used appropriately, it helps weed out the culprits most of the time and is fairly easy to work with.

Treating IBS

The treatment of this condition actually gets started as you do the diagnosis: Eliminating the food starts the ramping down of the immune response. After you identify all the offending agents, you remove them from the diet for three to six months. During this time, you can use anti-inflammatories, such as fish oil, glutamine, rosemary, turmeric, and other supplements, to restore the gut wall to health. Then, after sufficient time has passed to have all IgG die off, you can reintroduce the foods one by one, usually with good success.

Most folks with IBS immediately recognize that the symptoms are worse when they feel stressed. During periods of high stress, your body produces higher levels of *cortisol,* the hormone most in play during the fight or flight response. It causes blood to be shunted to muscles and the brain, so you can think fast and get away from danger. It has also been shown to shunt blood away from the GI tract; the gut doesn't get the usual amount of oxygen and nutrients, so the function changes and the cells get damaged. More IBS. Also, cortisol itself produces inflammatory chemicals, such as cytokines, which also contribute to the damage.

Over time, another stress hormone, DHEA, which had originally gone up as part of the stress reaction, tends to fall. Part of DHEA's job is to clean up inflammatory chemicals in cells while you sleep. Most people under chronically stressful conditions start to develop interrupted sleep. So between not sleeping enough and not having enough DHEA, the inflammatory cleanup process doesn't happen, leading to even more residual inflammation in the gut wall.

To treat the stress and get the hormones back in balance, several processes have been shown to help, starting with getting your levels tested. For cortisol, either an early morning blood level or a saliva level taken four times during the day is appropriate. For DHEA or DHEA-S (a related hormone), stick to the blood levels. Ideally, both the cortisol and DHEA will be in the midline of the lab's reference range at the same time.

For treatment, options include techniques perfected by the Institute of HeartMath, long-term Transcendental Meditation (TM), or long-term Loving Kindness meditation. The Institute of HeartMath has shown that changing emotional states has a direct influence on cortisol and DHEA levels and subsequently on the function of the immune system (see Chapters 5 and 11 for details). You can reach these same states over time via TM or Loving Kindness.

Acne and Chronic Skin Conditions

How well the immune system is functioning makes a big difference in how the skin looks and feels. Some of this influence is an indirect effect, and some of it is very direct. Either way, improving the immune function improves chronic skin conditions, such as acne, psoriasis, eczema, and contact dermatitis, which we discuss in the following sections.

Acne

Acne is a disorder of the pilosebaceous unit, which is made up of a hair follicle, sebaceous gland, and hair, all found within the skin. These units are found in greater abundance on the face, chest, and back but can be located anywhere except the palms of the hands and soles of the feet. The sebaceous gland is supposed to create sebum, which keeps the skin lubricated and protected. Sometimes, a blockage occurs in the gland, and the sebum can't get out, creating a plug and leading to inflammation in the entire area.

Inciting events are changes in hormone status, dietary issues, and a change in how the immune system handles a friendly bacterium, *P. acnes.* As you may imagine, these inciting events actually all interact and influence each other. And, as is usually the case with immune issues, the end result is an inflammatory reaction.

Here are the specifics: Increased androgen hormones (testosterone, DHEAs, and androstenedione) increase the production of sebum. If increased faster than the gland can transport it, the gland may become clogged. In men, puberty and its associated rapid rise in androgens often triggers acne formation. The use of anabolic ("building") hormones by some body builders and other athletes also leads to acne via the induction of higher androgens from the anabolic steroids. In women, any time unbalanced estrogen and progesterone occurs, such as during puberty and perimenopause, the "excess" estrogen can be converted to androgens in the skin, leading to increased acne. Stressful events also tend to lead to acne, via the increase in DHEA.

Diet is also an issue. Although many foods have been pointed to as problems, studies indicate that only a few actually contribute to acne. Too much sugar, harmful fats, and cow's milk have all been shown to raise the chances of developing acne.

✔ **Sugar:** A high glycemic diet (one that raises the blood glucose levels higher than average) leads to increased insulin levels because the insulin has to go up to keep the glucose levels in check. Higher insulin levels are known to be inflammatory, which raises the chance of developing acne. (The good news is that dark chocolate hasn't been associated with acne, as long as it's eaten in low quantities.)

✔ **Harmful fats:** Harmful fats found in processed foods are also known to be inflammatory and compete with healthy omega-3 fatty acids.

✔ **Cow's milk:** A small amount of cow's milk may not cause much trouble, but think about it: It's designed to grow a baby calf. It's naturally filled with growth hormones, anabolic steroids, and insulin-like growth factors. Yes, even in organic, raw milk from happy cows. Cow's milk also includes a good bit of sugar in the form of lactose. So if you can drink milk and not get acne, go ahead. If you have a lot of acne, it's worth going dairy free to see whether it helps.

P. acne and *S. epidermidis* are two bacteria commonly found on the skin, but they can also be a source of acne. The immune system must have the ability to maintain the correct balance of these bacteria, because too much leads to acne and too little can lead to other, even more dangerous bacteria taking over their space. If the immune system is functioning improperly, the bacteria cause infections within the sebaceous glands and increase acne formation.

Common treatment for acne includes topical benzoyl peroxide, which kills the *P. acne,* antibiotics either topically or orally, and topical or oral retinoids. Retinoids are related to vitamin A and are used to normalize the follicle cell life cycle, which helps avoid clogging of the sebaceous gland. The retinoids, although effective, have significant side effects: dry skin, changes in liver enzymes and triglycerides, and birth defects if used during pregnancy.

Obviously, if overgrowth of bacteria is one cause of acne, then boosting your immune system will stop this particular effect. Studies show that using a good probiotic helps fight acne because normal bowel flora changes immune function (see Chapter 2 for details). Other studies show that additional vitamin D also causes improvement, presumably due to immune-boosting and anti-inflammatory mechanisms. A good night's sleep has also been shown to improve acne, and good sleep is associated with a healthier immune system.

Psoriasis

Psoriasis is a skin condition that creates patches of red, itchy skin covered with flaky, silver scales. It's an immune-mediated condition in which activated T cells move from the dermis to the epidermis of the skin, triggering the production of inflammatory cytokines. Increased growth of the dermis causes the scales; the inflammatory process causes the skin areas to look red and raised and to itch.

Psoriasis tends to have a genetic component and run in families. It's diagnosed simply by visual inspection; no specific test is available, although a skin biopsy may rule out other conditions. Various things cause flares: too little or too much sunlight, stress, bacterial or viral infections (even something as simple as an upper respiratory infection), and excess alcohol intake.

Essentially, the three kinds of treatment for psoriasis are

- **Topical creams:** Topical creams are aimed at improving the skin barrier to improve moisture or to improve immune function directly. Creams for barrier improvement include moisturizers, mineral oil, or petroleum jelly. Creams for inflammation include coal tar, retinoids, and corticosteroids. Creams for immune enhancement include vitamin D look-alikes.

- **Systemic treatments aimed at the immune system:** Systemic treatments include immunosuppressant drugs, like methotrexate and cyclosporine, or biologics, which target specific portions of the immune reaction. T cell inhibitors include alefacept. Monoclonal antibodies target cytokine production; they include drugs such as Remicade and Humira. Although these drugs are effective, they have a large number of side effects because they completely suppress cytokine production rather than simply modulate it.

- **Phototherapy:** UVA and UVB light are both used to treat psoriasis. Occasionally, the drug psoralen is used first; the light appears to activate the drug in the skin so it more effectively interacts with the immune system in the skin. Unfortunately, long-term side effects of phototherapy include the development of skin cancers.

 Rather than resorting to prescription medications, several studies show that much of the immune-boosting lifestyle changes we discuss throughout this book can alter the course of the disease and decrease flares. Omega-3 fatty acid supplementation, vitamin D supplementation, and a healthier overall diet prove helpful, as does stress management.

Eczema

Eczema, also called *atopic dermatitis,* is a skin condition with redness, swelling, itching, and flaking or blistering. It's directly related to the function of the immune system, most often seen in children whose immune systems aren't yet fully mature. Many people grow out of it, but those who also have other allergic conditions (asthma or contact dermatitis) are more prone to continued eczema.

In Chapter 3, we cover the causes of eczema and its treatment. In short, eczema is an allergic reaction and can be managed by modification of the immune reaction. Conventional medicine relies on drugs that stifle the immune response, and natural medicine relies on substances that boost the immune response. Things to try from a natural medicine standpoint are probiotics (especially helpful in moms and infants), gamma linoleic acid from evening primrose oil or borage oil, licorice root gel, and an immune-boosting diet.

Contact dermatitis

Contact dermatitis occurs either from irritants in the substance you're exposed to or from an immune response to a substance. The resulting skin rash, irritation, and itching look the same no matter the cause. In immune-mediated contact dermatitis, antibodies are formed to specific chemicals in the object causing the reaction, which leads to the production of inflammatory cytokines, histamine, and other inflammatory reactive intermediates. Contact dermatitis is a chronic skin condition simply because it occurs whenever an individual is exposed to the inciting agent. With care, though, the actual rash can be avoided.

For example, a common allergen is poison ivy. Many individuals develop this reaction at a young age; others develop it when they're older, especially if the immune system is already "turned on" by an autoimmune condition or other immune system abnormality. When the immune system is primed to react to poison ivy, any exposure produces a rash, which can proceed to oozing sores, irritation, and possible secondary bacterial infection of the area. Typically, conventional medical treatment consists of steroid hormone prescription. Although this treatment is effective, it has side effects, from ovarian hormone imbalance to insulin dysregulation to mood instability.

A different approach to treating contact dermatitis is homeopathy. *Homeopathic remedies* are a form of energy medicine; their job is to stimulate the body's own healing system. Specific remedies are used for specific conditions; the remedy Rhus tox is used for exposure to poison ivy and several other allergen-producing vines. Homeopathic remedies can be used after exposure or even prophylactically before exposure to a known allergy-producing substance.

When an allergic reaction has been triggered, the substance will generally always trigger a reaction in any given individual because the memory cells have been made and don't go away. Therefore, try to keep a healthy immune system that doesn't respond to allergens and also to avoid the things you know you're allergic to.

Part III
Laying the Groundwork for Super Immunity: Nutrition, Lifestyle, and Detox

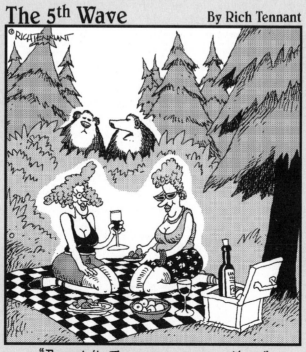

The 5th Wave   By Rich Tennant

"Forget it. Too many preservatives."

In this part . . .

The foundation of boosting your immunity is discovering how to fill your plate with the most nutrient-dense foods available. This part makes understanding how to eat for immunity easy. In addition to a primer on nutrition, the chapters in this part also cover nutrient-packed super-foods, supplements, and herbs. Understanding how to live an immune-friendly lifestyle goes a long way in providing you with a lifetime of good habits that move you toward health, give you strength, and help you fight aging naturally. We also look at your detox options; exploring detoxification is your best defense against environmental and internal toxins, giving you a cellular cleanse that will make you healthy, energetic, and ageless.

Chapter 8

Improving Your Immunity with Nutrition

In This Chapter

▶ Boosting your immunity with foods

▶ Building an immune-boosting plate

▶ Getting familiar with the "proceed-with-caution" food list

▶ Leaving some foods off your plate for good

▶ Figuring out whether common foods you love make the grade

*I*mproving your nutrition is the fastest way to boost immunity. The key is to eat foods that have a high nutrient density with *naturally* lower calories and to omit foods with a low nutrient density and wasted calories.

When you eat refined, processed, denatured foods, you suppress your immune system, leaving the floodgate open for disease and infection. Eating low nutrient-dense foods also causes you to become overfed and malnourished. You get all the excess calories and none of the nutrition, which may cause weight gain, bloating, fatigue, skin problems, joint pain, or a million other symptoms. Over time, this nutritional deficiency lowers your immune system to the point where it may lead to more serious life-threatening problems.

That's why eating foods with beneficial antioxidants, vitamins, minerals, and nutrients that create a state of nutritional sufficiency and immune defense is crucial to your well-being. When your body has all the nutrients it needs, it's like you're wearing an anti-disease, anti-aging shield.

This chapter explains how to meet your macronutrient needs, without consuming excess calories, while flooding your body with nutrients. In other words, this chapter is the fast track to building a healthy immune system. In this chapter, we also highlight foods to stay away from and special considerations surrounding old favorites, such as salt, dessert, and alcohol.

Calling in Nutrition's Big Guns

You'll love how you feel when you start putting real, nutrient-dense foods first. When you start eating foods that boost your immunity, you flourish in every way. You say goodbye to illness, aches, pains, and fatigue. You lose excess weight, and inflammation and bloating disappear. You look and feel younger. You burst with energy, and enthusiasm floods back into your life.

To be as healthy as possible, your cells need *macronutrients,* such as proteins, fats, and carbohydrates. Macronutrients are just larger sized *nutrients* — chemical substances that your body uses to build, maintain, and repair tissues and conduct natural functions, such as breathing, seeing, tasting, and thinking — that your body uses to function at its best. When you focus on these three macronutrients as the foundation to your immunity-boosting plate, you get healthy — fast.

How are these macronutrients used in the body?

- ✔ Proteins help build and replenish your body.

- ✔ Fats help every structure and function of the body work, from your brain to your muscles.

- ✔ Carbohydrates give you that quick source of energy to cook a meal, run to catch a train for work, do homework with your kids, or take your dog for a walk.

The key to macronutrients and boosting your immunity is to know which sources of protein, fat, or carbohydrates will serve you and your cells the best. When you're equipped with the strategies you need to know to purchase and consume the best foods in these categories, you have your road map to super immunity.

In the following sections, we explore the best (and worst) types of proteins, fats, and carbs and how they affect your health.

Powerful protein: Making you healthy (and thin!)

Protein builds you up. Growth and repair are protein's major roles: Your body uses the protein you take in as food to build cells, synthesize new proteins, and keep your tissues healthy. Eating adequate protein supports your physique and satisfies your appetite.

Macronutrient bonus: Protein burns fat!

When you eat sufficient amounts of protein, you can increase the rate at which your metabolism burns calories. Your body requires more energy to break down protein because it isn't as readily available to use for energy as carbohydrates are. This promotes fat burning. Protein is also required for growing and repairing lean muscle mass. Couple this with exercise and movement, and your body soon becomes more efficient at laying down lean muscle and burning fat. Protein is a great blood stabilizer, too. The less spikes you have in your blood sugar, the more efficient your body will be at keeping fat from ending up around your waist. When your blood sugar is stable, your immune system functions better as well, so protein is important all the way around!

Our earliest ancestors were meat eaters, and scientists estimate that our genes have changed only about 0.02 percent since then. Influencing genes takes a long time, so your body has a nutritional blueprint for healthy meats as a powerful protein.

Protein is a nutritional powerhouse in that it provides important immune-boosting nutrients — essential fatty acids (good fats), vitamins, and minerals. Among these minerals is zinc, which helps in the production of infection-fighting white blood cells. Even a mild deficiency in zinc can open the door to many diseases and infections. So sufficient amounts of protein are wonderful in supporting a healthy immune system.

In the following sections, we outline the best kinds of proteins you can get from both meat and veggie sources.

Traditional sources of protein: Meat, fish, and eggs

The protein in meats strengthens your body by building strong muscle, providing fuel storage for bursts of energy, and even helping your body burn fat, which keeps you healthier.

The healthier your food source is, the healthier you'll be. A direct relationship exists between the quality of the foods you eat and your overall health. Quality is especially important when it comes to protein, so we recommend you buy the best quality protein possible. Here are our suggestions:

✔ **Meats:** Buy the leanest, organic grass-fed, free-range meat as possible. Beef, buffalo, lamb, goat, turkey, chicken, organic organ meats, pasture-raised pork, nitrite- and gluten-free deli meats, and nitrite- and gluten-free sausages are all good sources.

Where deli meats, pork, organ meats, and sausages are concerned, if you can't buy pasture-raised or organic, we recommend giving them the ol' heave-ho. They're just too unhealthy and toxic to eat otherwise. You're better off choosing another protein source.

✔ **Wild meat (game):** This type of meat is the best kind, if you can get it, because it's full of good fats. Venison, rabbit, pheasant, quail, and even boar are all good choices.

✔ **Conventional meats:** If a super tight budget means store-bought meats, don't stress about buying conventional meats; just be sure you know how to prepare them for the best health benefit. Do what you can and know that you can still vastly improve your health by having sufficient meat prepared in the healthiest way. Choose the leanest cuts and trim all visible fats before cooking. Make sure you drain as much of the fats released before you cook.

When buying conventional meats, look for the symbol shown in Figure 8-1, which indicates food has been *irradiated* (exposed to ionizing radiation to kill bacteria, viruses, or microorganisms). Purchase the best quality meat that *hasn't* been irradiated with chemicals, which is counterproductive to your boosting immunity efforts.

✔ **Fish:** The benefit of fish is that healthy fish are loaded with healthy fats. Purchase wild-caught, sustainable fish when you can. Fattier, deep cold-water fish are your best choices. Salmon, sardines, mackerel, cod, and herring are all great for boosting your health. Tuna packed in olive oil is another choice to add to your grocery list.

Fish can have pollutants and pesticides. Freshwater fish have a higher concentration of toxins, which are definitely not immune building. Visit the Monterey Bay Aquarium Seafood Watch online at `www.monterey bayaquarium.org/cr/cr_seafoodwatch/sfw_recommendations. aspx?c=ln` to find the cleanest, healthiest fish in your area and check out its downloadable pocket guide or nifty smartphone app as well.

✔ **Eggs:** Eggs are amazing: They're rich in key nutrients, especially fat-soluble vitamins A and D, and the egg yolk is also loaded with brain food and immune-fighting nutrients. Capture as much of this immune-building nutrition as possible by buying the best quality. Organic pastured eggs have the best fatty acid profile. If you can find a farm that carries pastured eggs, you're sure to get an explosion of nutrients!

Many people have eliminated eggs or egg yolks from their diets because of the possibilities of raising cholesterol and, therefore, making them more susceptible to heart disease, which is simply based on untrue and misguided information. Studies show that *dietary* cholesterol has very little effect on *blood* cholesterol. Actually, the egg yolk contains *choline,* which is a natural fat transporter, keeping cholesterol out of the blood! Dietary cholesterol is simply not a good indicator of heart disease.

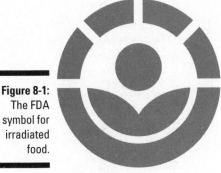

Figure 8-1:
The FDA symbol for irradiated food.

Illustration by Wiley, Composition Services Graphics

If you don't eat meat because you're concerned about animal welfare, sustainability, or environmental concerns, check out the following resources for ethical ways of sourcing animals:

 ✔ www.sustainabletable.org/home.php

✔ www.eatwild.com

✔ www.grasslandbeef.com/StoreFront.bok

Vegetarian protein options

Eating nutrient-dense animal-based foods provides a lot of health benefits; however, we understand that some people choose not to eat meat for religious or spiritual reasons or simply because they've chosen a vegetarian path.

If you choose to eat vegetarian protein sources, the most optimal choices are organic, non-GMO (genetically modified organisms, which have had changes introduced into their DNA by genetic engineering techniques), plant-based foods, such as the following:

✔ Beans

We recommend lentils, black beans, pinto beans, and red beans because they have the lowest impact on blood sugar (and having your blood sugar spike up and down causes you to become unhealthy and overweight). If you buy canned beans, be sure to rinse them a couple of times before eating. If you're preparing dried beans, soak them for at least 12 hours before cooking. Rinsing and soaking remove the starch (and salt, if canned) and reduce the gassiness that beans cause for many people.

✔ Full-fat yogurt and kefir from milk of pasture-raised cows

Don't look to string cheese, cottage cheese, or conventional yogurt or dairy products as your protein sources. The proteins *whey* and *casein* may cause an overreaction of the immune system, causing congestion or inflammation in the body.

✔ High-quality protein powders, such as hemp or pea protein

✔ Natto

✔ Tempeh

Healthy fats: Protecting your body

Understanding and embracing that healthy fats do a spectacular job at making you healthy is one of the most important principles in nutrition. Eating healthy fats protects you against heart disease; melts away inflammation; aids in conditions, like skin disorders, arthritis, high cholesterol, high triglycerides, diabetes, and depression; and can help you lose weight. Healthy fats make all the structures and functions of your body flourish. They're needed for hormone production and the growth and development of the brain, immune system, nervous system, heart, and blood vessels.

Healthy fats also make you look younger; they nourish the skin and give it a beautiful sheen, make your hair shiny, diminish wrinkles, and give you a beautiful, healthy appearance.

So what are these healthy fats? Essential fats (omega-3 and omega-6 fatty acids) are healthy fats. Your body doesn't produce these fats on its own, so you must consume them to get the benefits (which, lucky for you, healthy fats make foods taste better and help you feel satisfied). You should include some essential fats with every meal to give you immune-boosting power.

With fatty acids, it's all about the ratios. The ideal ratio is about 1:1, omega-6 to omega-3, but getting that balanced ratio is easier said than done. The normal ratio of omega-6 to omega-3 in the modern diet is between 15:1 and 22:1. People consume about 15 to 20 times too much omega-6! Omega-6 fatty acids are found just about everywhere in the form of processed foods and refined oils, which causes these off-kilter ratios.

All the fats in food are a combination of fatty acids, depending on how many hydrogen atoms are attached to the carbon atoms in the chain. The more hydrogen atoms, the more saturated fatty acids. Depending on which fatty acids are in the majority, the fat content in a food is likewise characterized as saturated, monounsaturated, or polyunsaturated. We discuss these three types of fats and healthy options of each kind, along with a few you should avoid, in the following sections.

Saturated fats

Saturated fats have single bonds only and contain mostly saturated fatty acids. Saturated fats are solid at room temperature and get harder when chilled. Good sources of saturated fats include coconut oil, coconut flakes, coconut milk, coconut butter, and organic clarified butter from grass-fed cows. (Clarified butter is the full butter fat after the milk solids and the water have been removed from the butter, so even if you're lactose intolerant, this may be a good option for you.)

Changing what you know or changing a habit is never easy to do. However, when it comes to saturated fats, we recommend that you try your hardest. Saturated fats have been on the "no" list because of the reputation they've had for causing heart disease. However, researchers are finding more evidence that higher saturated intake does *not* increase the risk of developing heart disease.

Not only are saturated fats powerful antiviral and antifungal agents and key players in immune health, but they can also do the following:

- ✔ Allow for proper nerve signaling
- ✔ Build stronger bones
- ✔ Fight autoimmune disease
- ✔ Lower (yes, lower!) cholesterol
- ✔ Ward off cancer

So to add some healthy saturated fats to your diet, grab a handful of coconut flakes for a great snack or add some full-fat coconut milk to your coffee for a delicious, creamy taste — but always make sure it's not sweetened. Full-fat coconut milk is most often found in cans. For a lighter taste in an easy-to-use carton, try unsweetened coconut milk (coauthor Kellyann likes So Delicious brand). Just be aware that coconut milk sold in a carton isn't full-fat milk, so don't look to it as your only fat source.

Monounsaturated fats (MUFAs)

Monounsaturated fats, or MUFAs, contain one double bond and have mostly monounsaturated fatty acids. These fats are liquid at room temperature and get thicker when chilled. Good sources of this type of fat include olives (green or black), olive oil, avocado, avocado oil, macadamia nuts, macadamia oil, cashew nuts, cashew butter, and hazelnuts. MUFAs are super healthy and fantastic on salads.

Olive oil is best used uncooked, added at the end of cooking for a burst of flavor, or drizzled over salad. It's also okay cooked at low to medium temperatures, but cooking it at a high temperature ruins the oil and makes it no longer good for you.

To find out how to use oils to boost immunity, figure out the *smoke point* of that oil — the point where the oil starts to break down and starts to burn or smoke. When the oil has reached this point, it becomes rancid and will derail your attempts to consume healthy fats. You can find a handy smoke point chart at `www.goodeatsfanpage.com/collectedinfo/oilsmoke points.htm`.

Polyunsaturated fats (PUFAs)

Polyunsaturated fats (PUFAs) have more than one double bond and contain mostly polyunsaturated fatty acids. Polyunsaturated fats are liquid at room temperature and stay liquid when chilled. Good sources of polyunsaturated fats include almonds, almond butter, Brazil nuts, pistachios, pecans, chestnuts, walnuts, pumpkin seeds, sesame seeds, sunflower seeds, sunflower butter, and pine nuts.

PUFAs are just a bit higher in omega-6 ratios than MUFAs, so consume PUFAs in moderation. For example, avocado, which is a MUFA, has an omega-6 to omega-3 ratio of 12:1. Walnuts, on the other hand, which are PUFAs, have a ratio of 53:10.

Refined fats and oils to avoid

What's popular isn't always right. For example, industrial and seed oils may be common, but they're not naturally occurring and certainly not immune building, so they're not healthy. They have a high propensity for turning rancid, which creates free radicals and inflammation.

Avoid these refined (often or easily rancid) oils:

- ✔ Canola oil
- ✔ Cotton/cottonseed oil
- ✔ Palm kernel oil
- ✔ Partially hydrogenated oil

✔ Peanut oil

✔ Safflower oil

✔ Soybean oil

✔ Sunflower oil

✔ Trans-fats

✔ Vegetable shortening

Carbs your body will love: Getting your charge back

Carbohydrates give you the fuel your body needs for bursts of energy. Whether you eat a chocolate bar or kale, your body transforms the carbohydrate into glucose. Your brain and your cells use this glucose for fuel for your daily activities.

Controlling insulin is an issue with carbohydrates. Here's the lowdown: Your pancreas produces insulin, which lowers sugar in your blood, called glucose. High levels of glucose signal insulin release; low levels suppress this release. If you can maintain low levels of insulin release, your body can more readily use stored fat as fuel (in other words, it keeps your body in a fat-burning state). If you eat bad carbs or too many carbs, your pancreas produces more and more insulin. Over time, this excess insulin production can cause *insulin resistance,* which is the precursor to many serious diseases, such as diabetes and obesity. Choosing healthy carbohydrates is an absolute must for keeping your immune system strong and you healthy.

But how do carbohydrates affect your immunity? Healthy carbs contain micronutrients (vitamins and minerals), antioxidants, and fiber. Healthy carbs flood your cells with nutrition and keep your blood sugar stable and your calories naturally low, which improves immune function and makes your body resistant to diseases. In contrast, unhealthy carbs cause blood sugar problems and leave you deficient of fiber and nutrients. Unhealthy carbs are fattening, void of nutrition, and suppress your immune system, leaving your body wide open for diseases.

When it comes to choosing carbohydrates, remember the "big three," which guarantee that you get the nutrition you need to boost your immunity without extra calories and the injection of glucose in your system — in other words, *nutrient-dense foods.* The carbohydrate "big three" include

✔ Carbohydrates that have only minimal effects on blood sugar

✔ Carbohydrates that are naturally loaded with fiber

✔ Carbohydrates that are filled with protective antioxidants, vitamins, and minerals

Of all the macronutrients, you have to be really in the know when it comes to carbohydrates. Certain carbs can raise insulin, which always lay down fat and make you unhealthy like nobody's business! So knowing which carbs to eat, such as the ones we list in the following sections, is key. You may notice that we don't list foods that have chemicals, additives, added sugar, sugar substitutes, or are processed or denatured in any way, such as candy, baked goods, prepackaged meals, and junk food. If you want your immune system to sing, you've got to get your carbs from *real foods.*

The most beneficial nutrients are lost the more heavily refined a food is. All the white foods, such as white flour, white rice, white pasta, white potatoes, white bread, croissants, packaged cereals, bagels, cakes, waffles, and pancakes, are highly processed and void of nutrients. More important, these foods suppress the immune system, and when you eat them, you increase your risk of diseases. All you have to do is remember this catchy phrase: "The whiter the bread, the quicker you're dead." Now that's motivating!

Healthy carbohydrates: Vegetables

Eating vegetables gives you lower-starch carbohydrates that are full of nutrition. Locally grown, organic, in-season vegetables are always preferred. For a handy guide to show you which vegetables you can get away with buying conventional, check out the Environmental Working Group's Dirty Dozen and Clean 15 list at www.ewg.org/foodnews/guide.

Have as much variety of these healthy, lower-starch vegetables as you can and always go for the *rainbow effect* and include a colorful plate of vegetables with your meals. Think *variety, color,* and *in season* whenever possible.

A quick word on white potatoes

White potatoes don't have a place on the boosting-immunity plate because they contain a ton of sugar and starch, which releases too much insulin. If that isn't enough, white potatoes also contain antinutrients. (See "Staying Away from Foods on the Proceed-with-Caution List." You'll get much more bang for your nutrient buck and boost your immunity with sweet potatoes and yams.

- ✔ Artichoke
- ✔ Arugula
- ✔ Asparagus
- ✔ Bell peppers
- ✔ Broccoli
- ✔ Beets
- ✔ Bok Choy
- ✔ Brussels spouts
- ✔ Cabbage
- ✔ Carrots
- ✔ Cauliflower
- ✔ Celery
- ✔ Chile peppers
- ✔ Cucumber
- ✔ Eggplant
- ✔ Endive
- ✔ Escarole
- ✔ Green beans
- ✔ Garlic
- ✔ Greens: Beet, collard, mustard, turnip
- ✔ Kale
- ✔ Kohlrabi
- ✔ Leeks
- ✔ Lettuce
- ✔ Mushrooms
- ✔ Nori (Seaweed)
- ✔ Okra
- ✔ Onion
- ✔ Parsnip
- ✔ Pumpkin
- ✔ Radish
- ✔ Shallots
- ✔ Snow peas
- ✔ Spaghetti squash
- ✔ Spinach
- ✔ Sugar snap peas
- ✔ Summer squash
- ✔ Sweet potatoes/yams
- ✔ Tomatoes
- ✔ Tomatillos
- ✔ Turnips
- ✔ Winter squash: Butternut, acorn

Healthy carbohydrates: Fruits

Don't let fruits push vegetables off your plate. Vegetables come first; however, fruit adds a side of sweetness and nutrition and fiber your body will love. Berries are always considered the gold standard in fruit for their incredible immune-building potential — without causing blood sugar swings (see Chapter 9).

- ✔ Apple
- ✔ Apricot
- ✔ Banana
- ✔ Blackberries
- ✔ Blueberries
- ✔ Cantaloupe
- ✔ Cherries
- ✔ Clementine
- ✔ Cranberries
- ✔ Date
- ✔ Fig
- ✔ Grapefruit
- ✔ Grapes
- ✔ Honey dew
- ✔ Lychee
- ✔ Kiwi
- ✔ Kumquat

- ✔ Lemon
- ✔ Lime
- ✔ Mandarin
- ✔ Mango
- ✔ Nectarine
- ✔ Orange
- ✔ Papaya
- ✔ Peach
- ✔ Pear
- ✔ Pineapple
- ✔ Plum
- ✔ Pomegranate
- ✔ Raspberries
- ✔ Strawberries
- ✔ Tangerine
- ✔ Watermelon

Be careful when eating dried fruit and fruit juices. They're easy to overconsume and have a lot of concentrated sugars, so enjoy them, but just be mindful. You don't want to inject your body with too much glucose in a sitting. Also the fruit sugar *fructose* causes increased belly fat, insulin problems, and a long list of chronic diseases, all leading to becoming overweight and unhealthy, and can accelerate the aging process.

Building Your Plate for Everyday Wellness and Robust Immunity

The key to immune-building meals is to eat the foods that give you the nutrients you need without too many calories or blood sugar swings. You have to get enough food to feel satisfied in between meals and not feel deprived. Eating the right foods in the right amount will normalize your weight and give you more energy. You'll get sick much less (if at all), and you'll fight aging. Sound good?

When deciding what and how much to eat, erase the idea of calories in, calories out. The concept that a calorie is a calorie is a calorie is dead. What's more important than the calorie is the *source* of the calorie. You can eat 200 calories that provide you with a nice, nutritious steady stream of fuel, or you can eat 200 calories that cause insulin to be released and are void of nutrients, which in the end won't provide you with anything nutritional or sustaining — just calories. See the difference?

The most fattening foods at your local store aren't the ones highest in calories but the foods that cause your blood sugar to do somersaults. The key here is quality foods. Keep your foods simple and real.

Instead of worrying about calories, we show you how to build a plate at a glance and know, just by looking at your food, whether it's enough to satisfy you or whether it will indulge you! If you stick to this guideline most of the time, you'll stay healthy, live longer and stronger, and fight aging.

In the following sections, we show you how much food you should have, what foods go beyond the macronutrients that boost your immunity and give you some flexibility in your meals, and how to fight sugar cravings (also known as the sugar monkey).

Finding the right portion sizes

Just by eyeballing your food, you can determine how much is the right portion size. Meeting your daily needs, however, depends on three personal factors, which you have to gauge daily: how hungry you are, how much energy you have, and what your activity level is for that day. We give you the foundational tools to build a plate. Your personal gauge determines how many meals or snacks to have that day.

Check out the immune-boosting plate in Figure 8-2 and notice that the meal is based around protein. You fill the rest of your plate with a minimum of two vegetables — raw, steamed, baked, sautéed, boiled, roasted, or grilled — and one or two servings of fat (notice the avocado and olive oil in Figure 8-2). If you built three meals a day that looked like this (with variety, of course), you'd say goodbye to illness and fat and fight aging big time!

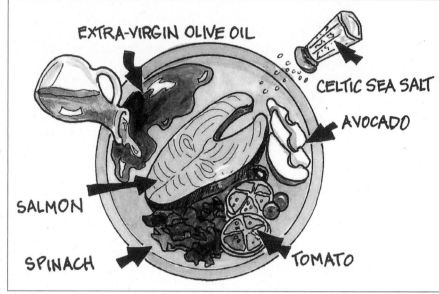

Figure 8-2:
The immune-boosting plate pairs protein with lots of vegetables.

EXTRA-VIRGIN OLIVE OIL

CELTIC SEA SALT

AVOCADO

SALMON

SPINACH

TOMATO

Illustration by Elizabeth Kurtzman

So many people blame poor soil quality for nutrient deficiency and malnutrition problems. Although poor soil quality is certainly part of the problem, the bigger problem is that people just simply don't eat enough (if any) vegetables. Adding two vegetables per meal may seem daunting at first, but it really does get easier as you develop new habits.

Pick two days a week to prepare some of your proteins, veggies, and fruit for that week. This preparation, called *batch cooking,* keeps you from being unprepared — and hungry. We all know too well that not having food available is a recipe for disaster. (See Chapter 13 for details on preparing and keeping food on hand.)

Here are some simple guidelines for appropriate portion sizes:

✔ **Protein:**

• Meat or fish should be about the size and thickness of your palm (see Figure 8-3). That's 3 to 4 ounces for women and 5 to 6 ounces for men.

• For organic, gluten- and sulfite-free deli meats, fold the slices over, and the serving size should measure up to the thickness of your palm (see Figure 8-3).

• A serving of eggs is as many as you can hold in your hand. That's usually about three for women, four for men. If you choose to eat egg whites, just double the amount of whole eggs.

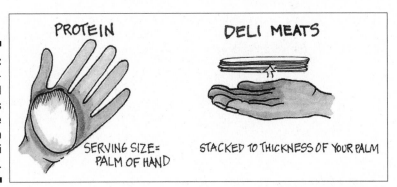

Figure 8-3:
Recommended portion sizes at a glance for protein and deli meats.

Illustration by Elizabeth Kurtzman

✔ **Vegetables:** You can't have too many vegetables on your plate! Pick two per meal, and fill your plate up, leaving room for the protein in the center.

✔ **Fruit:** Eat small amounts of fruits and only between meals. A serving size is half an individual piece or a closed handful of berries.

✔ **Healthy fats:**

- For oils and nut butters, a serving is 1 to 2 thumb-size portions (see Figure 8-4).

- Half of an avocado is an easy serving size.

- For coconut flakes or olives, an open handful is a serving (see Figure 8-4).

- Measure one closed handful of nuts or seeds for a serving (see Figure 8-4).

- One-third to one-half a 13.5-ounce can of coconut milk is an appropriate serving size.

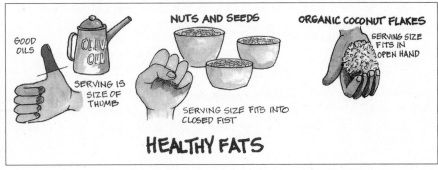

Figure 8-4:
Recommended portion sizes for some healthy fats.

Illustration by Elizabeth Kurtzman

✔ **Snacks:** Snacks typically are about half the size of a regular meal — or half the plate shown in Figure 8-2. When you snack, always be sure you include a protein and a fat. (For some great snack ideas, see Chapter 18.)

How much you eat depends on how hungry you are, your energy level, or your activity for the day. Some people do great on three meals a day; others need more. If you feel a little weak from working out or if you're just one of those people who need more than three meals a day, adding some healthy snacks can help.

Satisfying your thirst

A good rule to follow when it comes to drinking is to stay away from liquid nutrition. Get your nutrition from foods, and hydrate with liquids. Stay away from sports or energy drinks, fruit drinks, and sodas. These liquids do nothing more than inject glucose into your system and overload your body with stuff it doesn't need, making you overweight and unhealthy. When it comes to your immune-building drinks, stick with the basics:

✔ Water (filtered water is best)

✔ Coffee: Black or with coconut milk

✔ Teas: Black, white, green, herbal or Yerba Mate (for more on boosting teas, see Chapter 9)

Try adding slices or wedges of orange, lemon, or lime to water. Throw in a mint leaf for an extra splash of flavor. Trust us: No one in your house will be missing the other sugary juices.

Eating before and after you exercise

Some people don't need to eat before a workout; others do. Whether you eat before working out is completely subjective. If you're one of those people who need pre-workout fuel, be sure to eat about 30 to 90 minutes before you get going. Also, your best bet is to choose a meal that consists of protein and fat, which allows your body to start burning fat for fuel while you exercise. Avoid carbohydrates before a workout.

After you exercise, you want to eat the more dense carbohydrates, like sweet potatoes or squash, with lean protein, like eggs or salmon. This post-workout meal is the only one where you don't need to add fat. Instead, you should concentrate on carbohydrates to refuel your muscles so they can recover from your workout. Recovery is key to get the most out of your hard work.

Staying Away from Foods on the Proceed-with-Caution List

We've given you lists of healthy, immune-boosting foods in the preceding sections of this chapter. If you stick with these foods between 70 and 80 percent of the time, *you will* get results because you're boosting your body and flooding it with foods rich in nutrients.

What you find in the following sections are common, everyday foods that aren't immune building. Some of these foods are even notorious health foods. Sometimes, it's not what you do but what you *don't* do that makes all the difference. Staying away from these foods — most of the time — will start changing the way you feel, think, and look.

Most of the foods in the following sections contain *antinutrients,* which are chemical compounds found in the food that interfere with the absorption of nutrients. They have toxic effects to the body. Specifically, they include phytic acid or phytates, protease inhibitors, and lectins. What you need to know about these antinutrients is that they can cause digestive distress and bloating. Long term, however, they can permanently damage your intestinal track, which leads to internal inflammation and all types of health problems.

If we had to pick the top three bad guys when it comes to weakening your immune system, we'd have to go with the following troublemakers: grains, sugar, and processed foods with bad oils. In the following sections, you discover foods in these categories and others that can be toxic to your body and why you need to just say "no."

Unhealthy grains

Nope. No typo. This section is appropriately called *unhealthy* grains. We've been told for so long that grains are a necessary part of the diet to provide nutrients and energy. The cold hard truth: Grains contain antinutrients, which prevent your body from absorbing the nutrients it needs. Grains — all of them — trigger the release of insulin, which tells your body to start storing fat. Grains also create autoimmune and intestinal irritation. In fact, they're counterproductive to a healthy diet and boosting immunity. No recommended daily allowance exists for grains, and you don't need grains to sustain a healthy existence.

If you do have a known autoimmune disease or suspect you do, ditching all grains should be your first order of business, because they're a major irritant.

If you want to have super immunity, all grains and gluten have to go, including the following:

- ✔ Amaranth
- ✔ Barley
- ✔ Buckwheat
- ✔ Bulgur
- ✔ Corn
- ✔ Millet
- ✔ Oats
- ✔ Quinoa
- ✔ Rice
- ✔ Rye
- ✔ Sorghum
- ✔ Spelt
- ✔ Teff
- ✔ Wheat

Don't fret! Tasty alternatives to using grains include coconut flour and almond meal. With these alternatives, you can eat muffins, bread, and spaghetti that are immune building and not immune suppressing. Discovering how to make the foods you love while omitting unhealthy grains won't take long. Plus you'll start looking and feeling so much better that grains won't even be on your radar.

Beans and legumes

This one may shock you. However, beans have antinutrients similar to grains. Careful preparation by presoaking, spouting, or fermenting these foods can reduce or even eliminate these antinutrients, but they're still a high-carbohydrate food and with that comes insulin response on the higher side. Beans are also difficult to digest.

The items in the following list are beans and legumes you should restrict as much as possible:

- ✔ Black beans
- ✔ Broad beans
- ✔ Garbanzo beans
- ✔ Lentils
- ✔ Lima beans
- ✔ Mung beans
- ✔ Navy beans
- ✔ Peanuts and peanut butter
- ✔ Peas
- ✔ Soybeans: Tofu, tempeh, natto, soy sauce, miso, edamame, and soymilk
- ✔ White beans

We make an exception for snow peas, sugar snap peas, and green beans because they're more of a pod than a pea and contain very little of the antinutrients. So chomp away!

The only exception to this list is if you're a strict vegetarian. If you choose to not eat meat, fish, or eggs, you need to expand your protein sources as much as possible. (See the section "Vegetarian protein options," earlier in this chapter.)

Dairy and stuff

Some people can't tolerate dairy products. Bloating, gas, cramping, or diarrhea are often the indications of this intolerance. The following conditions may be irritated by consumption of dairy:

- ✔ Asthma
- ✔ Colitis and ulcerative colitis
- ✔ Crohn's disease
- ✔ Digestive problems
- ✔ Inflammatory bowel disease (IBD)
- ✔ Irritable bowel syndrome (IBS)

- Joint aches
- Leaky gut syndrome
- Premenstrual symptoms or menstrual discomfort
- Yeast infections

Why the problems? Being lactose intolerant or allergic to the milk protein *casein* causes most irritation problems related to dairy. Therefore, even though full-fat foods in general are good for you and even though some dairy has beneficial CLAs (*conjugated linoleic acids,* which are anticancer agents), we prefer you get these benefits from other sources, like full-fat coconut milk, grass-fed or pasture-raised meat, or egg yolks. For vegetarians, mushrooms are a great source of CLAs (also see the section "Vegetarian protein options," earlier in this chapter).

The following dairy products can do more damage than good, so we suggest you do without:

- Cheese, string cheese
- Cream
- Half-and-half
- Milk
- Sour cream
- Yogurt

We give the green light on only one dairy product: Clarified butter from a cow that's organic and grass fed.

Worried about getting your calcium without dairy? No need. You can get plenty of calcium from plants, sardines, seafood, and some nuts. Here are some options:

- Plant sources of calcium:
  - Bok choy and cabbage
  - Collard, mustard, and turnip greens
  - Green beans
  - Kale
  - Seaweed, like kelp and dulse
  - Spinach
  - Watercress

✔ Fish sources of calcium:

- Canned mackerel

- Salmon (with bones)

- Sardines (with bones)

- Shrimp

✔ Fat sources of calcium:

- Nut and seed butters: Almond, sesame, and sunflower

- Nuts: Almonds, Brazil nuts, cashews, and chestnuts

- Seeds: Sesame and sunflower

✔ Other sources of calcium

- Olives

- Sulfite-free dried dates

- Sulfite-free dried figs

Avoiding Certain Foods at All Cost

Certain foods should never touch your lips. They cause such havoc, inflammation, and damage to your system, that they shouldn't even be on your radar — ever. Damaging foods, such as artificial sugars, food additives, and the others listed in this section, make your body run about as good as a car runs on dirt. You're only as good as the food you digest. Your energy comes as a byproduct of your digestion. When you eat the foods listed in this section, your body simply doesn't recognize them as food but rather a food product of some type. As a result, you simply can't properly digest these foods. Eating these foods can cause long-term damage to your health, particularly in regard to organ damage.

Always read the ingredients of the foods you eat and ask yourself, "Is it worth it?"

"Frankenfoods"

Frankenfoods are the worst of the worst of processed foods. They've been genetically engineered, and they're full of allergens, preservatives, additives, or maybe flavor enhancers. In a word, *yuck!*

Frankenfoods are processed soy and meat alternatives. Unlike soy foods, such as edamame, tempeh, and traditional miso, which are closer to their natural state, these foods are a far cry from anything real.

We understand that some vegetarians don't eat any meat, eggs, or fish and are looking for ways to expand their protein sources — okay, that's smart; you have to get your protein somewhere. But look past these food products for your options. This stuff just isn't healthy for anyone. Period. In fact, these options aren't even foods. They're food products, usually a mixture of a wheat protein with a subpar oil.

The following foods get the *frankenfoods* label and should be avoided:

- ✔ Soymilk
- ✔ Tofu hot dogs
- ✔ Veggie bacon
- ✔ Veggie chicken
- ✔ Veggie chicken wings
- ✔ Veggie loafs
- ✔ Veggie patties or boxed veggie burgers
- ✔ Veggie "sausage" links

If you're choosing to eat soy because you're a vegetarian, be sure to stick with the fermented products that are closer to their natural state, such as those listed in the earlier section "Vegetarian protein options."

Soy-processing techniques destroy any possible benefit you can gain. In fact, you can even be at risk for estrogen dependent tumor growth — definitely not immune boosting!

Here are some hidden words for processed soy:

- ✔ Hydrolyzed vegetable protein
- ✔ Lecithin
- ✔ Monodiglyceride (who knew?)
- ✔ Protein isolate
- ✔ Soy isolate
- ✔ Soy protein
- ✔ Soya

- ✔ Textured soy flour (TSF)
- ✔ Textured vegetable protein (TVP)
- ✔ Vegetable fat
- ✔ Vegetable oil
- ✔ Vegetable protein

Sneaky food additives

When you eat processed foods, you run the risk of encountering "sneaky stuff" — the unsuspecting additives that find their way into your foods. The marketing of the product may lead you to believe that you're getting something wholesome when, in fact, you're not.

Additives are designed to make a food look good, taste good, and last longer. Here's the kicker: Now, more than 400 additives are perfectly legal to put in your food. If that stirs you, just wait; there's more — many substances used for flavor enhancers don't even have to be listed on the ingredient label. These additives put an unnecessary burden on your immune system to make additives immune suppressors.

Here are the many faces of sneaky food additives:

- ✔ Artificial coloring
- ✔ Artificial sweeteners
- ✔ Emulsifiers
- ✔ Flavor enhancers
- ✔ Glazing agents
- ✔ Preservatives
- ✔ Stabilizers

Monosodium glutamate (MSG) is a common food additive with many different names. It's also what we call a *neurotoxin,* meaning it can have a toxic effect on your nervous system. Headaches, nausea, anxiety, or sleeplessness are all among the side effects of MSG. If you see any of these names on your food label, steer clear:

- ✔ Autolyzed yeast products
- ✔ Glutamate

✔ Anything "hydrolyzed"

✔ Soy protein

✔ Yeast extract

Added corn or maize in a food is something you really have to watch out for. This food isn't immune building, is often genetically modified, and is high on the allergen list. What makes this challenging is that corn and its processed derivatives "sneak" into just about anything packaged — which makes it one of the most overused foods. Look for corn or its derivatives under the following guises:

✔ Corn flour

✔ Corn starch (mazena)

✔ Corn syrup solids

✔ Dextrin

✔ Dextrose

✔ Food starch

✔ High-fructose corn syrup

✔ Maltodextrins

✔ Modified gum starch

✔ Sorbitol

✔ Vegetable gum

✔ Vegetable protein

✔ Vegetable starch

Here's a great way to avoid the sneaky stuff. If you choose to buy packaged or processed foods, look for ingredients that you recognize or know. Also, avoid any foods with too many ingredients. The problem with processed foods are they often have long ingredient lists. When you start getting past five or so ingredients, they're often preservatives, sugars, poor quality oils, and other additives, all of which are terrible for your health. Be careful of snacks, soft drinks, French fries, cured meats, candy, desserts, frozen foods, and fast foods — these foods are highly processed and where additives are frequently found.

Sugar: The monkey on your back

If you want to boost immunity, this section is a must read. It's the bare-bones foundation of how to begin building your immune system.

Ever wonder why some people seemingly have no trouble eating "clean"? Do you think they possess a certain strength or power that most people don't have? Probably not. What they've done is quiet that unrelenting gnawing feeling that can be a monkey on their back. That monkey is your constant desire for sugar or sugary carbohydrates. We've all been there. We know all too well: The more we have, the more we want.

Here's the part of the equation that's so important to understand: Eating sugar releases insulin to reduce your level of blood sugar, which can cause your blood sugar to fluctuate too low. Whenever anything in your body gets a low signal, your brain tells you to do something about it. In this case, it signals you to eat more sugar. Enter the unrelenting cycle that can make you fat and sick.

How does sugar affect your immunity anyway? Sugar is an immune suppressor. As little as 3.5 ounces can suppress your immune system up to 50 percent. The American Journal of Clinical Nutrition published research as early as 1973 that showed these effects start within an hour of consuming sugar and can last up to five hours. Most sugar is void of nutrients, and get this: It actually requires nutrients to metabolize sugar and, therefore, pulls minerals from your body. So sugar can actually deplete your body of vitamins and minerals. Sugar also impairs your white blood cells from doing their job, which is to scavenge up bacteria that can make you sick.

The absolute best way to reprogram your body to not reach for sugar or sugary carbohydrates is to go completely without sugar for 30 days — no cheating, no wavering — just 30 days of cleaning your body, letting yourself get rid of weak, unhealthy cells, and building healthier cells for a more youthful, strong body. The process is scary and difficult, yes, but we promise you it's well worth the effort. It's one of those game changers in life that's worth doing.

We recognize that slaying this sugar monkey on your back may be difficult (breaking any addiction is). However, conquering diseases like cancer, diabetes, and heart disease, which can result from a weak immune system, is probably more difficult.

Sugar can also create the following problems:

- Accelerated aging by oxidative stress, which is an unhealthy state for your cells
- Cancer cells
- Food addictions
- Inflammation in the body
- Insulin resistance
- Less good cholesterol (HDL), more bad cholesterol (LDL)
- Weight gain

Wiping out sugar entirely is nearly impossible, because all carbohydrates are essentially sugar, even the healthy carbohydrates. However, you can control the added sugar. Here's the hit list of added sugars to watch for:

- Agave
- Artificial sugars
- Aspartame (Nutrasweet or Equal)
- Brown sugar
- Corn syrup
- High-fructose corn syrup
- Maltodextrin
- Maple syrup
- Molasses
- Raw sugar
- Rice syrup
- Sucralose (Splenda)
- Sugar cane
- White sugar

After you do your Boosting 30 (see the section "Restarting Your Health and Nutrition with the 'Boosting 30,'" later in this chapter), and you want something sweet, we recommend choosing raw, organic honey once in a while because at least it provides some nutritional benefits and has vitamins, minerals, and amino acids. You can also sweeten recipes with fruit juices. Try to wean yourself off anything that causes you to crave sugar, that is, if you want to boost your immune system, live leaner and stronger, and fight aging.

Having to Say Goodbye to Foods You Love, or Do You?

When you embark on a new food or lifestyle journey, such as the road to boosting your immunity, you often have to change your habits, mindset, or maybe your paradigm. Doing so is well worth the effort. And when something works, people become agents of change. When people find better health and energy, enjoy better body compositions, and start reversing diseases and aging, they're excited to share how they made the change. People also want to be sure they're making the right choices so they continue to flourish.

As people transition their lifestyle to a healthier paradigm, they often want to know whether they have to say goodbye to the foods they love, such as salt, desserts, and alcohol. We address these foods in the following sections.

Salt: Friend or foe?

Nothing is quite like a pinch of salt. It brings out the flavors in just about any food. Thankfully, your "salt tooth" isn't something you have to do without. Your body needs and thrives from salt. Salt is vital to both your nervous system and your glands. Whether salt boosts your immunity or makes you sick completely depends on the source of the salt.

Run-of-the-mill table salt is a heavily refined food. It's chemically cleaned with bleach and then mixed with toxic anti-caking agents to make sure the salt flows properly. Nothing immune boosting about that!

Healthy salt is a different story. These salts are loaded with trace minerals, including magnesium and potassium. These two minerals allow fluids to flow in and out of your cells, letting your cell walls become permeable. When your cells are permeable, your body naturally releases what it doesn't need. Fluids flow in and out, and you don't have fluid retention that causes the high blood pressure you hear about with salt intake.

We do have a salt we love: Fine Ground Vital Mineral Blend of Celtic Salt (www.celticseasalt.com) is rich in minerals and trace elements and has no additives. Very pure, very delicious.

Iodine in salt is actually not natural. Therefore, when you buy unprocessed salt, you won't find iodine in the product. Because you need iodine for your thyroid, hormones, and immune function, make sure you get iodine from other sources, such as the following:

- ✔ Protein: Eggs, meat, poultry
- ✔ Seaweed: Kelp and dulse
- ✔ Strawberries
- ✔ Vegetables: Swiss chard, asparagus, spinach

Another great way to get iodine is from a delicious product called SeaSnax (http://store.seasnax.com). You can use these roasted seaweed sheets, which are naturally rich in iodine, as a snack just by themselves, or you can crumble them up in soups or salads.

Are desserts on the menu?

Dessert doesn't have to be a forbidden word. You don't have to avoid desserts; you just have to get savvy to what kind of desserts are best to boost immunity — and guess what? They can put any bakery to the test.

What you have to know is that you're hard-wired to have desserts from time to time. The problem doesn't arise from the fact that you eat something sweet once in a while; the problem comes from how *often* and *what kind* of sweets you're eating to satisfy your sweet tooth.

These days, desserts are wrapped in packages and loaded with sugar (both artificial and real) and contain artificial flavorings, preservatives, and colors. Even going out for ice cream can land you in a world of artificial ingredients because "new and improved" methods and tastes are always being born. If you opt for a baked good to tantalize your sweet tooth, your trip to the bakery will most likely leave you reeling into a massive sugar-a-thon. For a real look at what sugar does to your system, refer to the section "Sugar: The monkey on your back," earlier in this chapter.

The answer is not to give up on desserts but to *redefine* desserts. You simply need to temper your natural craving for sweets with modern sugar in its most natural form: fruits and nuts.

We promise you won't be disappointed. Boosting desserts will blast your body with not only scrumptious good taste — we know they have to taste amazing — but also phytonutrient immune-boosting power. Going with berries and other low-sugar fruits, eaten slowly to really give you their honest-to-goodness homegrown taste, is the way to go. The transformation happens when you add natural seasonings that turn fruit into decadence. Dessert is born!

None of the desserts we recommend will suppress your immune system. Vanilla, coconut flakes, crushed nuts, and lemon zest are all miraculous taste twisters that add that wow factor! (See our recipes for boosting desserts in Chapter 18).

A great way to reprogram your taste buds and calm that need for super sugary sweets and carbohydrates is to try putting together an immune-building plate for 30 days. Watch your overactive sweet fix get slayed! See "Restarting Your Health and Nutrition with the 'Boosting 30,'" later in this chapter.

How about happy hour?

Enjoying moderate amounts of alcohol while socializing does have some positive aspects. And ingesting small amounts of alcohol is said to have some health benefits, such as lowering risk of cardiovascular disease. However, alcohol is toxic to the liver, it's a known carcinogen, and, because it's a drug, alcohol has addictive qualities. So make wise choices, and don't over-consume. The best scenario is no alcohol, but when you make the choice to drink, proceed with caution.

If you decide to have a glass of wine or spirits (for special occasions), try to make the best choices. Here are some suggestions:

- Organic red wine
- Organic sparkling wine
- Organic white wine
- Potato vodka
- Rum
- Tequila

The drier the wine, the less sugar content it has. Try pinot noir, cabernet sauvignon, and merlot for the red wines, and sauvignon blanc and albariño for the whites.

Mix spirits with soda water, ice, and a squeeze of fresh lemon or lime juice. Avoid sodas, juices, or tonic water, all which are very high in sugar. Also, when you indulge, get plenty of fat and protein in your belly!

When choosing to celebrate, steer clear of grain-based drinks that can also include gluten. These spirits are off limits 100 percent of the time:

- Beer
- Bourbon
- Gin (some brands are processed with grain-based alcohol)
- Grain-based vodka
- Whiskey

Restarting Your Health and Nutrition with the "Boosting 30"

For 30 days, stick to all the foods we mention in the section "Calling in Nutrition's Big Guns," earlier in this chapter, and build your plate according to our advice in the section "Building Your Plate for Everyday Wellness and Robust Immunity," also earlier in this chapter. Sticking to these basics for 30 days — no cheating, hedging, or going back and forth — will dramatically reduce your cravings for sugar.

During the 30 days, you begin to break habits, diminish food cravings and food addictions, detoxify your body in the most natural way possible, and flood your body with nutrition. This process won't be a walk in the park, mind you. You may feel lousy at first, which is to be expected. Some people may even experience "the carb flu" symptoms — exhaustion, mental fuzziness, fatigue, headaches, and shakiness — for up to three weeks, when their body goes from burning those sugary carbs for energy to burning fat for energy.

Healthy fats are a helping hand in conquering the symptoms of the carb flu. Try a handful of coconut flakes or nuts or have some full-fat coconut milk.

You start to change as your cells start regenerating. You become leaner, your skin looks healthier, and your eyes become brighter. Just give the rest of your body time to catch up! ***Remember:*** The length of discomfort varies from person to person. Just know that if you stick with your boosting 30, the magic *will* happen. Your body will be cleaner, leaner, stronger, and you'll become more and more disease free.

Chapter 9

Tapping the Immune Properties of Superfoods

***

In This Chapter

▶ Understanding the nutritional powers of superfoods

▶ Looking at everyday superfoods that can improve your health

***

*N*othing beats deep nutrition. *Deep nutrition* is when your foods start healing you on a cellular level. When you experience true nutritional excellence, your immune system becomes solid, you no longer have to fear diseases, and you age gracefully.

A nutritionally competent immune system is like a sturdy, dependable battleship. It protects you through storms of illnesses that come your way and guards you against all the serious potential invaders. Your body begins to operate on a different level. You have more energy, look younger, and feel stronger.

The purpose of this chapter is to get you in the know about certain superfoods that have powerful immune-building effects. These superfoods are easily available and can heal and protect against acute and chronic diseases. What's more amazing is that even in moderate amounts, these superfoods can make a big difference in your health.

In this chapter, we explain why superfoods are different from the pack; we introduce you to everyday superfoods and how they may help you lose weight. Add these foods to your immune-building plate, and take your health to a new level!

Getting the Scoop on Superfoods

Superfoods can heal, protect, and make you look and feel younger. They do these things so well because they have a *high nutrient density,* meaning that you get a high amount of nutrition for the amount of calories they contain. In other words, you get a lot of nutrients without costing you much in terms of calories.

Understanding nutrient density is important because so much malnutrition and obesity exist today from people eating too many packaged, processed, or refined foods that are high in calories and low in nutrition. These types of food have *low nutrient density* and should be avoided.

In the following sections, we fill you in on how and why superfoods differ from other foods. We also explore a bonus to eating superfoods: weight loss.

Separating superfoods from the rest of the pack

Superfoods give you nutrients galore. The information these foods provide to your cells sets you up for health and longevity.

What are these superfoods? Certain berries, tree fruits, root vegetables, leafy greens, spices, teas, and other deep healing foods (see the section "Robust, Everyday Superfoods with the 'It' Factor," later in this chapter). These nutrition-packed foods benefit you by doing the following:

✔ **Keeping your heart healthy and reducing blood pressure:** Your body is so amazing; it operates daily — breathing, digesting, and even your heart beating — without you ever having to think about it. Even though you may not feel it happening, it's a lot of work for your heart to pump 2,000 gallons throughout your body every day. To keep up with the workload, your heart has to be healthy. Eating superfoods helps lower your cardiac risk factors in the following ways:

   • You get the vitamins and minerals you need without all the calories and the sugary carbohydrates from low nutrient-dense foods, which can cause elevation in triglycerides and eventually lead to plaque buildup. (See the nearby sidebar "Cholesterol and triglycerides in a [big] nutshell" for an explanation on triglycerides.)

   • You get natural disease-fighting substances called *flavonoids,* which reduce blood pressure and inflammation in your arteries. Flavonoids come with an even bigger bonus: They stimulate antioxidant activity, which repairs damage done to your cells by smoking, pollution, fried foods, and poisons as well as damage done as a byproduct of normal metabolism.

   • Some superfoods contain healthy fats, such as polyunsaturated fatty acids (PUFAs; see Chapter 8), which regulate your heartbeat and blood pressure.

   • Fruits and vegetables contain dietary fiber, which keeps you feeling full and prevents overeating, thus preventing a rise in triglycerides.

Cholesterol and triglycerides in a (big) nutshell

Cholesterol is a fatty-like substance that your body needs for cell membranes and hormones to function. Two forms of cholesterol exist: LDL (bad) and HDL (good). LDL stands for low-density lipoprotein — think *lousy* cholesterol — and is bad because it gets stuck in arteries and causes blockages. The good cholesterol, high-density lipoprotein (HDL) — think *happy* cholesterol — works like a sweeper. It sweeps away all the bad cholesterol and takes it to the liver for disposal. The key is to keep the balance between these two in order. Also, the actual size and the number of cholesterol particles are important. The bigger the molecule, the better. Studies show that the small-particle LDLs can raise a person's chances of a heart attack by a factor of about 3, because the smaller particles have a way of wedging themselves into the arterial wall. Because only 50 percent of the people with coronary artery disease have high levels of LDLs or any other risk factors, measuring the percentage of LDLs with a standard cholesterol screening test may not be enough. You may want to get an additional test called a *subfraction analysis.* It usually costs about $100 and may not be covered by insurance.

Tip: If you want a detailed analysis of your cholesterol, be sure to have your *percentages,* *size,* and *particles* of cholesterol evaluated. You can ask your healthcare practitioner to do this test, called a *CV Health Test,* or you can go through the lab we recommend, Genova Diagnostics, who will also include other valuable testing for cardiac risk factors, such as how much inflammation you have or how your body processes insulin. Another option,

which isn't as extensive but certainly a viable alternative, is called the *VAP Cholesterol Test* from Quest Diagnostics. This simple blood test is often covered by insurance and is easily accessible through your healthcare practitioner.

Triglycerides are a function of eating too much of the wrong foods, such as nutrient-poor, sugary carbohydrates. Your body turns these extra calories into triglycerides that are then stored in your fat cells for later use. High levels of these triglycerides lead to plaque buildup in the arteries. Researchers are always on a quest to understand exactly how triglycerides affect the body. Testing for triglycerides involves a simple blood test that your healthcare practitioner can administer. In fact, when you get a comprehensive cholesterol screening, such as the CV Health Test or VAP Cholesterol Test, your triglycerides will be tested as part of the panel.

The importance of these two fatty substances is that, when elevated, triglycerides and cholesterol work together to damage the heart. Many people with high triglyceride levels have low HDLs and high LDLs. Often, they go hand in hand. When all these fats build up, they restrict the networks to your heart, and your risk of heart disease increases. Although both of these fats are naturally occurring in the body, most instances of high cholesterol and triglycerides are from outside factors, such as lifestyle. Eating sugary carbohydrates and unhealthy fats and not exercising are often big contributing factors, which is why an immune-building lifestyle is also good for your heart!

✔ **Providing immunity against cancer:** Many superfoods have cancer-fighting properties. Foods rich in nutrients help prevent you from getting cancer — and help you beat cancer. The largest cancer research center in the United Kingdom, World Cancer Research Fund (WCRF), asserts that between 35 and 70 percent of cancer is related to eating an unhealthy diet. A diet rich and sufficient in nutrients provides the opposite — a strong defense against cancer. Tomatoes with *lycopene* (a healing phytochemical), berries with *antioxidants* (phytochemicals that neutralize damage done to your cells), broccoli with a phytochemical known to slow down the progression of cancer, and garlic with its cancer-fighting properties are all examples of how these powerful superfoods can protect you and your family against cancer.

✔ **Calming inflammation:** When your body is exposed to stresses, it becomes inflamed. Pollution, processed foods, smoke, mental or physical stress, and illnesses are some of the triggers that open the gate for inflammation to set in. When you eat foods rich in nutrients that boost your immunity, you put the fire out on a lot of the inflammation in your body and lower the probability that you'll have ongoing or chronic inflammation, which can lead to more serious health problems.

✔ **Lessening digestive disturbances:** If we had a dime for every person who came in to see us for problems stemming from digestion, such as constipation, gas, bloating, hemorrhoids, abdominal aches, and discomfort, we'd be buried in dimes. Digestive disturbance is a very common (and unnecessary) ailment. Eating superfoods improves your digestion a great deal. When you boost your fiber intake naturally by adding some of the fiber-rich superfoods, like almonds, avocados, and broccoli, your digestion starts to wake up and your body absorbs nutrients and water better. The more nutrient-sufficient state your body is in, the better it will run and provide you with superimmunity.

✔ **Building a strong defense against disease:** Superfoods are continuing to show evidence of their potent ability to fight and prevent disease. They contain great properties to strengthen the body's immune system. Garlic, for example, has been used as a natural antibiotic for more than a century. Studies have shown garlic to kill bacteria. When you add super-foods to your plate, you can say goodbye to all those sick days.

✔ **Building healthy cells with antioxidant power:** Antioxidants are natural substances that fight cellular damage. These substances, called *bioflavonoids* (or vitamin P, which isn't really a vitamin; in fact, it's more powerful), give fruits and vegetables their color. That's one of the reasons it's so important to build your plate with "rainbow-like colors." Superfoods are power packed with these antioxidants and provide you with healthy cells and less cellular damage due to free radicals. Blueberries, broccoli, and spinach are all great examples of superfoods with a strong antioxidant power.

What are free radicals? Free radicals are unstable molecules that can travel throughout the body, trying to take particles from healthy cells. This process creates even more free radicals, which damages more cells, and causes inflammation and a chain reaction of damaged cells. One of the roles of antioxidants is to fight this cell damage.

✔ **Fighting aging:** These superfoods are a big piece of the "aging beautifully" piece. When you see someone that looks as though they're aging so gracefully, you wonder whether they might know something. Eating powerful superfoods may be part of their lifestyle habit that helps give them the extra youth boost. Superfoods promote a lean body through higher nutrient-dense foods naturally lower in calories, beautiful skin through eating the foods rich in antioxidants that build better collagen, and definitely more zoom in your step due to nutritional sufficiency. You end up with a youthful glow. You can even guard against the need for age-related visual correction by adding superfoods rich in nutrients like antioxidants and healthy fats.

✔ **Fighting blood sugar battles:** Superfoods are the perfect foods to balance blood sugar and prevent diabetes and high blood sugars. Superfoods are non-starchy and provide many nutrients and protective compounds that won't cause your blood sugar to have swings. Also, the fiber helps you feel full with fewer calories for longer periods of time. This slows the release of insulin. Controlling insulin is the lock and key to preventing and controlling blood sugar issues. When you build your plate with these superfoods, you start to notice how much more balanced you feel when your blood sugar is stable.

Tacking on a superfood bonus: Weight loss

Superfoods can make you stronger, disease proof, and feel and look younger, but a major bonus to adding superfoods to your life is the ability to lose weight and keep it off. One really fantastic natural side effect to being healthy is normalizing your weight.

Superfoods are your non-diet diet. You can eat these foods for a lifetime. When you begin to build your plate for immunity (see Chapter 8), you'll begin to lose weight without even trying to lose weight. Effortless weight loss and a youthful glow are the result of the nutrient-dense foods with crucial nutrients, which are low in calories, high in fiber, high in water content, and some even high in protein.

Another natural byproduct of eating superfoods is that you'll get refueled. For many, you'll feel energy on a regular basis for the first time in a long time. This energy catalyzes you to do much more with your day. This has a cyclical affect. The healthier you become, the more energy you have, the more your body moves, and the more you lose weight.

Superfoods also keep you hormonally balanced and burning fat. When you eat foods that cause you to release too much insulin (see Chapter 8), your body starts to become resistant to insulin, which is the precursor to diabetes and hormonal problems, both of which cause weight gain. However, when you eat superfoods, insulin release is kept at a low level, which causes your body to use stored fat for fuel. This is key — because this is what keeps you in a fat-burning mode.

Weight normalization is when your weight normalizes to its natural state. You become the weight your body is designed to be. Forget about being too skinny or overexercising. When you treat your body with superfoods, you'll see a change. Looking and feeling good becomes effortless — natural. Always remember the byproduct of healthy cells is looking good.

Robust, Everyday Superfoods with the "It" Factor

Most diets probably include packaged, processed, mineral-deficient food, foods sprayed with pesticides, antibiotic treated meat, hormonally altered dairy products, refined sugar, refined grains, and refined salt. Over time, these foods cause a dysfunctional immune system, low energy, and the inability to lose weight.

That's one of the many reasons these superfoods are so valuable. It's as if you push your body's compost button and start fresh. Superfoods detoxify you, replenish you with all the nutrients you need, and rebuild you with healthier cells, which paves the way for you to flourish in every way.

Robust with flavor and bursting with nutrition is what the "it" factor is all about. The food you eat is paramount in creating healthy cells. Think of it this way: Food is the raw material that builds your blood and cells, and your organs are made of cells. You really are walking food! Understanding what foods to make a part of your immune-boosting lifestyle is paramount in living a disease-free, strong, vibrant, and youthful life.

In the following sections, we introduce some of these magnificent superfoods (listed in alphabetical order) that all set the stage to boost your immunity.

Dark chocolate

Most of the time when people think of superfoods, chocolate isn't even on their radar. That's why we love to give patients the green light on dark chocolate. When you think healthy chocolate, you have to think "dark chocolate." This kind of chocolate contains more cocoa than milk chocolate, which is where all the healing powers come from.

Cocoa is rich in *epicatechin,* which is a type of flavonoid (antioxidants found naturally in plants) that reduces inflammation, improves vascular health, protects cells from damage that could cause disease, and reduces the pregnancy related condition called *preeclampsia.* It's also rich in magnesium, which is great for your nervous system.

Look for dark chocolate that's at least 65 percent cocoa to ensure that you get the flavonoids without all the sugar and fat. Store it in a cold, dark place at about 70 degrees Fahrenheit. Also, avoid Dutch-processed cocoa, which is processed in such a way that destroys its health benefits.

What's the telltale sign of a good, healthy piece of chocolate? When it breaks off evenly without little pieces crumbling off the edges. A good-for-you chocolate will break solid and clean.

Fruits

The health benefits of immune-boosting fruits come from the vitamins, minerals, and phytochemicals they contain, all of which help the body fight and prevent disease. Fruits also contain fiber, which is great for digestive health, as well as lutein, which is healthy for your vision.

Although fruits contain many healthful elements, keeping your serving size low is important. The fruit sugar *fructose,* while all natural, still causes insulin to rise too much, causing blood sugar problems, diabetes, heart disease, and obesity. Enjoy the following fruit superfoods in moderation, and don't let fruit push vegetables off your plate!

Apples, oranges, cantaloupes, grapes, and cherries are best purchased organic to reduce your exposure to pesticides that are toxic to your health.

✔ **Berries:** Blueberries, cranberries, raspberries, blackberries, cherries, and strawberries win our gold star of approval of the top immune-boosting fruits. These fruits contain phytochemicals (natural plant chemicals) that give them their vibrant colors, called *anthocyanins.* Berries are flooded with antioxidants, are an excellent source of vitamins and minerals, and are also high in fiber. They provide all this nutrition and are low in natural sugars to boot! They suppress the growth of several cancers and colds, reduce high blood pressure, and prevent strokes, arthritis, and osteoporosis.

✔ **Avocado:** Although berries win the award for our favorite fruits, avocado comes in a close second. What's unique about avocado is that it's one of the few fruits that contain fat. The fatty acids it contains are superior fats. This fat soothes inflammation, controls blood sugar balance, and is super healthy for your cells. In addition to being filled with nutrients, avocados are also a nutrient booster, enabling you to absorb other nutrients you take in from other foods you consume.

✔ **Lemon:** Lemons are super versatile and contain numerous health benefits. Lemons naturally cleanse the body, and the antifungal and antiseptic qualities help kill germs. Lemons provide a wealth of vitamins and minerals, including lots of vitamin C, and have been shown to slow the rate of cancer growth. Lemons also help balance the acidity in your body, which is great for boosting your immune system.

✔ **Lime:** Limes are also versatile, and they have the amazing ability to speed up your body's healing process. Limes contain antiviral properties that trigger the production of white blood cells, which gobble up all the harmful bacteria or dead and dying cells.

✔ **Apple:** Eating apples is like giving your body a mini-cleanse. Apples are rich in the fiber *pectin,* which binds cholesterol, toxins, and heavy metals to move them out of your body. Apples clean out your colon, keeping it healthy, which makes your skin glow.

✔ **Rose hip:** Rose hips are the berrylike fruits of the rose bush left behind after the bloom has died. Rose hips contain 20 times more vitamin C by weight than oranges. Rose hips also improve resistance to infection by stimulating white blood cells, making you resistant to colds, and are commonly used to make immune-building teas. Fresh rose hips are always more potent in vitamin C than the dried varieties.

✔ **Orange:** Most of us know that oranges are a top source of vitamin C. However, there's more to oranges than meets the eye. They contain *beta sitosterol,* which has been shown to prevent tumor growth and lower blood cholesterol. The versatility of oranges allows you to enjoy this high-fiber fruit on its own or in some savory dishes or drinks!

✔ **Grapefruit:** Detoxification is what grapefruit does so well. It also inhibits cancer growth and lowers cholesterol. It's an antifungal and an antiparasitic. Grapefruits have also been linked to weight loss.

- **Kiwi:** Kiwi is loaded with vitamin C, more so than the familiar vitamin-C-containing orange. Just one of these little guys contains 120 percent of an adult's daily recommended dose. Kiwi is also a great fruit for fiber.

   Kiwi can cause allergic symptoms in some children.

- **Mango:** Mango is a delicious tropical fruit that's loaded in beta carotene, the precursor to vitamin A. Vitamin A is antiviral and important for immune function. Mango is also one of the only fruit sources of vitamin E, which protects against cell damage and boosts disease-fighting antibodies.

- **Cantaloupe:** The healing ability of cantaloupe comes from its beta carotene. Vitamin A plays a big hand in producing white blood cells to fight disease. Also rich in vitamin C, this fruit helps protect against colds, cancer, and heart disease.

- **Pomegranates:** This fruit provides numerous benefits. Studies show that pomegranates have antioxidant, anticancer, and anti-inflammatory abilities. The juice and the seeds of this fruit stop tumor cells from growing, spreading, or creating blood supplies. Pomegranates lower blood pressure, improve heart health, reverses atherosclerosis, and improve depression.

- **Grapes:** Grapes strengthen your capillaries, so they're a powerful natural remedy to improve circulation and prevent heart disease. They're high in antioxidants, keeping your cells healthy and free from the damage that causes disease. Grapes are another detoxifying immune-building fruit, detoxifying the skin, liver, kidney, and intestines.

   When you buy grapes, reach for the red grapes instead of the white. Red grapes contain more *anthocyanins,* which are the antioxidants found in grapes that make them so immune building.

- **Cherries:** Cherries perform in your body in a similar way that berries do. They contain a powerful compound that blocks cancer cells from developing. Rich in antioxidants, cherries help you fight disease, viruses, and bacteria. The anti-inflammatory nature of cherries provides relief to inflammatory diseases like arthritis.

- **Pineapple:** The protein-digesting enzyme in pineapple called *bromelain* is responsible for all pineapple's wonderful qualities. Bromelain's power comes from reducing inflammation. Injuries, digestive discomforts, sinusitis, arthritis, as well as any inflammatory condition are supported by the use of pineapple. It tastes good, too!

Nuts and seeds

Nuts and seeds are nature's gift. They're crunchy, delicious, and a great snack in a pinch or between meals to balance your blood sugar. But that's not why they're superfoods. They also have many talents. They have healthy oils and vitamin E that help reduce heart disease, cancer, diabetes, cognitive decline, inflammation, and aging. They're filled with vitamin minerals (called *micronutrients*) that help all the interworking and connections of the body work better. Studies also show that people lost more weight when they consumed reasonable amounts of nuts and seeds than those who didn't.

The following are the gold standard in nuts and seeds in order according to their nutritional profile (see Figure 9-1 for a visual):

- ✔ First picks:
  - Cashews
  - Hazelnuts
  - Macadamia nuts
- ✔ Second picks:
  - Almonds
  - Brazil nuts
  - Pecans
  - Pistachios
- ✔ Third picks:
  - Pine nuts
  - Pumpkin seeds
  - Sesame seeds
  - Sunflower seeds
  - Walnuts

We talk a lot about food quality in this book, because the source of your food is directly related to how useful it is to building healthy cells. When it comes to nuts and seeds, this point rings loud and clear.

When you're buying nuts and seeds, be sure they're not rancid. When they're rancid, they lose their nutrients and can even be unhealthy. It's actually better to not eat nuts and seeds at all than to eat them rancid. Here are some tips:

- ✔ Buy nuts only in the shell. Don't buy nuts or seeds hulled or shelled.
- ✔ Purchase raw, not roasted nuts. Cashews are the exception here because in the raw state, the shell that surrounds the cashew nut contains a toxic chemical residue called *urushiol,* which can cause an allergic reaction, so be sure not to eat *raw* cashews.
- ✔ Purchase unsalted nuts. The salt covers up the rancidity and makes it hard to detect.

✔ Store in dark containers in cold places (the refrigerator is a great spot).

✔ Don't store in plastic (the oil combines with the plastic, making them toxic).

✔ Buy in bulk bins in a busy store where they move quickly. Farmers' markets are a good bet as well.

✔ Don't purchase more than a month's supply at once. You can freeze nuts and seeds for up to three months.

If you have trouble finding fresh nuts and seeds, try Sun Organic Farm (www. sunorganic.com). It supplies quality products delivered to your door.

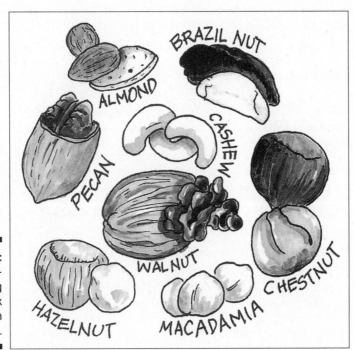

Figure 9-1:
Immune-
boosting
nuts pack
a punch in
nutrition.

Illustration by Elizabeth Kurtzman

Spices and herbs

Nothing perks up your food like the personality of spices and herbs. The wonderful bonus prize is that many of these spices also keep you well.

Although herbs carry amazing healing properties, they're a man-made medicine, and with any medicine, natural or not, you want to be careful not to overuse or misuse. Consult with a healthcare practitioner who can work with you and your personal needs for dosing concerns.

Spices and herbs are great for boosting the nervous system, respiratory system, and your glands. Here are our honorable mentions:

- **Cinnamon:** This warming and strengthening spice wins our golden seal for the number-one spice. Every household should have cinnamon. Here's why: A whopping 24 million Americans have Type 2 (adult-onset) diabetes. Another 57 million have blood sugar handling problems that are pre-diabetic. Researchers credit cinnamon's active ingredient *cinnamaldehyde* for its ability to decrease blood sugar, total cholesterol, and triglycerides as well as increase good cholesterol. Cinnamon balances blood sugar long term and stops spikes in blood sugar after a meal. It improves your body's sensitivity to insulin and lowers risk factors for pre-diabetes. Also, this wonderful spice is helpful in the treatment of cancer because it may slow the development of new blood supplies to tumors. Delicious and versatile, cinnamon is good stuff!

- **Cayenne:** If you have a ticker, you should have some cayenne. This spice provides amazing cardiovascular benefits. Cayenne lowers blood pressure and has even been known to stop a heart attack! Cayenne thins phlegm and eases its passage through the lungs. You can improve digestion, nausea, or gas with cayenne.

- **Black pepper:** This is a great spice to turbo jump your digestion. Pepper helps move food along the colon at a good pace, called your *bowel transit time,* and the quicker and smoother the ride, the healthier your colon. Black pepper's healing power is attributed to *piperines,* which are the compounds that give you that zing when you eat some. Black pepper also helps prevent and treat cancer and reduces the compounds known to worsen the inflammation of arthritis — providing much pain relief for arthritis sufferers.

  If you have digestive complaints, be careful about using black pepper because it can be irritating to the intestinal lining.

- **Turmeric:** The active ingredient in turmeric is *curcumin.* This ingredient is so diverse and so deep in its antioxidant power that it's been shown to protect and heal virtually every organ in the human body. Turmeric is a cornucopia of healing; it holds promise in about every area of disease prevention and healing imaginable. Turmeric protects against cancer, Alzheimer's disease, Parkinson's disease, heart disease, stroke, diabetes, eye diseases, depression, skin problems, and more. So amazing is this spice that research at Tufts University showed turmeric may prevent weight gain. Wow!

- **Curry:** This is a standard spice used in India to control diabetes, prevent or treat heart disease, infection, age-related memory loss, and inflammation. Curry has powerful antioxidants called *carbazole alkaloids* that are abundant only in curry leaf and are responsible for preventing cell damage, which causes disease and premature aging.

✔ **Oregano:** This herb is your natural protection against infection. The active compounds in oregano are *carvacrol* and *thymol.* These compounds have strong antiviral, antibacterial, and antifungal properties. Oregano helps get rid of intestinal parasites, kills the bacteria that causes food poisoning, heals ulcers, calms intestinal irritation, and aids in digestion. It has a lot of minerals, antioxidants, fiber, and omega-3 fatty acids. Does it get any better?

✔ **Parsley:** Parsley is the helping hand. It contains an antioxidant called *apigenin,* unique to parsley, which helps other antioxidants work better. Parsley has so many healing powers; it's amazing. Parsley is used as a diuretic, can reduce high blood pressure, and is a natural agent to fight cancer, heart disease, and Type 2 diabetes. As you can see, parsley is much more than a garnish!

✔ **Thyme:** If you need an antiseptic, the healing oil in thyme called *thymol* is what you're looking for. When applied to skin or the mucous membranes of the mouth, it kills germs. It's great for calming coughs, helping to prevent teeth decay, and helping to prevent infection.

✔ **Peppermint:** Peppermint relaxes your intestinal tract, which makes mint wonderful for intestinal discomfort, such as irritable bowel syndrome. It calms indigestion, and, because it's rich in menthol, it eases nasal congestion and respiratory discomfort to help you breathe easier. It also kills the bacteria that cause tooth decay and plaque buildup.

✔ **Ginger:** Ginger is the king of all natural digestive aids. It relieves nausea and vomiting, settles the stomach, and eases the discomfort from gas and bloating. Research shows that ginger is one of the most effective remedies available for motion sickness, even more so than over-the-counter medications. Ginger is a miracle for the nausea-induced morning sickness of pregnancy or post surgeries or the delayed nausea associated with chemotherapy treatment. Because ginger is rich in phytonutrients called *gingerols,* which are antioxidant, antibacterial, antiviral, and anti-inflammatory, ginger is a great helper in the treatment of migraine headaches, arthritis, and asthma.

For a warming winter drink, break off some ginger and throw it into a pot of water. Bring to boil, turn off the stove, and let the ginger sit for 20 minutes. It's not only warming and delicious but also a great digestive aide after a meal.

Hot stuff to the rescue

Hot foods like radishes, chili pepper, cayenne, hot mustard, hot peppers, garlic, and onion all contain substances called *mucolytics,* which thins mucus. If you have a lot of congestion in your sinuses or breathing passages, hot foods are the way to go!

Teas

Coffee may be the beverage of choice in America, but many populations consume tea more than any beverage, except water. Teas are inexpensive, have no calories, and are associated with relaxation and sense of community. People around the world not only enjoy the taste of teas, but they also reap the awards of the positive health benefits. Teas contain *polyphenols,* which are a broad class of antioxidants that stimulate immune system cells to make your body a disease-fighting machine. Tea helps prevent cancer and osteoporosis, lowers blood pressure, lowers risk for stroke and heart disease, and even fights aging. Teas also contain compounds that help you absorb fat, so you can even lose weight drinking tea. If you're not sipping on some tea — you may be missing out!

You can drink teas as you like them — hot or iced. You can prepare them the easy way from ready-made tea bags or you can use dried or fresh herbs. However you like them, the healing benefits are amazing.

You can find immune-building teas to strengthen your body's own natural defenses or to rebuild your body systems and strength. Here are our top immune-boosting picks:

- ✔ White tea
- ✔ Green tea
- ✔ Black tea
- ✔ Rooibos (pronounced roy-boss) tea
- ✔ Yerba Mate (great coffee substitute)

Vegetables

Adding immune-boosting vegetables to your diet is one of the most critical lifestyle changes you can make. The difference veggies make in your health is worth any effort. They reduce your risk of chronic diseases, such as heart disease and some cancers. Veggies help you not only get well and stay well but also look good! When your body gains nutritional sufficiency from vegetables, your hair, skin, and eyes all show the signs of health.

To avoid the toxicity, we suggest buying organic vegetables that are traditionally higher in pesticides, such as mushrooms, tomatoes, beets, spinach, red peppers, and sweet potatoes.

Don't hesitate to load your plate (with a minimum of two) of the following veggies:

✔ **Cruciferous vegetables:** These vegetables are the gold standard in immune-boosting vegetables and definitely our top pick. Although all vegetables have nutrients and some protective powers, for these vegetables, it's off the charts. Cruciferous vegetables have a special chemical composition: They have sulfur-containing compounds that are responsible for their pungent flavors. When they're broken down by biting, blending, or chopping, a chemical reaction occurs that converts these sulfur-containing compounds into *isothiocyanates* (ITCs). ITCs prevent and knock out cancer and have infinite proven immune-boosting capabilities. They contain antiviral and antibacterial agents that keep you disease free. Adding the following cruciferous vegetables to your daily plate is like taking an anticancer pill:

- Arugula
- Beet greens
- Bok Choy
- Broccoli, broccolini, and broccoli rabe
- Brussels sprouts
- Cabbage
- Cauliflower
- Collards

- Horseradish
- Kale
- Kohlrabi
- Mustard greens
- Radishes
- Red cabbage
- Turnip greens
- Watercress

Because the magic happens when cruciferous vegetables are broken down, try to eat as much of these in the raw state so you can chew, chew, and chew!

✔ **Garlic:** Garlic is surely one of the world's most potent medicines, and its potent smell is what makes it so powerful. The active ingredient *allicin* turns into *organosulfurs,* which are the compounds that keep your cells safe from all the destructive cellular processes that can cause major chronic diseases. Garlic is a natural antiseptic; it prevents cancer, fights infection, and prevents colds. Research also states that garlic may prevent or decrease chronic diseases associated with age, such as atherosclerosis, stroke, cancer, immune disorders, brain aging, cataracts, and arthritis. Even though garlic may "hang around" for a couple of days, it may be worth it!

To help get rid of garlic breath, try adding parsley to garlicky meals. After chopping garlic, washing your hands with lemon juice and water can help eliminate the smell from your hands.

✔ **Onion:** Onion has potent healing powers. Onions are rich in *quercetin*, a powerful antioxidant that may reduce the risk of cancer. Like garlic, onions also contain the amazing compound *allicin.* Red and purple onions contain *anthocyanins,* the same antioxidants that make berries so robust in healing powers. In addition to being extraordinary at preventing and healing cancer, the quercetin contained in onion makes them a safe therapy for allergies; it also helps prevent heart disease and reduce high blood pressure.

✔ **Mushrooms:** Although cruciferous vegetables are the top dog of healthy vegetables, mushrooms are a close second. The power of mushrooms comes from their ability to enhance the activity of natural killer T cells (NKT). These NKTs attack and remove cells that are damaged or infected by a virus. Mushrooms are associated with decreasing most cancers and significantly reducing the risk of breast cancer in women. They prevent DNA damage, slow cancer or tumor growth, and prevent tumors from acquiring a blood supply. To avoid pesticides, choose organic versions of these immune-building mushroom varieties (also see Figure 9-2):

- Cremini
- Maitake
- Oyster
- Portobello
- Reishi
- White

Make sure you cook all mushrooms because toxic effects from mushrooms have been noted in some animal studies.

✔ **Tomato:** Tomatoes are chock-full of vitamin C; in fact, one medium-sized tomato gives you 50 percent of your recommended daily dose of vitamin C. Tomatoes are also the richest source of the exceptionally potent antioxidant *lycopene,* a substance that prevents cancer, particularly cancer of the prostate. Tomatoes also have high levels of beta carotene, an antioxidant that supports the immune system. They have high dietary fiber and taste delicious raw or cooked.

Cooking tomatoes releases the potent healer lycopene. Try making some immune-building tomato sauce to get your dose of lycopene!

✔ **Beets:** Beets are an amazing blood purifier. They're rich in iron and produce the disease-fighting white blood cells. They also stimulate red blood cells and improve the supply of oxygen to the cells. Beets prevent cancer and heart disease, and the detoxifying properties make them good for your organs. Beets are also high in fiber and nourishing for digestive health.

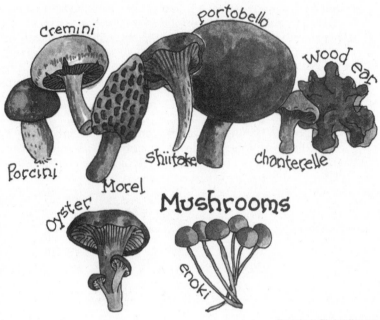

Mushrooms

Illustration by Elizabeth Kurtzman

Figure 9-2:
Pick from
mushrooms
for immune-
boosting
qualities.

✔ **Spinach:** Spinach is rich in beta carotene, which the body transforms into vitamin A, triggering your immune response to keep you well. Spinach prevents cancer and heart disease and is rich in the disease-fighting mineral *zinc.* The vitamin C helps you resist colds and infection and keeps your skin healthy; the B vitamins keep you calm and more energetic.

✔ **Asparagus:** Asparagus's biggest talent is its ability to encourage the body to flush out toxins, due to its natural diuretic abilities. It's both cleansing and anti-inflammatory to the body. It has the antioxidant *glutathione,* which can lower your risk factor for heart disease and cancer. It's useful for all inflammatory conditions, such as arthritis and irritable bowel syndrome.

✔ **Artichoke:** This vegetable supports the liver. The substance *cynarin* gives artichoke its detoxifying qualities. Artichokes' B vitamins increase mental alertness and strengthen your immunity.

Because of the protective effects of artichokes on the liver and it's diuretic capabilities, artichokes have been used traditionally as a remedy for the ill-fated hangover.

- **Red bell pepper:** This sweet and lively vegetable is bursting with vitamin C, making it a powerful immune builder. Red bell pepper's high level of beta carotene turns into vitamin A, making it a strong defense against disease. Although green and yellow peppers are certainly healthy, they're more superfood*ish*. Although they both have similar amounts of vitamin C, red bell peppers have quite a bit more of the superstar beta carotene.

- **Sweet potato:** Sweet potatoes are far superior than the run-of-the-mill white potato. The orange variety contains beta carotene, which makes them filled with robust antioxidant, antiviral, and anticancer abilities. They're also full of fiber and the vitamin E they contain is healthy for the skin.

Always buy sweet potatoes with the red skin because they contain the most beta carotene. The more beta carotene, the more vitamin A, which is a powerful antioxidant to fight cancer.

Chapter 10

Getting an Extra Kick from Supplements and Herbs

Sometimes your body just needs that extra kick. If your immune system has been in a slump for a while or if you're nutritionally deficient, boosting your immunity with supplements or medicinal herbs may give you that extra kick to move you toward health.

Getting the nutrition you need from lean protein, healthy carbohydrates, fats, and water should always be your goal. Nothing replaces real, wholesome food with deep nutrition. However, getting nutritious foods isn't always feasible. Food and environment don't always provide you with everything you need. Sometimes, supplementing with natural compounds found in the foods you eat can rev up your body and boost your nutrition.

You can't rely on supplementation as your sole means of nutrition. A poor diet eventually makes you deficient and malnourished — and quite possibly overweight. Think of supplementing as your *support system,* not as your sole source of nutrients. Remember that vitamins and minerals are responsible for all the reactions and interactions of the body, and they work synergistically to make them happen. Living healthy and boosting immunity always have and always will start with your diet.

This chapter introduces you to nutritional supplements and medicinal herbs that will support you in boosting your immunity. We also highlight a few more exotic additions to your diet that can have a positive effect on your immunity.

Adding Supplements for Better Health

When using supplements to support your immune system, you need to answer two important questions:

✔ Do you need that supplement?

✔ Is your supplement the highest possible quality?

The supplements we recommend help shore up your nutrition with their supporting compounds. If you feel as though your immune system or overall health needs some support or if you feel a cold or illness coming on, these supplements do show benefits. You may think that supplements or herbs aren't for you — whether they are is a subjective question. You have to evaluate your health history objectives to decide.

If you do decide to supplement, be sure you're using products made with integrity. You want wholesome products that move you toward health, not make you toxic. Make sure you're aware of brands known for quality, and check the ingredient list.

Check for the initials *USP* (U.S. Pharmacopoeial Convention; www.usp.org), which is a quality statement, meaning the supplement is easily absorbed in the body. Also to identify the quality of your supplementation, you can join *Consumer Lab* (www.consumerlab.com), which performs extensive third-party testing for toxic substances and contamination in supplements.

In the 1990s, the FDA introduced the consumer-friendly nutrition food label with its guide to nutrient content and complete ingredient listings. That label appears on supplements, too, so check the label to be sure the product doesn't contain unhealthy additives, such as fillers, synthetic ingredients, and coloring; any wheat, yeast, or corn; or preservatives.

Also check the expiration date and make sure the product is fresh. Purchasing from supplement companies that use organic ingredients and have high standards and values makes your experience buying supplements much easier. Your best insurance is to purchase supplements from a natural health store or through a healthcare provider preferably educated in quality professional supplements. You can also get affordable quality supplements from Vitacost (www.vitacost.com/vitaminsandsupplements).

The following sections explore supplements that may benefit you on your road to boosting immunity. And, as always, before beginning any new supplement program, check with your healthcare practitioner.

Fish oil

The omega-3 fatty acids contained in fish oil have many benefits for your overall health and immune system. Your body can't make these particular fatty acids on its own, so you have to get them from food or supplements.

Fish oil helps your immune system by reducing inflammation and improving your blood chemistry. Your cells love this healthy oil and perform better when you have enough omega-3s. Fish oil helps so many conditions that we could use every page in this book to mention them; here are the highlights: Fish oil promotes brain health and heart health, protects against cancer, depression, bowel disorders, and arthritis, and prevents or improves a myriad of skin conditions, such as psoriasis.

You can get this important omega-3 fatty acid into your body by consuming healthy meat, seafood, eggs, or fish oil supplements. The higher-quality food you buy — including grass-fed meat, wild-caught cold-water seafood, and organic eggs — the more omega-3 fatty acid it contains. If you eat a lot of non-organic sources of meat, fish, and eggs, we strongly recommend you supplement with a high-quality fish oil as an insurance because you're probably not getting enough omega-3 fatty acids in your diet. In fact, we feel so strongly about the benefits of fish oil, we recommend this supplement to all our patients.

Always be sure to get fish oil that's clear of PCBs and pesticides through your health practitioner or Consumer Lab. Fish oil is available as a liquid, capsule, and tablet. Some have an enteric coating to prevent the indigestion or burping that can accompany taking fish oil supplementation.

Choose your fish oil based on whatever form is more suitable for your needs and easier for you to take. For the liquid form, we recommend Stronger Faster Healthier (www.strongerfasterhealthier.com/products/omega_3-oil) because it's potent and pure and tastes great. Some people prefer the liquid form because of its fast absorption (because it's already been broken down). If you prefer capsules or tablets or need enteric coating to avoid indigestion, we recommend the brand Metagenics (www.metagenics.com/products/a-z-products-list/o); for softgel tablets, we recommend OmegaGenics EPA-DHA 720; for enteric-coated softgel tablets (for those who get the "fish burps" from ingesting fish oil), OmegaGenics EPA-DHA 500.

Fish oil can have an affect on blood clotting. If you have a bleeding tendency, are on blood-thinning agents like Coumadin, or have a surgery planned, make sure your physician knows you're taking fish oil.

General recommendation for fish oil supplements is 2 to 4 grams daily, but always check with your healthcare provider before you start taking any new supplements.

Magnesium

Magnesium is one of the most abundant minerals in the body. It's an essential mineral in your nerve cells, and over half of the magnesium in your body is in your bones. Where magnesium's partner, calcium, contracts or tightens muscles, magnesium does the opposite and relaxes muscles.

Although magnesium is critical for bone health, it also does so much more. In fact, magnesium is talented enough to be somewhat of a magic bullet for many. In addition to playing a major role in immunity, magnesium is also amazing for insomnia, hypertension, asthma, chronic fatigue, depression, chronic pain, constipation, irritability, menstrual cramps, rapid heartbeat, regulating blood pressure, and regulating blood sugar.

In our experience, many people are deficient in this essential mineral. In fact, about 80 percent of the population is probably deficient in magnesium. Processed foods and depleted soil are major contributors. Leafy greens, nuts, seeds, fish, meat, and seafood are all decent food sources of magnesium. If you feel like you need a little insurance with supplementation, we recommend Natural Calm (www.calmnatural.com).

An appropriate dosage for magnesium supplements is 1 to 3 teaspoons in water before bed.

Probiotics

You have approximately 25 feet of intestines filled with bacteria. In fact, you have approximately 1,500 different species of bacteria in your intestines that help you digest your food, absorb minerals, manufacture vitamins, and take up space so unhealthy bacteria can't take over. What you may not realize is that your intestines and these bacteria have much to do with your immune system. In fact, as much as 80 percent of your immune system is either strengthened or weakened by the health of your gut's bacterial population.

To have a healthy immune system, your intestines must have a balance of the right kinds of bacteria in the right amounts. These bacteria provide you with a physical barrier to microbes. When bacteria aren't in balance, *gut dysbiosis* can occur, which opens the floodgate to autoimmune disorders, cancer, diabetes, skin problems, and more. That's where probiotics come in. *Probiotics* are microflora (microscopic organisms) that help the body build natural immunity against many diseases (including cancer) and are nature's defense against allergies. Probiotics work by balancing the pH (acid-base balance) and the billions of microorganisms in your body to get you well and keep you well. *Probiotics* means "for life," and that's exactly what they do — increase healthy life inside your intestines.

You can get some of this immune-fighting protection by eating foods like raw, unpasteurized sauerkraut, kimchi, kombucha beverages, or coconut-based kefirs.

You can determine which probiotic is most suitable for you by getting a stool GI Effects Profile test done. This test measures your gut environment and gives you your microbial balance. Go to www.metametrix.com for more info and to find a practitioner in your area or a local lab that can perform the test for you.

If you're under stress, have had a history of infections or antibiotic use, or have had a diet with processed or sugary foods, you may want to try a high-quality multi-strain probiotic supplement in addition to your immune-fighting foods. We like Primal Flora from Primal Blueprint: www.primalblueprint.com/brands/Primal-Flora.html.

Take probiotic supplements as directed.

Vitamin C

Vitamin C is a healing agent. It's an antioxidant essential for the development and maintenance of all the tissues that connect fat, muscle, and bone — which is the framework of your body.

Vitamin C helps fend off colds and illnesses due to its ability to speed the production of new cells in wound healing, thus protecting your immune system and helping you fight off infection. Vitamin C also helps prevent cancer, reduce the severity of allergic reactions, protect against the harmful effects of pollution, produce anti-stress hormones, and play a role in keeping your hormones working.

The body doesn't manufacture vitamin C, so you must get it through diet or supplementation. Some natural sources of vitamin C include berries, citrus fruits, and green vegetables. However, if you get colds or bronchial infections frequently, experience prolonged healing time, bruise easily, have gums that bleed when brushed, or if you feel a cold or illness coming on, you may want to take some vitamin C supplements. If you're under chronic physical or emotional stress or don't eat enough fruits and vegetables, you're probably depleted of vitamin C and taking supplements may be useful. We love Emergen-C (www.emergenc.com/index.php/products/original#) for that extra vitamin C boost.

Take vitamin C supplements as directed.

Vitamin D3

Vitamin D3 is actually a hormone and a critically important one at that. An overwhelming amount of evidence supports the amazing, immune-fighting power behind D3. Proper levels of vitamin D3 can help you avoid many ailments, from cancer to colds. In fact, vitamin D3 is the holy grail of immune protection. So making sure your levels are where they need to be is essential. In addition to immune support, vitamin D3 is also important for bone health.

Because vitamin D3 is a hormone, you can actually get toxic doses. We rarely, if ever, see a healthy vitamin D3 level in our patients, so we suggest you get your levels tested before starting any supplement regimen. Getting a baseline vitamin D3 is a smart way to manage your health and can be very telling. It's just a simple blood test your practitioner can do for you.

To up your levels of vitamin D3 naturally, choose meat and eggs as your food sources, or you can go out in the sun with your arms and legs exposed for about 15 minutes daily, sunscreen-free. In the winter, the UVB rays that supply vitamin D aren't strong enough for you to get your D3 requirements, so you may need supplements.

To determine how much you need, get your levels checked (ask for a 25-hydroxy-vitamin D test) and work with your practitioner to find the right dose for you. Generally, it's from 3,000 to 5,000 IUs daily.

Zinc

Many studies have shown that a deficiency in zinc is linked to an increase in severity and incidence of infection. Studies also show that regular zinc supplementation decreases the duration and severity of cold symptoms and the incidence of antibiotic use.

Whether you should take zinc year-round or just when you're feeling a cold coming on depends on your zinc levels. If you have excellent zinc stores, taking a supplement year-round likely won't be effective, because you don't need it. But if your tank is running low, supplementation may help you avoid colds.

The RDI (recommended daily intake) for zinc is 15 milligrams. If you eat foods rich in zinc, such as oysters, egg yolks, fish, meats, poultry, sardines, sunflower seeds, pumpkin seeds, sesame seeds, kale, and broccoli, your stores may already be healthy. If, however, you're susceptible to colds and you don't eat many of these foods, you may be deficient and taking zinc on a daily basis may be right for you.

To check your zinc levels, you can try the screening method called Zinc Tally from Metagenics. After placing two teaspoons of Zinc Tally in the mouth, a lack of taste or a delayed taste perception suggests a zinc deficiency. An immediate taste suggests your zinc levels are adequate. The test is available only through authorized healthcare practitioners; visit www.metagenics.com/products/a-z-products-list/Zinc-Tally and click Find a Practitioner to search for one in your area.

For a zinc supplement, we like Zinc A.G. tablets from Metagenics (www.metasavvy.com/Zinc_A_G_60_Tablet_p/zn025.htm). Take zinc supplements as directed.

Mixing in Medicinal Herbs

Medicinal herbs really are nature's gift. They work wonders at alleviating and preventing many ailments, and herbs are an effective, inexpensive, and convenient way to manage your health.

Herbs can help many conditions. If you suspect vitamin or mineral deficiencies, lack proper rest, are under chronic stress, or get numerous colds or infections, you probably have a lowered immune system and medicinal herbs may help.

Nothing takes the place of putting real food first and making healthy lifestyle choices. As with nutritional supplementation, use medicinal herbs only as a support system to a healthy lifestyle. Medicinal herbs can be a great addition to your healing and prevention strategies.

If you're considering herbs to boost your immune system, discuss your particular needs with a health practitioner who understands your individual situation. Some herbs for the immune system may enhance or interact with the action of synthetic medications and should be monitored by an herbalist or a doctor who understands how herbs interact with other treatments.

In the following sections, we explore some of the best medicinal herbs for boosting your immunity and discuss their overall benefits.

Aloe vera

Aloe vera's healing powers are so impressive and so extensive that covering all its benefits would take an entire book. Here are just some of the healing powers of aloe vera:

- Contains *acemannan,* a natural immune booster
- Halts the growth of cancers
- Lowers high cholesterol
- Accelerates healing
- Replaces a dozen first-aid products
- Soothes arthritis pain and inflammation
- Ends constipation
- Hydrates and repairs skin
- Heals ulcers, irritable bowel disease (IBD), Crohn's disease, and other digestive disorders
- Nourishes the body with minerals

You can either keep an aloe plant at home or purchase aloe vera from a natural health store. You can use aloe vera topically or take it orally. If you've never eaten aloe before, start slowly. Any aloe vera plant you consume needs to go through quality assurance standards. Having certification by the International Aloe Science Council (www.iasc.org) and purchasing your aloe from a natural products retailer or health food store increase your probability of a healthier plant. However you include aloe in your healing arsenal, just include it! It's the wonder gel of herbal superfoods and deserves all the accolades it receives.

Astragalus

Chinese medicine has many little herbal gems. One of them is astragalus, an herb that's been used for centuries in China. This plant is harvested for its roots and has many healing properties.

Astragalus is one of our favorite boosting tonics and works by stimulating the immune system as well as carrying amazing antioxidant benefits. The root is said to infuse the body with energy and healing.

Make sure your astragalus root or herbals have been evaluated for heavy metals, whether you purchase it from Chinese grocers or health food stores. In fact, herbals should always have tight quality control and be screened for pesticides, heavy metals, sulfites, and bacterial contamination. Check out Health Concerns (www.healthconcerns.com), which has a wide variety of high-quality herbs. Also consider working with a healthcare professional educated in herbs who can guide you through the process of herbal supplementation.

You can buy the loose leaves and simmer slices in teas or soups. You can also get it in capsules, extracts, and powders. Astragalus can amp up the immune system and do the following:

✔ Help you beat the flu

✔ Stop a cold in its track

✔ Balance blood sugar

✔ Work as a support with cancer and chemotherapy drugs

✔ Improve fatigue symptoms

✔ Sooth arthritis pain and inflammation

✔ Accelerate healing

✔ Replace a dozen first-aid products

✔ End constipation

This herb is non-toxic and can be used long term to increase resistance. The next time you feel a cold or flu coming on, give this Chinese wonder herb a try!

Cat's-claw

The name *cat's-claw* actually comes from the thorns on the plant's leaves, which look like the claws of a cat. The root bark is used medicinally.

Cat's-claw contains chemicals that stimulate the immune system, helping you fight viruses. This medicinal herb helps lower blood pressure and acts as a diuretic, helping the body lose excess water. Studies show that cat's-claw may even kill tumor cells.

Cat's-claw is particularly useful against the aches and pains of arthritis. The anti-inflammatory nature of this medicinal herb may provide relief from both osteoarthritis and rheumatoid arthritis.

Cat's-claw comes in tablet, capsule, tea, dried herb, or tincture forms. We recommend that you purchase this herb from a company that knows how to harvest this herb correctly; otherwise it could contain *tetracyclic oxindole alkaloi,* which is toxic.

Echinacea

This herb has been used in many households for quite some time at the first sign of sniffles and colds. Even if you're unaccustomed to natural remedies, you've probably heard about the healing powers of echinacea and its use to treat or prevent colds, flu, or other infections. Even gargling with it for sore throats is effective. Some evidence suggests that echinacea may be used to treat or prevent upper respiratory infections.

Some people even use echinacea for success in treating skin conditions, such as skin wounds, burns, eczema, psoriasis, UV radiation, herpes simplex, bee stings, and abscesses.

Nine known species of echinacea exist; however, *echinacea purpurea* is the most common and is known to be the most potent. The aboveground parts of the plant and roots are used fresh or dried to make tablets, teas, squeezed juice, extracts, or preparations for external use.

Take echinacea at the first sign of cold or flu. The sooner you start taking it, the more affective it is. Also, don't take echinacea for more than three weeks at a time. It loses its effectiveness if you do because your body kind of burns out on it. If you still need echinacea after you cycle on three weeks followed by one week of cycling off, you can cycle back on again for another three weeks.

Elderberry

We love elderberry — and boy does this stuff work. Elderberry plus some zinc is like the dream team for colds and flu. This herb works amazingly to enhance the immune system and also reduce inflammation, lower fever, and sooth the respiratory tract, and it has powerful antioxidant power to boot.

Elderberry prevents the flu virus from attaching to the cell, so it shortens the duration and lessens the severity of the flu. One of the biggest bonuses of elderberry is its fantastic taste, making a sweet elderberry syrup or tincture.

As you soon as you start to feel a cold or flu come on, take elderberry. The sooner you begin taking it, the more effective this herbal remedy will be.

For an elderberry supplement, we love Sambucol (`www.sambucolusa.com/store`), which is available at most natural food stores. It's available in a syrup or tablet form and both forms are effective. Take as directed, and avoid the raw berries, which can cause vomiting

Ginseng

Ginseng gives you an extra zing. It's used as a tonic to combat weakness and fuel your body with extra energy. Of the number of different types of ginseng, panax ginseng is the most widely used species.

Although ginseng's superpower lies in its ability to give you energy, it has a host of other attributes, including the following:

- Heals bronchial disorders
- Gives you mental clarity
- Balances blood sugar
- Stimulates physical activity
- Improves fatigue symptoms
- Rejuvenates all systems of the body
- Fights aging
- Helps with inflammatory diseases, like arthritis
- Protects against the side effects of radiation

Ginseng is available as a whole root that you can slice and put into soups or tea and as a powder, extract, tinctures, tablets, or capsules. Make sure you get pure ginseng with no added sugars or colors.

If you have a supplement or a product with added ginseng, chances are the amount used is too low to be effective, so don't depend on this source for some good ginseng power.

Like echinacea, ginseng must be cycled on and off for best results. Take it for three weeks maximum and then cycle off for a week. Avoid long-term use of high doses.

Hyssop

Hyssop is cultivated for its flower tops, which are often steeped in water to make an infusion for use as an expectorant to thin and loosen mucus. The healing virtues of this plant are due to its oil, which has a stimulating affect that promotes expectoration (causes your mucus to thin and loosen in the lungs, throat, and bronchi so it's easier to eliminate).

Hyssop also helps with asthma, arthritis, and wound healing. It comes in tablet, capsule, tea, dried herb, or tincture forms. The most favored way to take hyssop is in warm water, such as in a tea, because it provides more of a catalyst to loosen mucus.

Hyssop definitely has its place in your home when you have congestion or sinusitis or when you're experiencing a cold. It works about as well as any expectorant you can use — with the benefit that it's all natural.

Licorice root

Scientists have identified many healing substances in licorice root. The herb's key compound is called *glycyrrhizin* (which is super sweet — about 50 times sweeter than sugar, in fact). Here are some of the amazing things licorice can do for you:

- Prevent the occurrence of and heal ulcers
- Cleanse the colon
- Lower stomach acid, relieving heartburn and indigestion
- Lower cholesterol
- Enhance immunity
- Improve menopause symptoms
- Stop the growth of viruses, such as the flu
- Promote adrenal gland function (to help your body deal with stress better)

✔ Increase the fluidity of and thin mucus in the lungs and bronchial tubes

✔ Soothe, heal, and reduce irritation and inflammation in the respiratory system, making it useful in treating irritating coughs

Before taking licorice root, consult with a healthcare provider who understands your individual needs. If you have high blood pressure or a history of stroke, are pregnant, or have diabetes, glaucoma, or heart disease, don't use licorice root. Prolonged use may cause high blood pressure, fluid retention, and symptoms related to loss of potassium. For these reasons, we don't advise taking licorice for more than seven days in a row. Side effects are especially dangerous for those who already have high blood pressure, heart disease, diabetes, or kidney disease. For those needing long-term use or who have chronic diseases, the deglycyrrhizinated (glycyrrhizin free) form may be an option.

Nettle

Nettle, also called *stinging nettle,* may be your answer if you have hay fever or other allergies. Nettle is a great natural alternative to antihistamines — which don't actually change the allergic process but just block its expression. Steroid nasal inhalers used for treatment of hay fever and other seasonal allergies can be effective, but some of the steroids are bound to get into the rest of the body, and these hormones weaken the immune system. That's why nettle is so valuable. It's effective and has no negative effects on the immune system.

Nettle has also been used as the following:

✔ Anti-inflammatory

✔ Expectorant (thins mucus)

✔ Diuretic

✔ Pain reliever

Nettle is available freeze-dried in capsules and cut and dried for infusion (teas). Herb Pharm has a good nettle product that's great to have on hand for seasonal allergies. Keep in mind that the leaves and stems are better for allergies. Check it out at www.herb-pharm.com/store/product_info.php/ products_id/332.

St John's wort

More people than ever are turning to antidepressants to deal with the stresses of day-to-day life. In fact, Prozac, Paxil, and Lexapro are now the three most widely prescribed drugs in the United States. That's why the medicinal herbal St John's wort, also called *hypericum perforatum,* is such a welcome and useful herb.

St John's wort acts as a natural antidepressant. In some countries, St John's wort is commonly prescribed for mild depression, especially in children and adolescents. Studies show that this herb is superior to placebo in patients with major depression and is as effective as standard antidepressants. Another huge benefit is that St John's wort has fewer side effects than standard antidepressants. There have also been benefits in using St John's wort as a pain reliever for nerve pain.

When taking St John's wort, you may have heightened sensitivity to sunlight, especially if you're fair-skinned. Also avoid taking St John's wort if you're on any medications because it's contraindicated with the use of many pharmaceuticals.

Seeking Out a Few Exotic Superfoods

Sometimes, the best food choices are under the radar — more unknown than some of the superfoods you can find in Chapter 9. Exotic superfoods are more mysterious, perhaps even harder to find, but well worth your efforts.

The exotic superfoods we mention in the following sections have been used successfully in other parts of the world for their powerful healing punch. We recommend that you get to know some of these unusual superfoods and figure out how to implement them into your overall superfood regimen.

Acai berries

Acai berries (pronounced ah-sigh-*ee*) are grown on the palm trees in the Amazon rainforest of northern Brazil. The name of the game with acai berries is pure antioxidant and nutrient power. Studies show extracts from acai berries may destroy cancer cells, particularly those associated with leukemia.

The acai berry is dark purple to almost black in color and the size of a blueberry. The dark, rich color of the acai berry is the giveaway that it's filled with flavonoids. The healing flavonoids in acai berries are called *anthocyanins*. Just one serving of these potent berries gives you large amounts of these anthocyanins as well as calcium, vitamin A, and amino acids.

Here's how acai berries help you stay healthy:

- ✔ **They fight leukemia.** A well-known study, done by the University of Florida, found that extracts of the acai berry destroyed human cancer cells grown in a lab. More studies are needed to confirm its effects, but this step is definitely in the right direction.

- ✔ **They reduce inflammation.** One of the best things that acai berries can do for you, due to the large amounts of anthocyanins they contain, is reduce inflammation associated with chronic diseases. Heart disease, cancer, diabetes, arthritis, fatigue syndromes, digestive discomforts, aches, and pains are all helped by reducing inflammation.

- ✔ **They shield your heart against disease.** The pulp of acai berries has deep healing agents that contain antioxidants and fiber that reduces cholesterol — and keeps your digestive system healthy to boot!

Acai berries are too fragile to ship in their raw state, so you often see them as juice, pulp, in supplements, or in food bars. You can add the juice or pulp to smoothies or blend it with other foods or teas. This magical Brazilian fruit is on the pricey side, but the benefits are priceless.

Goji berries

Goji berries (pronounced *go*-gee), which are the commercial name for wolfberries, have been used for thousands of years in Chinese medicine. These berries are richly immersed in antioxidant power (some experts believe even more so than blueberries, which are always a top-ranked antioxidant source).

These superfood berries are a member of the nightshade family, which includes tomatoes, peppers, eggplant, and potatoes. Because of the delicate nature of goji berries, they're not shipped as fresh fruit. Instead, you can find them in the form of juice, tea, or dried (like other dried fruits) in health food stores, the health food section of grocery stores, and online stores. They look like raisins, except they have a reddish color with a bit of a sour taste.

Here's what goji berries can do for you:

- **Battle cancer:** The phytochemicals in goji berries may have powerful anticancer effects. A 1994 study published in the *Chinese Journal of Oncology* stated that goji berries have a positive effect on treatments when used in conjunction with other cancer therapies.

- **Support weight loss:** Goji berries contain natural compounds that are *lipotropic,* meaning they help carry fat away from the liver and burn those extra calories.

- **Protect your heart:** Goji berries have compounds to lower cholesterol, are natural defenders against free radical damage, and release levels of *homocysteine,* a protein associated with heart disease and inflammation.

- **Prevent age-related eye problems:** Goji berries have a high level of antioxidants, like beta carotene and zeaxanthin, which are important for vision. Zeaxanthin protects the eyes, specifically the retina, and may reduce the risk of age-related macular degeneration.

- **Boost your libido:** This amazing superfood not only raises your spirits, but it also raises your libido! Goji berries raise testosterone levels, and, therefore, your sex drive goes up.

Wondering what to do with this magnificent superfood? You can use goji berries anywhere you'd enjoy raisins. Mix them in a recipe, or eat them right out of the bag as a snack. Another great use of these beautiful berries is to throw 10 to 20 berries into your tea, or you can just drink goji berry tea all by itself. You can ice it on a hot day for a refreshing way to accentuate your health!

Sea vegetables

Sea vegetables have long been appreciated as a healthy staple in Asian cuisines and consumed for hundreds of years in many countries. You've probably had some sea vegetables without even knowing it. Food manufacturers use processed sea vegetables as thickeners or stabilizers in all types of common foods, like pudding and even toothpaste!

Sea vegetables are extremely good for you. They have many vitamins, minerals, essential fatty acids, and other natural food chemicals with antioxidant properties. Minerals are particularly important in your diet because they regulate just about every system and function of the body, and when it comes to providing minerals, sea vegetables really shine. The salty taste in sea vegetables comes from a balance of sodium and other minerals from the sea. Sea vegetables also give you a good dose of fiber.

Here are some of the other wonderful things sea vegetables can do for you:

- ✔ Bind heavy metals and toxins and escort them safely out of the body
- ✔ Purify the blood and digestive tract
- ✔ Nourish the thyroid (which keeps your body's internal thermostat on track — and helps you control your weight)
- ✔ Support the treatment of anemia
- ✔ Support the treatment of degenerative nerve diseases (such as Alzheimer's)
- ✔ Promote healthy skin and hair
- ✔ Naturally increase energy levels
- ✔ Promote a healthy immune system
- ✔ Help you maintain a healthy cardiovascular function
- ✔ Support a healthy digestive system
- ✔ Keep your body in a state of nutritional sufficiency rather than deficiency
- ✔ Help prevent breast cancer

Just who are these superstars? Here are some of the more common sea vegetables you may find in natural food stores, in the natural foods section at the grocery store, online, or in Asian food stores that you can add to your superfoods repertoire:

- ✔ **Dulse:** Dulse is reddish brown and comes in whole leaves, powdered, or as a condiment. This sea vegetable is chewy with a salty finish. Dulse flakes give a great flavor to salads. You can also eat it right out of the package!

- ✔ **Hijiki:** Called the "beauty vegetable" in Japan for the shiny hair and beautiful skin it gives to those who indulge, this sea vegetable looks like black angel hair pasta and requires soaking before adding to your dishes. Hijiki goes well with fish.

- ✔ **Kelp:** You can find virtually every nutrient in sea kelp. It's a great source of iodine, which is a vital nutrient that many are deficient in. Kelp noodles are delicious and a wonderful way to add sea vegetables to your diet.

- ✔ **Kombu:** Kombu is a type of brown algae that has a beautiful dark purple hue. You can find kombu fresh, frozen, or dried. It comes in thick strips or sheets. It has a savory taste and can be used as a food flavoring, food topping, or a nice salty addition to soups.

Superfood bonus: Iodine in sea vegetables

Iodine is an important trace element that's pretty rare on the earth's crust, but you can find it in sea water. Your body needs iodine to have a healthy, functioning thyroid gland. If you go a long time without iodine, you can get a swollen, underactive thyroid called a *goiter*. People who have a goiter look like they have a large, thick neck. Children who have an iodine deficiency have even bigger problems because the deficiency causes stunted growth and mental delay. Because iodine is added to table salt, iodine deficiencies are now uncommon in Western societies, although the U.S. population has been showing a decrease in iodine intake. The RDA for iodine is 150 micrograms, but people probably need more.

Iodine was added to table salt to avoid iodine deficiency. However, table salt is processed with unhealthy chemicals and anti-caking agents, added to make the salt flow freely. So when you eat table salt, you take one step forward and two steps back. We recommend using a natural unprocessed salt that's mineral rich (see Chapter 8) and supplementing with sea vegetables to feed your thyroid the iodine it needs. Seafood also has iodine as do vegetables grown in iodine-rich soil.

Warning: If you've been diagnosed or suspect you have Hashimoto's thyroiditis, Graves' disease, or any thyroid disease, take caution when ingesting iodine and always check with your doctor first.

✔ **Nori:** Nori is the most popular sea vegetable because it's used to make sushi. You can find nori in colors from dark purple to marine green. You can use it as a condiment for soups, salads, and casseroles or cut into strips.

✔ **Wakame:** Wakame (pronounced wah-kay-may) is a tender grayish green sea vegetable, and when you soak wakame, it expands many times its original size. Eat it raw as a snack, add it to soups and stir-fries, or roast it and sprinkle on salads and stews. Wakame becomes soft and melts in your mouth when cooked. What a great way to add minerals to your foods!

Chapter 11

Living an Immunity-Friendly Lifestyle

Getting nutrients is essential. Your nutrient levels decide how healthy you are or how open you are to illness and aging. What's often not so readily understood is the many ways to deliver these nutrients to your body.

When most people hear the word *nutrient,* they think of supplements or foods. However, other things can make your body healthy, ageless, and strong. Certain habits can provide your body with a healthy flow of nutrition and balance, creating an environment that allows your body to flourish.

When you give your body what it needs, it responds by giving you more energy, better sleep, better skin, less ailments, and fewer cold and illnesses. You look and feel better all around.

This chapter has advice on how to give your body the nutrients it needs. We cover ways to get more from your routine through sleep, sunshine, water, and exercise and how to manage stress, which are all part of your immune-boosting lifestyle!

Getting More from Your Daily Routine

When you give your body the right raw material, it flourishes. The right food is the foundation, but there's more. You can move yourself toward health by your daily habits — what you *do,* as opposed to just what you *don't* do. You can take an active role in making choices that can help your body heal, become strong, and help all the structures and functions of your body work their best.

Map out your day and start looking at some of your habits as ways to give your body that extra burst of nutrition. Sleep, sunshine, water, and exercise are all habits you can use to your benefit to build the best body you can. These simple, free nutrients can make a big difference in your cells and, therefore, in your ability to fight aging, get well, and stay well.

Sleep

Sleep is one of the most powerful tools for health. Think of sleep as the foundation for everything. When you're deprived of sleep, nothing else you do right matters. Your body can't heal and regenerate, and your cells become sluggish.

Sleep deprivation has a pretty powerful overall affect on your body. When you lack sleep, you risk a lowered immune system. In fact, your number of white blood cells decrease when you're low on sleep. But that's not all. Here are some other potential outcomes that may surprise you:

- ✓ **Illness:** Going to bed too late doubles your risk of breast cancer.

- ✓ **Weight gain:** You can lose 14.3 pounds a year by getting one more hour of sleep a night. Sleep deprivation causes you to gain weight; proper sleep causes you to lose weight.

- ✓ **Earlier death:** In 2004, a study in the journal *Sleep* found that women who averaged less than five hours of sleep per night had a higher death rate than those who slept seven hours.

- ✓ **Hormonal shifts:** When you don't get enough sleep, hormones shift, causing your appetite to change. The sugars you crave shoot your insulin up and create blood sugar problems, which cause weight gain and health issues.

- ✓ **Heart disease:** When your hormones shift causing you to eat more sugar, you get insulin resistance. Insulin resistance causes you to get fat. During this process, you convert all your carbohydrates into bad cholesterol, and you retain water, which alters your blood pressure and paves the way to heart disease.

- ✓ **Pre-hibernation messaging:** When you expose yourself to unending artificial light, your brain registers that it's a long summer day. Long summers are followed by cold, dark winters, so your body naturally puts on a fat base preparing for the winter. Your body can't metabolically resist craving carbohydrates to prepare. These excess carbs cause blood sugar problems and weight gain.

- ✔ **Altered brain power:** Memory, concentration, and creativity are all impaired with lack of sleep.

- ✔ **Premature aging:** The body decreases its growth hormone needed for ongoing tissue repair, healing, cell rejuvenation, and bone function. Growth hormone can reverse the effects of aging; therefore, sleep deprivation causes aging.

- ✔ **Sugar handling problems:** When you're sleep deprived, the ability to metabolize sugar decreases, turning sugar into fat.

- ✔ **Decreased regenerative powers:** Sleep is needed to regenerate the body, especially the brain. When you don't have enough sleep, your body doesn't heal or regenerate.

- ✔ **Prolonged high cortisol levels:** When you're awake for long periods of time with the lights on, the stress hormone cortisol doesn't naturally drop like it's supposed to. High cortisol occurs in nature when you need it to run fast or deal with pain from an injury. This constant high cortisol causes people to become panicky and depressive.

Sleep deprivation is cumulative. Your body doesn't adapt to sleep deprivation. You only get more tired and, eventually, unhealthy and overweight.

Without sleep, you can't get well, stay well, or fight aging. But just how do you get those much-needed zzz's? Here are some tips to help you get the most out of your shut-eye:

- ✔ **Go to bed at the same time every night.** If you don't give yourself a scheduled bedtime, you'll get distracted. Before long, your awake time will be squeezing it's way into your much-needed sleep time.

- ✔ **Go to bed by no later than 10 p.m. and be up by no later than 7 a.m.** Set your phone, watch, or an alarm clock to remind you to close down shop for the night. Most of your body's repairing goes on before 1 a.m., and you get more growth hormone. Your circadian rhythm will also be in sync with your sleep-awake cycle.

- ✔ **Rise with the sun.** The sunlight regulates your hormones for the day.

- ✔ **Unplug one to two hours before bedtime.** Make sure you're not doing anything but relaxing, journaling, or reading one to two hours before bed. Doing so releases the hormone *melatonin* to get you to sleep. That means no TV, no computer, or anything stimulating. Dim the lights if you can to allow your body to start producing even more melatonin. Move away all alarm clocks or electrical devices at least three feet from your bed.

✔ **Black out your bedroom completely.** Melatonin is produced when it's dark, so cover the windows to prevent any light from coming in. Use blackout shades if you need to. How dark does your room need to be? Dark enough that you can't see your hand when you hold it in front of your face. Otherwise, hormone production slows down.

✔ **Keep your bedroom cool and well ventilated.** Keep your room at a temperature that's comfortable for you, but make sure it's on the cooler side. About 68 degrees works for most. Some people also like an air purifier in their bedroom, which can improve the way you breathe, thus improving your sleep.

✔ **Limit caffeine.** Drinking caffeine prolongs the time it takes you to go to sleep and decreases the amount of deep sleep you get. It takes about three to five hours for about half of the caffeine you've had to clear out of your system, so plan accordingly. Caffeine limitations vary greatly from person to person, so see what works for you.

✔ **Limit alcohol.** Alcohol may make you fall asleep quicker, but your quality of sleep is diminished. Deep sleep and REM sleep are both greatly reduced, so even if you fall asleep quicker, you'll probably wake up feeling tired.

Sleep-inducing foods are ironically also powerful, immune-building foods. These foods include turkey, almonds, bananas, spinach and other leafy greens, as well as seasonings and spices like nutmeg, turmeric, and garlic. Calcium and magnesium are also helpful sleep aids. Some of these foods are high in tryptophan, which is an amino acid that helps induce sleep. When eating close to bedtime, be sure to watch your portion size, and avoid eating heavy meals because the digestion process may disturb your sleep. We recommend just a light meal or snack in the hour leading up to bedtime.

Sunshine

Sunshine is like sleep. It's one of those nutrients that isn't known as a necessity yet is imperative to your health and well-being. Just as eating immune-boosting foods are important, so is getting sun exposure.

Reaping the benefits of sun exposure

Sunshine is a fantastic way to ward off cancers and other diseases. It also helps your body keep the hormonal rhythm of your natural light-dark cycle. Early morning exposure to sunlight activates your hormones and sets your biological rhythm for the day. This healthy burst of morning sunshine also provides you with a healthy blast of vitamin D.

Here are just a few of the fabulous benefits of sunshine:

- ✔ **Increases immunity:** Exposure to sun increases your vitamin D production, which is an integral part of proper function of the body's T cells, the immune systems first line of defense. Vitamin D decreases your risk of many cancers, colds, and the flu.

- ✔ **Promotes better sleep:** Exposure to bright light has a positive effect on sleep cycles. Sleep deprivation causes many health problems for which sunshine is protective.

- ✔ **Treats depression:** A dose of sunlight works magic on depression, especially Seasonal Affective Disorder (SAD). Sunshine increases the hormones that help you sleep and regulates the circadian system that affects sleep.

- ✔ **Strengthens bones:** Sunshine produces more vitamin D, better calcium absorption, and therefore stronger bones.

- ✔ **Reduces risk of stroke:** Studies show that folks who live in areas with less sun exposure have a higher stroke risk.

- ✔ **Lowers blood pressure:** That warmth that you feel from the sun increases circulation. That, along with increased vitamin D production, is an effective way to reduce hypertension.

Even with all these benefits, people fear the sun today. There's no doubt, however, that your body needs sunlight, so you can't completely avoid it. You have to work within nature's boundaries and find intelligent ways to approach sunlight.

Sorting out UVA and UVB radiation, sunscreen, and sunblock

Most of the fears people have about sun exposure are due to sunburn and skin cancer. In an answer to this fear, sunscreen manufacturers tell us that their sunscreens protect against cancer.

The truth is, no evidence shows that sunscreens prevent the main skin cancers, cutaneous melanoma and basal cell carcinoma. Sunscreens protect against sunburn. Sunscreens aren't an anticancer remedy. In fact, because they allow you to have prolonged exposure to the sun, using sunscreen actually gives you a heightened risk of melanoma.

Is the sun dangerous? The part of the sun that causes damage is ultraviolet (UV) radiation. This UV radiation is broken into two categories, A and B:

- ✔ **UVA:** Sunscreens often don't block out UVA rays. Although no conclusive evidence exists, scientists are strongly postulating that UVA rays increase your risk of melanoma. These rays are strong and deeply penetrate your skin throughout the entire day.

✔ **UVB:** This portion of UV radiation causes the burn (or redness) in your skin, which is why most of the sunscreen you buy blocks out these rays. These rays are low in the morning and later in the day, while strong midday.

Blocking UVB rays isn't a solution but actually causes another problem. UVB rays manufacture vitamin D production in your skin, so think of UVB as your "buddy." If you block UVB, you block vitamin D from 97.5 to 99.9 percent. Vitamin D is absolutely one of the most anticancerous types of nutrients your body produces. Blocking UVB really takes away one of the best cancer- and disease-fighting shields your body has to offer.

The problem doesn't stop there. Not only does no evidence suggest that sunscreens are protective against cancers, but they also contain toxic ingredients that actually *cause* cancers.

Unfortunately, the FDA guidelines for sunscreens don't help consumers. The guidelines fail to establish the ingredients that are safe and effective for sunscreens. They also don't address the claim that the "higher the SPF, the higher the protection" has in fact negligible benefits. What they do claim, however, is that you should lather this rather toxic substance on your skin every two hours.

What are the solutions when it comes to sunscreens? First, understand your options.

✔ **Sunscreens** are chemicals absorbed by the skin (going directly into the body). When they're absorbed, they form a sun barrier. They do, in fact, prevent sunburn, but no evidence suggests that they're effective in reducing skin cancer. Some statistical evidence shows that the toxins many of these sunscreens contain may actually increase your risk of cancer. Always avoid mists and sprays whose ingredients have been broken down into small particles that are more dangerous internally, especially when you breathe these mists into your lungs.

When you do need sunscreen, choose a natural brand that doesn't contain toxic ingredients. The Environmental Working Group (EWG) is a nonprofit consumer advocacy group that investigates products like sunscreen. Its investigation on sunscreen shows that many of the brand-name sunscreens contain unsafe ingredients. As a solution, the EWG offers a rating system on more than 1,700 sunscreen products on the market. Check out its sunscreen ratings to help you purchase a safe product at www.ewg.org/skindeep.

✔ **Sunblocks** are designed so that the ingredients literally lay on top of the skin to form a barrier against the sun. (This type of product is what people lathered on years ago before sunscreens hit the market.)

Sunblocks don't enter the bloodstream. If you purchase wisely, you can avoid the chemicals that some sunblocks may contain. Buying mineral sunblock whose active ingredient is zinc and/or titanium dioxide is a safe bet.

What causes skin cancer is intense, infrequent exposure to the sun that leads to burning, followed by little to no sun. These short blasts of sun may cause melanomas and many other cancers. What you don't want, then, is to burn.

Controlling your sun exposure to boost vitamin D

Start practicing the *slow immersion* process without sunscreen. When you get frequent, short periods of exposure, you build a protective layer. Build up your tolerance on a regular basis, gradually and early on in the springtime to prep your skin for the stronger sun. Try to get sun earlier in the morning where you have less chance of burning and overheating.

A huge benefit to going in the sun without sunscreen and building a base through slow immersion is that you're welcoming the production of vitamin D. This vitamin (which is actually a hormone) helps your body ward off countless diseases, including the following:

- Cancer
- Diabetes
- Heart disease
- Hypertension
- Multiple sclerosis
- Osteoporosis
- Psoriasis
- Rickets

How much exposure you need to get your dose of vitamin D depends on how dark your skin is and environmental factors (such as how close you live to the equator or what time of day you're sunbathing). The darker your skin, the more exposure you need. Just underscore in your mind that regular sun exposure is grossly understated as a vitally important barrier to disease. Think of it this way: Regular exposure to the sun protects against skin cancers, and intermittent exposure actually increases your odds.

The benefits of UVB exposure far outweigh any adverse effects. Vitamin D is extremely protective. Have your levels checked by getting a simple blood test. In our experience, we find that most people's levels are considerably low. You may need to supplement to "catch up" on vitamin D levels.

A skin cancer secret that shouldn't be

Most people don't realize that the type of oils in your body can either increase or decrease your risk of sunburn or cancer. A study from the National Academy of Science found that low omega-6:3 ratios was the key to prevention of skin cancer. Omega-3 fats decrease cancers, while omega-6 fats increase risk. That's another score for immune-boosting healthy fats!

Water

Your body is made up of about 60 to 70 percent water. Just as your body needs macronutrients (such as healthy protein, carbohydrates, and fats) to function, it also needs water. Pure, clean water is the most essential of all nutrients. You can live for weeks without consuming food, but you can't go for more than a couple of days without water.

Appreciating what water can do for you

Proper intake of water is so vital to your being that a deficiency of even 1 percent can present signs of dysfunctions in your body. Slightly more dehydration and you get exponentially more health risk.

You also need water to maintain the chemical balances in your body, such as these important functions:

- Balancing acid-base levels
- Eliminating waste from the lungs, skin, and colon
- Getting nutrients to the cells
- Regulating hormones

Avoiding dehydration

Many times, people confuse the signaling in their body. People often think that they're hungry, but really what they need is water. One of the main problems with this "signal confusion" between thirst and hunger is not understanding how much water you really need or not recognizing the signs of dehydration.

The biggest roadblock is waiting until you feel thirsty to drink. Your brain center doesn't send a message until you're almost 2 percent dehydrated. By then, you've likely already suffered some effects of dehydration. Your kidneys receive the low signal before you do, so it responds by decreasing urine output. This is a big sign that you need more water — fast. Other effects of dehydration include

- ✔ Arthritis pain
- ✔ Chronic hunger
- ✔ Depression
- ✔ Excess body weight
- ✔ Headaches
- ✔ High blood cholesterol
- ✔ High blood pressure
- ✔ Intestinal pain

How do you know whether you're dehydrated? The biggest "tell" is if you're not urinating at least six to eight times a day. Also, look at your urine. Is it bright yellow? If so, you need more water. Your urine should have a fairly clear to slightly yellow color.

You've probably heard that you should be drinking about 6 to 8 glasses of water daily. This recommendation is actually on the low side. You need at the *very least* 6 to 8 glasses. Here's the other surprise. Alcohol, coffee, tea and caffeine-containing beverages don't count as water.

The optimal water intake should be half of your body weight in ounces. So if you weigh 100 pounds, you need 50 ounces of water daily. If you exercise, you need to consume even more water. Get in the habit of drinking water before, during, and immediately after exercise.

Pre-hydrate in the morning by having some water as soon as you get up. It's a good way to get your blood moving and transporting all the good stuff to your body!

When you get used to water as your main source of liquid, it helps a great deal. Also, when you're not feeling well, feeling low energy, or feeling hunger, your first line of defense is always drink water first.

Ensuring you're getting clean water

Having clean water sources in your home is essential. Remember that water that gets into your body isn't just coming from your tap. It's also coming from all the water sources in your home like your bath water or shower.

You need pure clean water without all the chlorine, fluoride, and toxins. The best way to get pure water is to use a water filtration system. Knowing what's in your water and what needs to be filtered out is a good place to start. You can either test your water or, if you don't want to test, at the very least make sure the filtration removes the following:

- ✔ Arsenic
- ✔ Chlorine
- ✔ Chloroform
- ✔ E. coli
- ✔ Fluoride
- ✔ Nitrites and nitrates
- ✔ Parasites
- ✔ Radon

You can choose from a system that filters the water in one area of your house, or you can choose a whole house filtration system. The best-case scenario is to make sure all water in your house is filtered, including bath water, cooking water, and faucets. Choosing a system depends on what your personal needs are and what you can afford. You have many products on the market to choose from; just make sure they filter out the chlorine, fluoride, and toxins.

Beware of filtered water that's packed in plastic. The chemical Bisphenol A (BPA) and phthalates contained in plastics are dangerous for your health. Even low levels of these chemicals cause disease and can create hormonal disturbances. If you come up empty handed in your quest to find filtered water in BPA-free plastic bottles, look for glass bottles of water to avoid the BPAs. Also, be sure to find out the source of the water because 40 percent of bottled water is simply taken from municipal tap water, so most bottled water is really nothing more than tap water in toxic bottles.

Exercise

Daily physical activity is essential for good health and strong immunity. You won't be able to utilize your nutrients efficiently if you don't exercise. You can't think of physical fitness separate from all the other requirements for a healthy cellular function. Just as water, sunshine, and sleep are necessary for a healthy internal environment, so is exercise.

Physical inactivity makes your genes express an unhealthy state. If you're deficient in anything that's required for healthy cell function, you'll eventually express disease. Exercise is certainly no different.

Here's the good news: Just as a deficiency in exercise can make you sick and obese, the reverse can work as well. You can use exercise to create healthy cells and robust health. In fact, exercise is like taking a cure-all pill every day. Here are some of the medications that regular exercise may help you avoid:

- ✔ **Cold and flu meds:** The average adult has two or three colds or flu viruses each year. But if you're active, studies suggest that you'll have fewer colds than those who aren't active.

- ✔ **Cholesterol meds:** Being active boosts your good cholesterol and reduces unhealthy triglycerides, keeping a clear pathway for blood to flow naturally and preventing diseases like diabetes, stroke, and heart disease.

- ✔ **Antidepressants:** If you work out three times per week hard enough to sweat, you can reduce depression as well as an antidepressant. The connections made between nerve cells behave in your body as a natural antidepressant.

- ✔ **Respiratory meds:** Breathing becomes deeper, allowing more oxygen and nutrients to become more readily available.

- ✔ **Digestive aides:** Digestive juices are stimulated when you exercise, which create movement through your bowels and help with constipation.

- ✔ **Alzheimer's meds:** The Archives of Neurology published a report that a daily walk or run could lower the risk of Alzheimer's or tame it's impact once it's begun.

- ✔ **Sedatives:** During exercise, your body releases a chemical called *endorphins.* This chemical acts as a sedative and creates feelings of happiness and joy. Endorphins also decrease the perception of pain.

Exercise also increases the brain chemicals, which make the connections that help you learn better, reverse the aging process, reduce your body fat, improve muscle tone, and help the heart become stronger and more efficient.

Even though exercise is good for you and there's overwhelming proof of its benefits, too much is counterproductive and can make you weak and sick. David Nieman, PhD, a health and exercise science specialist in Boone, North Carolina, who has conducted studies on exercise and stress states: "Exercise creates stress on the body. In most cases, that's good. Putting your body under frequent, mild doses of this stress improves it over time. That's why people who do regular, moderate exercise get half as many colds as people who are sedentary. The immune system really likes activity. When you exercise . . . immune cells circulate at a higher rate. It is like taking the Marines out of the barracks and having them travel through the bloodstream."

Overexercising (called *overtraining*) has the opposite effect. Dr. Nieman found that the tipping point is 90 minutes or more of continuous activity at moderate to high intensity. At that point, stress weakens the immune system, making you more prone to illness. The effect can last up to 72 hours. If you work out too much one day, you may get a cold. If you do so day after day, you can run into far more serious problems.

How do you know whether you're overtraining? Signs include a drop in performance, longer recovery time, sore muscles, loss of appetite, headaches, and trouble sleeping.

Modern medicine has developed wonderful ways to save lives in emergencies. Drugs may make you feel better, but they'll never make your cells function better. Medicine isn't designed to help you live a longer, healthier life. Developing healthy living patterns is. The next time you think about taking a prescription, ask yourself, "Have I tried everything? Will changing some of my existing lifestyle patterns make the difference I'm looking for?" Exercise may help your body make that shift it needs to get well and stay well.

See Chapter 22 for some healthy, invigorating boosting movements you can do anywhere!

Exploring Ways to Reduce Stress

Almost everything you do rises and falls on how much stress that activity places on your body. In fact, even when you're doing something to boost your immunity, like getting sunshine or exercise, if you get too much, it becomes a *stressor* to your body and creates havoc instead of health.

There are all kinds of stress, from physical stress to emotional stress. Some stress is short term and can be positive (called *nu stress*) if it gives you that short burst of adrenaline to move you closer to your purpose. It's the stress that's adverse to your physiology that's dangerous.

Managing your stress needs to be on your radar. Your body is designed for short spurts of stress, not long-term, unrelenting stress. The purpose of your stress response is to get you out of an immediate crisis, such as if a tiger was chasing you or you needed to dart away from a moving car. But if your body needs to constantly churn out these stress hormones, you get in trouble — and fast.

Stress ages you like nobody's business. It's also a major contributor to illness, disease, and an unhappy life. Ask yourself these questions before you make any decision: "Is this decision going to add a lot of stress in my life? Is it going to simplify my life or bring complexity to it?" With complexity, stress follows. Always have your litmus test ready, and ask: "Is it worth it?"

In the following sections, we cover ways that we've seen patients manage stress successfully. Through massage, yoga, meditation, HeartMath, and chiropractic and energy work, you may find solutions.

Massage

Most people get a massage because it feels so good. Human touch is something we're hard-wired for. It's relaxing and reduces stress levels. But you'll be pleasantly surprised to know that getting a massage boosts your immunity, too!

Researchers from Cedars-Sinai Medical Center asserted that a single massage produced measurable changes in the immune system and endocrine system of healthy adults. The researchers, led by Dr. Mark Rapaport, studied 29 healthy adults who received a 45-minute Swedish massage and 24 healthy adults who had a 45-minute session of light touch massage, a much milder exercise that served as a comparison to the more vigorous Swedish massage. Blood samples were taken before the massage began and at regular intervals up to one hour after the massage was completed.

The study found several changes in the blood tests of the Swedish massage group that indicated a benefit to the immune system. The Swedish massage showed decreases in hormones that cause aggressive behavior and the stress hormone, cortisol, that results in lifted spirits and often lower blood pressure. Also, Swedish massage increased lymphocytes, the cells that help the body fight anything threatening to the body. This study gives us proof of the body's heightened immune response after a massage, and here are some other benefits:

- ✔ Boosts neurotransmitters serotonin and dopamine, which are involved in reducing depression and anxiety
- ✔ Reduces pain and stiffness
- ✔ Reduces blood pressure
- ✔ Heightens immunity
- ✔ Improves circulation and posture
- ✔ Relieves stress and relaxes muscle
- ✔ Relieves headaches

Yoga and meditation

Yoga is a wonderful way to heal the body and increase immunity. The health benefits of yoga are numerous, and combining some meditation with your yoga practice is an even more amazing way to heal and relax the body.

Here are just some of the health benefits of yoga, no matter what kind of yoga you do:

- Mental calmness
- Improved immunity
- Increased energy
- Peace of mind
- Improved breathing
- Improved muscle tone
- Anti-aging benefits
- Healthier and stronger body

Finding ways to calm your body and eliminate stress is priceless. Yoga does both for your body and does them well. The healing benefits are so great that some feel better after just one yoga session. The difference you feel in your energy and stress levels makes this practice worth the effort. If you can incorporate some yoga into your life, you may find a more relaxed, healthier you!

Meditation is another goldmine when it comes to stress relief. It brings you to a deep state of relaxation and inner stillness. Nowadays, you can find many smartphone apps and CDs with guided meditations that you can follow in the comfort of your own home.

Here are some things guided relaxation/meditation does for you that we just love:

- Increases happiness
- Reduces stress
- Teaches you to control your thoughts
- Creates healthier cells because of stress reduction
- Introduces feelings of calmness

Getting started with meditation isn't easy for everyone. Quieting your mind may be difficult at first, but with practice, it becomes second nature. Soon enough, you'll look forward to mediating. We share some of our favorite meditation and yoga exercises in Chapter 22.

Meditating for 20 minutes twice a day is ideal if you can do it. If once a day is all you can manage, try meditating first thing in the morning while your mind is relaxed.

The HeartMath solution

HeartMath is based on 30 years of research by cardiologists, physicists, and psychologists who studied how the heart's intelligence can influence your emotions and your well-being when it comes to handling stress. This program works on what you can do to balance your heart's rhythm, reduce your body's stress hormones, and boost your immunity.

The heart's intelligence is the nucleus of the program, and it refers to the heart's innate "brain." The heart has 40,000 neurons, and the signals that these messages send are intuitive ones, such as feeling love and gratitude. These positive emotions carry with them a certain pattern of activity, which is the pattern you want your body to capture and repeat. Because, when you can tap into this pattern, you have less cortisol (stress hormone) and more youth hormones (DHEA), making you younger, stronger, and healthier.

The technique outlined by the Institute of HeartMath (www.heartmath.org) involves teaching you how to harness the power of the heart's intelligence, including ways to manage your emotions and keep energy levels high. There are also techniques for calming the nervous system and other positive mind-body connections. The HeartMath technique isn't difficult to figure out, and we've seen many patients benefit from applying the research involved in the HeartMath Solution.

Chiropractic

Chiropractic care has been around for more than 115 years. It's a discipline that encourages people of all ages to work on lifestyle changes to improve health. Chiropractors look at the spine and evaluate the signal from the brain, going down the spine and out to all the end organs. With regular chiropractic adjustments, you'll experience many health benefits, including stress relief.

But isn't chiropractic just soft science?

Henry Windsor, MD, did a study about chiropractic and published some interesting findings in the *Medical Times* in the 1940s. Studying 50 cadavers from the University of Pennsylvania, Windsor examined the end stage disease that caused them to die (for example, if it was a heart problem, he looked at the heart) and traced back that organ to the segmental level (the level of the spine) and found involvement almost 100 percent of the time.

In 50 cadavers with disease in 139 organs, Windsor found a curve of the vertebrae (back bone) belonging to the same segments of the diseased organs 128 times. The discrepancy of 10 had a curve in adjacent vertebrae.

What this study tells us is profound: It's imperative that the spine is in alignment and functional to prevent disease from happening. Prolonged abnormal spinal posture stretches the nervous system, causing reduced blood supply to the organs, resulting in illness in that organ. Bottom line: Abnormal spinal curvatures are the prelude to organ diseases.

Dr. Windsor's study and his results justify chiropractic care and dispel the myth of chiropractic being a soft science. Chiropractic is grounded in solid, proven scientific principles, and millions of people, from infants to seniors, are benefiting from chiropractic care around the world.

Here are some of the other benefits of chiropractic:

- Reduces stress
- Improves immunity
- Improves nervous system function
- Maintains healthy organ function
- Increases circulation
- Increases flexibility
- Improves breathing
- Reduces chance of injury
- Removes lactic acid from the body
- Helps foster a healthier and stronger body
- Assists the body in the repair and recovery between training sessions
- Reduces muscle spasms, soreness, and pain

Maintaining the health of your spine and nervous system is where chiropractors truly shine. A healthy spine and nervous system are the cornerstones of prevention. Chiropractic is primarily aimed at restoring proper spinal mechanics, which will, in turn, influence the function of the nervous system. Chiropractors are driven by restoration and rehabilitation of normal structure and function, and not just for pain! What chiropractors do for your spine is similar to what dentists do to your teeth: They provide health and longevity to your spine, which is the key to prevention.

Chiropractic is aimed at making your body as healthy and vital as possible, so you get well and stay well. The philosophy is rooted in wellness care and in the understanding that you have an *innate intelligence* — your body's ability to heal itself, given the right raw material.

Research shows this innate intelligence can be measured through cell signaling that occurs in your body. Your cells literally communicate with each other by using various biochemical signals. As long as you provide the body with positive lifestyle practices, these cells will communicate, and your body's innate healing power will be strong. Bad choices can block this cellular communication. The better choices you make, the better this innate intelligence network works for you.

Look for a chiropractor that practices using "The Insight Subluxation Station." Created by the visionary Dr. Patrick Gentempo and Dr. Christopher Kent, this test is the most advanced technology to access the spine. It checks for the following:

- ✔ **Heart rate variability (HRV):** This shows a chiropractor how your nervous system is working and how your body handles stress.
- ✔ **Thermal scan of the spine:** This tells a chiropractor whether there's inflammation at different segments of the spine.
- ✔ **Surface EMG:** This tells the chiropractor whether any muscle spasms occur at different segmental levels of the spine.

What's so great about these tests is that you actually get measured results about the functioning of your spine. Remember: What gets measured gets managed! To find a chiropractor who uses this technology, go to www.findagreat chiro.com.

Meet Dr. "Fab"

The legendary Dr. Fabrizio Mancini, author of *The Power of Self-Healing: Unlock Your Natural Healing Potential in 21 Days!* (Hay House) was 33 years old when he became the president of Parker University in Dallas, Texas, making him the youngest president of a college or university in the United States — ever. His leadership abilities and vision for health and wellness has made him one of the world's experts on chiropractic and wellness care. He states:

"Chiropractic allows the body to be as stress free as possible. In other words, while many people live on the stress roller coaster, people who stay well adjusted find that they experience a steady road to better health through better living. That's why a chiropractor analyzes your body for nerve interference that occurs as a result of stressful lifestyles."

Naturopathy

The best way to understand what a naturopathic doctor (ND; or naturopath) does is to think of your family medical doctor. Although a medical doctor usually focuses the treatment plan on drugs or surgery, an ND's core philosophy is to dispense natural treatments and remedies to remove barriers to good health. NDs are trained to utilize prescription drugs, however, their concentration is on natural remedies to help their patients heal and create health.

Naturopaths focus on comprehensive diagnosis and treatment, so visits are often much longer than your family medical doctor. NDs often dig deep into all your lifestyle habits (smoking, stress, diet, chemical exposures, and so on) to find a comprehensive diagnosis, prevention, and treatment plan. NDs can treat many conditions, such as cancer, heart disease, diabetes, hormonal problems, dietary and weight concerns, fatigue, chronic issues, digestive problems, and allergies.

If you favor a holistic approach with noninvasive treatments and approaches, naturopathic medicine is right up your alley! It's a paradigm that will get you well and keep you well naturally. To find a naturopathic doctor in you area, consult the American Association of Naturopathic Physicians at www. naturopathic.org.

Energy work

Energy work is based on the philosophy that your body is infused with energy fields and that humans aren't just skin and bones but also atoms and molecules. Throughout this matrix of atoms and molecules, you have a multi-body system of energy and energy patterns. Things you say, think, and do don't just affect you physically; they affect you on all levels.

You have storage centers for these energy patterns, and a practitioner may manipulate these fields to affect health. The core belief is that diseases, illness, and duress are a result of being energetically out of balance in some way, and the key to healing is to balance, revive, or sedate these energy fields to heal. We're both big proponents of this healing methodology, because we've seen energy work provide deep healing to many patients.

Your body's *life force* (also called *prana, chi,* or *Qi*) is at the center of all energy work. Tapping into and balancing that force within your body gives you deep healing and strength — true health, or *vitality*. When you have vitality, you have life's golden ticket!

Here are different techniques that use energy work as the foundation:

- ✔ Chinese medicine (acupuncture), in which the energetic pathways are called *meridians*
- ✔ Qi Gong
- ✔ Reiki
- ✔ EFT (Emotional Freedom Technique)
- ✔ NET (Neuro Emotional Technique)
- ✔ Shiatsu
- ✔ Chakra healing
- ✔ Therapeutic touch
- ✔ Crystal healing

If you want to experience deep healing, relaxation, and calm, it's worth trying energy medicine to bring your body back to balance. See how it works for you!

To find a practitioner or technique in energy medicine in your area, ask friends, family, and those you trust who they feel comfortable with and are getting results with, using energy medicine. Or ask your holistic practitioner (holistic MD, naturopath, or chiropractor) who knows your history and approach him about his recommendations. These doctors are often well connected and have recommendations on techniques and individual practitioners that will suit your needs.

If you want to get started implementing energy medicine immediately, take a look at Chapter 22, where you'll find boosting movements that work like energy medicine. These exercises shift your energy and create healing throughout your body.

Chapter 12

Exploring Detoxification to Refresh Your Immunity

*T*he immune system works best when it has fewer distractions to its work. One major distractor is a body fighting with toxins and other cellular debris that aren't getting disposed of correctly. Normal detoxification processes in the body are elegantly planned and usually work well, but in modern culture, the system can get overwhelmed with the vast amount of material that needs filtered out, making the body work harder to eliminate toxins and perform smoothly. Sometimes, planning a purposeful support of the detoxification process helps get the system moving again and removes a drain on the immune system.

Regular detoxification is to immune health what brushing your teeth is to good dentition. Can people be lazy with teeth brushing and be okay? Sure. Can you never do a detox in your life and stay reasonably healthy? Sure. But given a choice of okay immunity versus fabulous immunity without a lot of work, why would you skip it?

In this chapter, we discuss why to detox, various ways to do so, and how to detox your environment as well as your body. We provide additional techniques to enhance your detoxification experience on Dummies.com. Go to www.dummies.com/extras/boostingyourimmunity to find information on hydrotherapy, skin brushing, and massage.

Deciding to Detox

The term *detox* is thrown around so much and used for so many things that sometimes knowing what people mean when they use it is difficult.

Technically, *detoxification* refers to the breaking down and elimination of potentially dangerous substances to prevent damage and disease. The human body does this naturally in a number of ways (see "Meeting the Key Players in Detoxification," later in this chapter), and you can help these processes work optimally by doing a few things. In the following sections, we walk you through the detoxification process and help you decide whether it's a path you want to take to help refresh your health.

What is a detox, and is it right for you?

Detoxification protocols have been around for millennia. Traditional Chinese medicine, ayurveda, and other ancient healing systems all have their own version of helping the body purify itself of toxins, allowing it to return to normal balance and boosting immunity in the process.

Detoxification can take many forms, but before you choose your detox plan, you need to know what detoxification is *not*. Because the liver and kidneys are the main organs of detoxification in the body, detoxes consist of really only those protocols that help those two organs. The bowel and kidneys then excrete the toxins (and the skin and lungs help a bit), so if a protocol is aimed at those organs alone, it's not a detox — it's just an enhancement of elimination.

Detoxification protocols can vary widely. Some last a month or more and involve specific dietary changes alone aimed at providing nutrients to the liver and kidney. Some use diet and herbs to do the same thing. More modern versions usually involve diet changes and nutritional supplementation in the form of powders to make a medical food shake. These types of detoxes are usually listed as *metabolic detoxification protocols* to distinguish them from traditional food-only protocols. Many supplement companies provide these; some are worthwhile, some aren't. Find out what to look for in the section, "Detoxing with supplement powder and medical foods," later in this chapter.

Weighing the pros and cons of detoxing

In traditional healing systems, detoxification can be prescribed as a treatment to regain balance and also as a preventive. In practical terms in our culture, we use it mostly as a preventive. We weigh the pros and cons of detoxing in the next sections.

The pros of detoxing

The good thing a detox does for you is provide nutrients to your liver to help it do its job. That may sound odd, because you're supposed to provide nutrients to your body anyway, but in these protocols, the dietary changes are designed to provide a higher proportion of liver-specific nutrients over the course of several days or a week, while eliminating those things you often expose yourself to that make the liver work overtime. At the same time, the protocols ask that you drink a lot more water than you may usually, while eliminating most dehydrating fluids like coffee and alcohol, so your kidneys get more fluid to work with and are more efficient.

Detoxification also helps you refocus on eating a clean, unprocessed, healthy diet. Even when striving to eat clean, most folks end up making a few concessions here and there; the detox protocol gets you back on track. Without the distraction of any added sugars and such, you get a chance to really taste whole foods again. By the end, most people feel lighter and more clear-headed.

In the process of detoxification, your elimination pathways get a renewal as well. The kidneys get flushed out, both with the extra water and the extra work. Most detox protocols require more vegetable intake than you're probably used to in a typical day (animal products are generally eliminated during this time), so the extra fiber helps move things through your bowels, giving them a scrubbing as well. Your other elimination organs — the skin and lungs — don't specifically get targeted during most protocols, though we usually add specific things to our own detoxes to help those along.

Generally speaking, a detox is a good idea if you want to rev up your detoxification and elimination systems, get your immune system up to speed, and refocus on eating well and getting bad habits (such as too much caffeine or too much alcohol) back under control. You'll be rewarded with a few days of fatigue during the process and perhaps some mild GI distress initially, but by the end, you'll likely feel more clear-headed and lighter and will be wondering why you don't always eat this way!

The cons of detoxing

So what's the downside of detoxification? Well, on a practical level, it takes a good bit of planning and a certain amount of discipline — not something everyone is willing to do! If you're used to cooking with even *some* processed foods, a ten-day detox protocol of cooking exclusively from scratch may sound tough. In the particular protocol we use, three days in the middle of the ten-day scheme have a pretty restricted diet (along with the medical food; see "Detoxing with supplement powder and medical foods"); and for some, the thought of three full days of only cruciferous veggies, salad greens, apples, and pears sounds out of this world. However, after you've done it the first time, you see how easy it can actually be.

Detoxification is a pretty energy-sucking process for the body, so don't do it during a time of great physical or mental/emotional stress. Detox also isn't appropriate during an illness or pregnancy. (Technically, women can do a few modified versions during pregnancy, but whether you choose to is an individual decision based on individual health concerns. Check with a holistic physician before attempting a detox during a pregnancy.) Any individual who is older or more frail physically may need to modify a protocol so as not to overtax the liver, kidneys, and other organs involved.

Meeting the Key Players in Detoxification

Detoxification is the job of a whole team. The main work is done by the liver with some help from the kidneys. The gastrointestinal (GI) tract is important in elimination of the breakdown products, and elimination via the skin and lungs also occurs.

✔ **Liver:** The liver is a large organ in the upper right-hand side of the abdomen. It actually has a number of jobs in addition to detoxification. A vein called the *portal vein,* which you can see in Figure 12-1, connects the digestive tract to the liver, allowing drugs, alcohol, and toxins found in food to be delivered this way. The liver also filters blood, removing toxins found there.

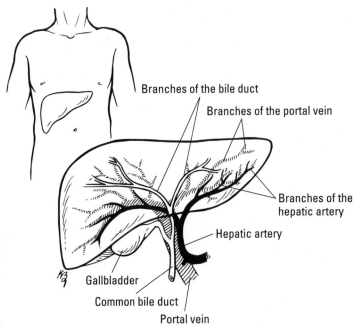

Figure 12-1:
A closer
look at the
liver.

Branches of the bile duct

Branches of the portal vein

Branches of the
hepatic artery

Hepatic artery

Gallbladder

Common bile duct

Portal vein

Illustration by Kathryn Born

Liver lobules (see Figure 12-2) are made up of individual liver cells formed into groups. In the liver cells, a host of enzymes work on the chemicals they find, helping break them down. In general, these compounds aren't water-soluble, so they need to be converted into another form that's both nontoxic and water-soluble to remove them from the body via stool or urine. The enzymes use a set of chemical processes referred to as *Phase I reactions* and *Phase II reactions.* Both of these sets of reactions need to work properly for full detoxification to occur. When the products are broken down, they're shunted to the bowel for elimination.

✔ **Kidneys:** The kidneys filter blood and do the bulk of detoxification of blood-borne toxins. Your kidneys reside just below the ribs on the back, one on each side; they're shaped like kidney beans. Blood flows into the kidney via an artery, gets filtered in the tiny capillaries of the nephrons, and then flows back out via the veins, which you can see in Figure 12-3. Byproducts and water that have been filtered out get transferred into the ureter and flow to the bladder for elimination. In addition to doing the work of detoxification, the kidneys remove other metabolic waste and balance out pH of the blood. Because this whole system is based on fluid, keeping hydrated is important so the functions remain intact.

✔ **GI tract:** The gastrointestinal (GI) tract doesn't really do any detoxification per se, despite what you may read in ads and see on the Internet. The GI tract does the work of breaking down food, absorbing nutrients, and eliminating waste, including what it receives from the liver. However, if it doesn't work well, then the byproducts of detoxification get backed up, so keeping it working smoothly is still vital. Any malfunction (such as constipation or diarrhea) impacts the elimination of the toxic byproducts and impacts health.

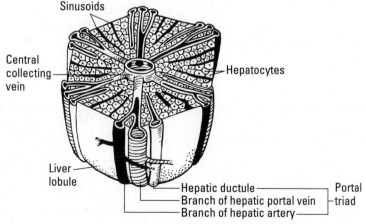

Figure 12-2:
A detailed
look at a
liver lobule.

Sinusoids

Central
collecting
vein

Hepatocytes

Liver
lobule

Hepatic ductule
Branch of hepatic portal vein
Branch of hepatic artery

Portal
triad

Illustration by Kathryn Born

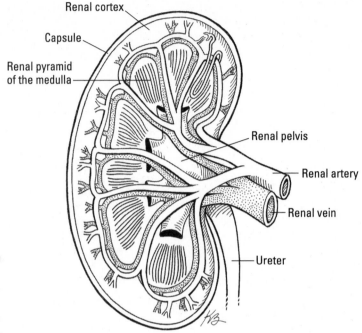

Renal cortex

Capsule

Renal pyramid
of the medulla

Renal pelvis

Renal artery

Renal vein

Ureter

Figure 12-3:
A close-up
of the
kidney.

Illustration by Kathryn Born

↙ **Lungs:** Lungs are primarily involved with respiration. As part of the process, they also help maintain blood pH and expel chemical vapors under specific conditions. One example is the sweet smell of a diabetic person's breath in ketoacidosis, a severe condition. The excess ketones in the blood are partially expelled in the exhaled breath and can be picked up by their distinctly sweet smell. Keeping the lungs working well helps keep the detoxification processes working smoothly. See Figure 12-4 for a detail of the anatomy of the lungs. In addition, conscious control of breathing patterns stimulates the immune system (see Chapter 21 for details).

Why nutrition is so important for detox

Each step of the detoxification process requires nutrient cofactors to proceed. Without these nutrients onboard, the processes get sluggish. That's why all detoxification protocols focus on improving nutrition. Some of the best foods to eat during detox include cruciferous vegetables, like broccoli, cauliflower, turnips, and kale. Apples also supply much of the nutrients needed, as does green tea.

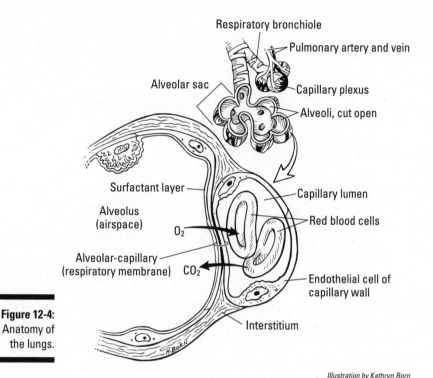

Respiratory bronchiole

Pulmonary artery and vein

Alveolar sac

Capillary plexus

Alveoli, cut open

Surfactant layer

Capillary lumen

Alveolus (airspace)

O_2

Red blood cells

Alveolar-capillary (respiratory membrane)

CO_2

Endothelial cell of capillary wall

Interstitium

H. BORN

Figure 12-4:
Anatomy of
the lungs.

Illustration by Kathryn Born

Technically, skin isn't really part of detoxification because it isn't capable of breaking down toxins into something harmless. However, excess fluid and a waste product called *urea* are excreted in the form of sweat. These two processes are vital to maintaining appropriate fluid balance and pH, so by extension, the skin helps to maintain the body in a detoxified state.

Our Immune-Boosting Detox Strategy

You can approach a detox in many ways. Ideally, you'd do a detox over weeks of rest, healthful eating, massage, accelerated elimination protocols, and supportive herbs — the way it's done in traditional ayurvedic practice. But who has time to do that in real life? We prefer to make this process practical so you can undergo a detox regularly, just the way you routinely tune up your car.

In this section, we outline how we, your authors, approach detoxification — both for ourselves and for our patients. Check with a holistic care provider before starting a detox to be sure it fits with your own health conditions.

Setting yourself up for detoxing success

To be successful detoxing, you need to know what to expect and how to prepare. Here are some guidelines to get you going:

1. **Pick the right time.**

   If you're sick, don't detox unless you do so under the guidance of a qualified care provider. If you're training for a big athletic event, it's probably not a good time. If you're pregnant, think twice. Historically, detoxification is done either at the fall and spring equinoxes (as coauthor Wendy does) or once each season (as coauthor Kellyann does).

2. **Plan ahead.**

   You'll probably be modifying your diet quite a bit, so be sure to shop for what you need and have it on hand. (See the discussion of specific foods in the "Detoxing with foods and drinks alone" section.) If you're detoxing during your usual work week, you may want to cook ahead so you don't have to think too hard about what to eat each day.

3. **Revise your exercise schedule.**

   Your energy level may very well be different during detox, so extreme exercise routines are often difficult to do during this time. Be prepared to do less.

4. **Get a journal and write about how you feel each day.**

   This step is actually really important because, as the days pass, you'll forget how you felt earlier in the detox process. You'll likely want to compare notes during your detox because different phases may stir up different things. As you add back any eliminated foods, write down any reactions you get.

5. **Tell your friends and family and ask for their support.**

   Sticking with a detox by yourself can be difficult. Having others to talk with, or at least to cheer you on, can make a big difference. Coauthor Wendy teams up with a group of patients, and they all start their detoxes on the same day. They become a support for each other and stay in touch by e-mail to ask and answer questions, share ideas on what to eat, and generally keep the fun in it.

Detoxing with supplement powder and medical foods

Many companies provide supplement powders and medical foods to assist in detoxification. All of them contain nutrients designed to help improve the Phase I and Phase II detox pathways. Most also suggest a partial elimination diet, meaning that over the course of several days, you remove certain categories of food from your diet. Each day, you remove another category of food until you're eating primarily only those foods that boost the detox processes specifically and that aren't likely to cause immune reactions. After a few days, you start adding the eliminated foods back in. All the while, you're taking the supplements.

We both use a medical food called UltraClear Renew by Metagenics. It contains not only the detox nutrients we need but also enough protein, carbohydrates, and healthy fats to help make up for the foods we eliminate. This product has both a 10-day and 21-day protocol. The good news about the longer protocol is that it's less demanding in terms of food elimination, but the bad news is that it's longer. (We usually do the 10-day version.)

Many other supplement companies make similar products. If you decide to detox with supplements, keep the following in mind when looking for a quality product:

- The product should contain protein, fats, and carbohydrates to maintain your energy as you eliminate foods. The protein should be low allergy and easily digestible.

- The product should contain nutrients specifically designed to boost Phase I and Phase II reactions, including vitamins A, D, and the B complex, among others. Minerals, such as magnesium and zinc, are also important.

- Avoid products that are really just helping elimination. These products contain herbs and fiber for the gut, and although they can be helpful for elimination, they're *not* detoxifying your system.

Detoxing with foods and drinks alone

In addition to using a prepared medical food to assist a detox protocol, you can do a mild detox, using food alone. These protocols do have a milder effect, but they still work if you stick to the eating plan. Again, many versions exist, but the following lists provide what foods and drinks to use and then the appropriate protocol to fit them in.

The following foods directly aid the liver's detoxification pathways:

- Cruciferous vegetables, such as broccoli, cauliflower, Brussels sprouts, kale, turnips, and bok choy
- Green leafy vegetables, such as spinach, salad greens, mizuna, arugula, and escarole
- Citrus, such as oranges, lemons, and limes (skip grapefruit because it contains naringin, which affects some of the liver enzymes)
- Sulfur-rich foods, like onions, garlic, and eggs (including the yolk)
- Foods with chemicals known to support the liver directly: asparagus, artichoke, beets, dandelion greens, and burdock root

The following foods support the colon and elimination:

- Apples
- Berries
- Carrots
- Pears

These liquids are approved for detoxing with food and drink alone:

- Water, water, water! Drink at least one half of your body weight in ounces each day of the cleanse.
- Green tea, not decaffeinated: The process of decaffeination removes a good many of the beneficial chemicals in the tea, so it's a bit of a waste. If the caffeine is too much for you, you can also take green tea extract capsules or liquid.

Don't forget protein. The detox process takes a lot of energy, and protein helps you get through the day. You need two, 3-ounce servings of clean, lean protein a day; here's what to look for:

- Try to get meat from pasture-raised animals, because these farmers tend to never use any antibiotics or hormones and often don't supplement with any grain at all, so the omega–fatty acid ratio is still optimal in the meat. Don't feel shy about asking how the animal was raised.
- Look for sustainably wild-caught fish. A fabulous source is the online company Vital Choice (www.vitalchoice.com).

You also need several teaspoons of oil daily.

✔ Organic extra-virgin olive oil is best.

✔ Flax oil for salad dressing is nice (and adding vinegar is okay!).

A few items aren't helpful to your immunity, especially during a detox, so be sure to avoid the following:

✔ Any processed foods whatsoever (no boxes, bags, or cans)

✔ Any added sugars, including honey and maple syrup

✔ Any artificial sweeteners, such as NutraSweet and Splenda

✔ Gluten in any form (the grains that are okay include rice, quinoa, millet, amaranth, teff, and buckwheat)

✔ Alcohol, caffeine (other than green tea), and over-the-counter drugs, unless absolutely necessary

Here's a step-by-step process for putting it all together:

1. **Follow the eating guidelines for seven to ten days.** This diet prepares your body for any toxins that get released; otherwise, you'll simply feel worse as the toxins get freed up from fat cells and start floating around in the system.

2. **Do one day of a juice fast to bring the toxins out.** During this day, drink lemon water copiously as well as organic vegetable juices and fruit juices. No added sweeteners at all. Drink at least a cup of fluid every hour while you're awake, alternating between water and juice. Take it easy this day; a walk is fine, but skip the Zumba class!

3. **Eat as you did in Step 1 for at least three days.** During this time, add in naturally fermented foods, such as unpasteurized sauerkraut or other fermented veggies, plain unsweetened yogurt (the label should say only milk and active cultures — nothing else!), kefir, or kombucha. These fermented foods help support the colon's ability to eliminate the toxins you've flushed out.

4. **By this point, the detox is done.** You can now decide how to add any eliminated foods back in, but do so slowly. Add in only one missing food type in any given day so if you get a bad reaction to it, you know what to blame. Be especially careful about caffeine and alcohol, because you may react more strongly to them now.

Adding supplements to support detoxification

When detoxifying only with food, you may or may not want to use supplements to help support you. As we mention earlier, many companies provide all the supplements you need in powder form, ready to mix with water and drink. These products generally include protein, carbs, and fats and can be used as a snack or meal replacement. However, if you want to use mainly foods with just a bit of support, add in the following:

- ✔ **Vitamin C:** A major antioxidant, vitamin C helps protect you from the free radicals of the reactive Phase I breakdown products.

- ✔ **B complex:** Several of the B vitamins act to improve breakdown as well as protect from free radicals.

- ✔ **N-acetyl cysteine:** This is a precursor to glutathione, which is essential to the detox process (and nearly impossible to absorb when taken as a supplement itself).

- ✔ **Milk thistle:** The silymarin in milk thistle has long been used as a liver protector and has been shown in multiple studies to restore abnormal liver enzyme levels.

Detoxifying Your Environment

Just as moving toxins out of the body is important, moving toxins out of the areas where you live and work decreases your exposure and gives your body a break. No, removing everything isn't possible, unless you live in a sterile bubble and avoid the world, but changing your exposure is possible. In some areas, like at home, where you're in charge, it's rather easy. At work, it may be a bit more difficult because you may not be the decision maker, and your line of work may have inherent exposures. In the following sections, we show you how to detoxify your environment, from what you use in everyday life to different measures you can take at home and at work.

Starting with self-care products

The first part of the chapter covered the main detoxification of the body via diet and other treatments to remove toxins. You can also avoid even allowing the toxins in in the first place. For women especially, one of the main culprits is self-care products. It's estimated that by the time the average woman leaves the house in the morning, she has been exposed to several dozen chemicals, not all of them friendly. These chemicals range from products in soap to deodorants to moisturizers, from facial creams and shampoos to cosmetics and hair styling gels. Just because it's on the market doesn't mean it's safe. The FDA has no authority to require proof of safety before a product comes to market and has little ability to enforce what few recommendations it does make.

According to the Environmental Working Group (EWG), more than 500 self-care products available in America contain products banned in Japan, Canada, or the European Union. Nearly 100 products contain ingredients considered unsafe by the International Fragrance Association. Even 61 percent of lipstick brands tested contained lead residues! To check specific products, go to the EWG's database, which is updated regularly: www.ewg.org/skindeep. Although you have to decide for yourself what you're willing to allow into your life, our recommendation is to keep it as simple as possible; use few products, and make sure to avoid paraben, toluene, and formaldehyde at the very least, because each of these products has a negative effect on the immune system.

Improving your surroundings at home and work

If detoxification is a good thing, then limiting what toxins you're exposed to in the first place is a good thing. Here are a few steps you can take to eliminate or reduce your exposure:

- ✔ **Avoid stain-resistant coatings on furniture, carpets, and clothing.** These coatings usually contain the chemical triclosan as well as PFCs (perfluorochemicals), which are implicated in liver damage, disruption of thyroid function, elevated cholesterol, and weakened immune function. When triclosan gets into the water system, it's also highly toxic to aquatic life.

- ✔ **Stop using antibacterial soaps.** The same triclosan in stain-resistant coatings is also found in antibacterial soaps. These products are *not* a good idea in day-to-day life because they're not only toxic to the person using them but can also lead to resistant bacteria. The AMA (American Medical Association) recommends that they not be used in the home.

- ✔ **Avoid products containing PFCs, including paper plates, the lining of microwave popcorn bags, and nonstick pans.**

- ✔ **Avoid plastics marked with "7" and "PC," and don't microwave any plastic at all.**

✔ **Filter your tap water at home.** Buying bottled water is expensive, there's no guarantee that it's any better than tap, and it leaves a lot of plastic bottles for the landfill. Reverse osmosis or carbon filter systems — or systems with a combination of the two — are best for home use.

✔ **Use a HEPA filter vacuum, which picks up the most contaminants from the floor.** Toxins are often concentrated on the floor, where they land from the air and are tracked in on shoes. Leave shoes at the door.

✔ **Don't use pesticides on your lawn or garden.** Teach your kids to not walk on lawns barefoot if they see the little flags that companies are required to put out after a treatment.

✔ **Use greener cleaning products that contain natural ingredients.** If your grandmother used it, it's probably a good thing to try.

Not everyone is a decision maker at work, and some people feel as though they have limited ability to protect themselves from exposure to toxins. If you fit either of these categories, check out the following ideas:

✔ If where you work has new carpet or paint, consider renting a small air filter for the space around your work area; use it for at least as long as it takes to get rid of that new carpet smell.

✔ Keep a carbon filter water pitcher at work if your employer doesn't provide filtered water.

✔ Ask that your employer skip the routine pest control spraying in your area, or at least try to schedule a day off when that happens.

✔ Skip the antibacterial soap in the company washroom, unless you work in a hospital.

Some jobs simply expose people to more toxins than other jobs do. Some of the worst are field workers on commercial farms, who are exposed to pesticides; and hair stylists and makeup artists, who are exposed to hundreds of different chemicals in a day. Jewelers can be exposed to aerosolized metal vapors, and potters are exposed to chemicals in the glazes for their ceramics. You get the picture. When faced with exposure at work that's simply unavoidable, the need for regular detoxification becomes more clear. It also makes sense to be extra careful at home, to help make up for exposure elsewhere.

Part IV

Cooking Up Recipes for Immunity and Wellness

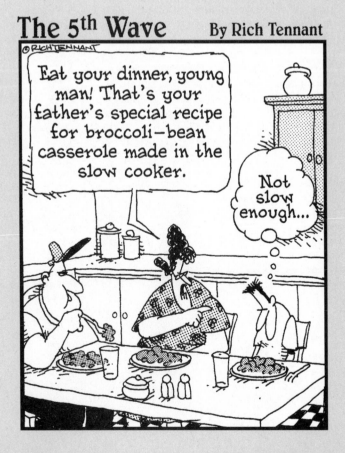

The 5th Wave   By Rich Tennant

Eat your dinner, young man! That's your father's special recipe for broccoli—bean casserole made in the slow cooker.

Not slow enough...

In this part . . .

*I*t's time to get in the kitchen! Modern life is filled with challenges, but we try to make your transition to an immune-boosting kitchen no sweat with a chapter on planning and stocking an immune-friendly kitchen. We share tips to help your family make the transition without a hitch (or a battle!).

The chapters in this part also contain 50 recipes to keep you satisfied and energized throughout the day. With the simplest of ingredients, you can cook easy, family-pleasing dishes for all times of the day and all tastes: breakfasts, lunches, dinners, side dishes, soups, and salads. We even include recipes for energizing teas and nutritional smoothies that will both cleanse and heal you.

Chapter 13

Planning and Stocking an Immunity-Friendly Kitchen

*T*his is where the rubber meets the road. You know that boosting your immunity starts with food. In fact, nothing influences your ability to get well and stay well more than the choices you make with food. Discovering immune-boosting foods and figuring out how to transform your kitchen into a place that moves your body toward health are the foundation to success.

One of the great things about living a healthy lifestyle is that you can make it really simple — nothing flashy or difficult; no hard-to-find or unusual ingredients; just simple, back-to-nature foods put together in a simple way without making you feel like you're missing out or, worse yet, on a diet.

Chapters 14 through 19 are packed with recipes designed to improve your immunity. If you're a newcomer to the kitchen, don't be intimidated. We've worked with enough people to know that if incorporating immune-boosting foods wasn't easy, not too many people would stick with it. We want to make your life easier, healthier, and more joyful — certainly not more overwhelming or exhausting.

But before you can start cooking, you need to first focus your attention on your kitchen, because what's in your cabinets, fridge, and freezer right now likely isn't the best fit for your new immune-boosting diet and lifestyle. This chapter gets you started on cleaning out and restocking your kitchen and shopping for healthier foods. We also share recommendations on food preparation, and at www.dummies.com/extras/boostingyourimmunity, you can find a helpful list of cooking tools to prepare you for your immune-boosting journey.

Getting Started: Cleaning Out Your Kitchen

Commit to living a healthier, immune-boosting life by going through your kitchen and taking inventory of what you have. Removing all the foods that don't move you toward health signifies the beginning of something positive — a healthier, stronger, and ageless you — which can be very motivating.

Cleaning out your kitchen makes everything easier. It's kind of like cleaning out your closet; after you're done, don't you instantly feel lighter, more inspired? Most of all, when you clean out your kitchen, you get clarity. You know exactly what you have to work with, and you don't have a bunch of clutter tugging at you. You're less tempted by foods that don't fit your new eating habits.

Not holding on to that "one last thing" or not holding on to foods because you don't want to waste them is difficult. But clear your mind of that thinking and just decide to commit and go!

Start with your cabinets and pantry. Brace yourself, because chances are you'll have to toss most of it. Read the labels and see what can be saved, but if you're like most people starting on a wellness journey, you're probably going to have to start from scratch.

Throw out anything that's opened. Separate items that are unopened for donation to a food bank, shelter, or any community of people that are in need of food. It may not be the best nutrition, but it can still help those in need.

Clear these foods out of your cabinets:

- ✔ All foods with flour, including breads, pasta, crackers, chips, and cookies
- ✔ Breakfast cereals
- ✔ All foods with grains and whole grains, including wheat, barley, rye, oats, spelt, corn, and quinoa
- ✔ Refined processed fats, such as canola (rapeseed), soybean, grapeseed, sunflower, safflower, corn oil, margarine, vegetable oil, and peanut oil
- ✔ Hydrogenated or partially hydrogenated oils (cookies, snack foods, Earth Balance, or other buttery spreads)
- ✔ All foods with artificial sweeteners, specifically Acesulfame K (Sweet One), aspartame (Equal and NutraSweet), saccharin (Sweet'N Low), and sucralose (Splenda)
- ✔ All foods with soy, including soy, teriyaki, and hoisin sauces

✔ Commercial condiments with sugars and artificial ingredients

✔ Foods with cornstarch

✔ High-fructose corn syrup and all other sugars except for raw honey and pure maple syrup, dark chocolate, and cocoa powder

✔ Packaged processed foods, like microwavable meals or food bars (check all processed foods carefully because most have additives and gluten)

✔ Sauces, soups, and stews (most have thickened flours)

✔ Dressings (most are thickened with flour)

✔ Canned foods with sugars and additives, such as canned fruits

Purge the following items from your refrigerator and freezer:

✔ Any leftovers that aren't part of your healthy food plan

✔ Commercial dressings and sauces

✔ Dairy products, including butter, margarine, milk, cheese, cream, half-and-half, and yogurt

✔ All soy frankenfoods, such as vegetarian burgers, hot dogs, and chicken nuggets

   Frankenfoods are processed foods that are made to look like a certain food product but are really made from wheat.

✔ Fruit juices or other sweetened beverages, such as soda or teas

✔ Lunchmeats, sausage, and bacon that contain gluten, nitrites, or sweeteners

✔ Commercial condiments with sugars and artificial ingredients

✔ Frozen waffles, pizza, macaroni, or other frozen meals

✔ Ice cream and frozen yogurt

✔ Popsicles and frozen fruit bars with sugar and artificial ingredients

What you should have left in your refrigerator are eggs, unprocessed meats, fresh fruits, vegetables, and condiments that don't contain sugar.

If you decide to have a sweet, you're better off going out and getting a single serving rather than keeping it in your house. That way, once you eat it, you're done, and you're not tempted by it lingering around the house.

Congratulations! The worst is over. You've said goodbye to those pesky foods that cause inflammation, fatigue, illness, and a lowered immune system to make way for foods that make you come alive. Now that's motivating!

Restocking Your Kitchen for a Boosting Future

Restocking your kitchen is like winning a marathon. You've already done the hardest part by deciding to move forward and committing to a healthy life by clearing out the old and making way for the new.

The foods you'll be restocking your kitchen with are full of nutrients and bursting with flavor. They're the foods your body was designed to eat. Immune-boosting foods help you get well, stay well, and fight aging. Enjoy making these foods your base and get excited about your healthy, vibrant future.

Picking proteins your body will love

When you read or hear that animal proteins aren't good for you, often the *quality* of that protein is in question, not the protein source. Factory-farmed meat is less healthy than animals raised humanely and sustainably. When you can, your best option is always to get meat from organic, pasture-raised, antibiotic-free sources. If doing so isn't in the budget right now, don't stress. Buying the leanest cuts you can find, removing the skin on poultry and the excess fat on red meat before cooking, and removing and draining excess fat after cooking are great strategies for making conventional meats as healthy as possible.

Follow this advice for making the best protein choices — from beef to wild game to eggs and everything in between — to restock your immunity-friendly kitchen:

- **Beef:** Grass-fed, organic beef provides you with the best balance of omega-6 to omega-3 ratios. In fact, when you buy grass-fed, you can eat all the fat — no need to cut or drain.

- **Lamb:** All cuts are good; pasture-raised is best.

- **Poultry:** All cuts of poultry are good. Organic, free-range or pasture-raised is best.

- **Pork:** If you can't purchase pastured-raised pork or wild boar to avoid the toxins and omega-6 fatty acids of conventionally raised pork, you may want to pick another, cleaner protein source. If you buy organic bacon, make sure it's free of sugar, and eat it in moderation.

- **Game meats:** Game meats, like elk, bison, duck, pheasant, and quail, are naturally low in fat and high in protein. If you can find them, they're great choices.

✔ **Organ meats:** Organic organ meats, such as liver, kidney, and heart, are rich in nutrition. Just keep in mind that organic and pasture-raised is your best bet. Conventionally raised organ meats can be toxic, so pass on those if you can't find a pasture-raised source.

✔ **Eggs:** Organic and pasture-raised eggs provide the healthiest omega-6 to omega-3 ratios.

When buying eggs, labels or cartons that read *vegetarian-fed* and *natural* have no impact on the quality of the eggs. Their titles sound like a breezy day at the farm but have no value.

✔ **Fish and seafood:** Wild-caught fish, seafood, and shellfish are healthier than farm-raised. Visit the Monterey Bay Aquarium Seafood Watch at `www.montereybayaquarium.org/cr/seafoodwatch.aspx` for a complete list of healthy fish in your area.

✔ **Nitrite- and gluten-free deli meats and sausages:** Look on the label for added sugar or other additives that could sabotage your healthy efforts.

Choosing produce with boosting power

Vegetables are a great way to reduce your chances of getting just about any disease, not to mention they keep you young and vibrant. They're also on the more alkaline side of the pendulum, keeping your body's acid-base balance in order.

Fruits in moderation are an excellent antioxidant source. The healthier your body becomes, the more fruit you'll be able to tolerate without blood sugar swings. One of the best qualities of fruit is its ability to satisfy your taste for sweet naturally while adding nutrition.

Local, organic, and seasonal produce is best. Frozen organic is a good choice as well because the produce is *flash frozen*, locking in all the freshness and goodness. Eat as much variety of produce as possible. Check out the section "Buying organic: Do's and don'ts," later in this chapter, for two lists: produce that you should always buy organic (the Dirty Dozen), and produce that's clean enough that you can buy conventionally (the Clean 15). For more on these categories, visit the Environmental Working Group at `www.ewg.org/foodnews/list`.

Healthy vegetables are an essential part of any immune-building plate. Take your pick from the list in Table 13-1. Just remember: Any vegetables are better than no vegetables, so eat your vegetables! Loaded with vitamins, minerals, and fiber, vegetables should be the superstar of your plate.

Table 13-1	Healthy Vegetables	
Artichoke	Eggplant	Parsnip
Arugula	Endive	Pumpkin
Asparagus	Escarole	Radish
Bell peppers	Green beans	Shallots
Broccoli	Garlic	Snow peas
Beets	Greens: Beet, collard, mustard, turnip	Spaghetti squash
Bok Choy	Kale	Spinach
Broccoli	Kohlrabi	Sugar snap peas
Brussels sprouts	Leeks	Summer squash
Cabbage	Lettuce	Sweet potatoes/yams
Carrots	Mushrooms	Tomatoes
Cauliflower	Nori (seaweed)	Tomatillos
Celery	Okra	Turnips
Chile peppers	Onion	Winter squash: Butternut, acorn
Cucumber		

Healthy fruits are as fabulous as can be — in small quantities. Even though fruit contains natural sugar, it's still sugar. So enjoy any of the fruits in Table 13-2 but in small doses. Most importantly, don't look to fruit as your main source of carbohydrates; they should never knock the vegetables off your plate!

Table 13-2	Healthy Fruits	
Apple	Grapefruit	Orange
Apricot	Grapes	Papaya
Banana	Honeydew	Peach
Blackberries	Lychee	Pear
Blueberries	Kiwi	Pineapple
Cantaloupe	Kumquat	Plum
Cherries	Lemon	Pomegranate
Clementine	Lime	Raspberries
Cranberries	Mandarin	Strawberries
Dates	Mango	Tangerine
Figs	Nectarine	Watermelon

Limit your consumption of dried fruit; it's easy to overeat and it lacks the nutrition of fresh fruits, while concentrating the sugars. You also have to be aware of the sulfites in dried fruits, which are toxic. Always opt for sulfite-free dried fruit when you indulge or choose to skip it altogether. Also, avoid fruit juices because they provide all the sugar of the fruit without the fiber and satiety of eating.

Selecting fabulous fats for a nourishing kitchen

Putting healthy fats on your plate makes just about everything you do better! Fats nourish every structure and function of the body — including your very important brain. Fats also help you absorb nutrients more efficiently and keep you feeling full.

The key when it comes to choosing fats is to get the healthiest fats you possibly can, such as the following:

- Avocado
- Butter: Grass-fed butter, from grass-fed, pasture-raised cows, and clarified butter (organic, grass-fed only)
- Coconut: Butter, fresh, flakes, and milk
- Nuts and nut butters: Almonds, Brazil nuts, cashews, chestnuts, hazelnuts, macadamia nuts, pecans, pistachios, and walnuts
- Oils: Macadamia oil, avocado oil, coconut oil, olive oil, and walnut oil
- Olives
- Seeds: Pumpkin, sesame, sunflower, and pine nuts
- Animal fats: From pastured-raised, grass-fed sources, such as tallow (beef fat), lamb fat, duck fat, and schmaltz (chicken fat)

When cooking with fats, you want them to be able to withstand high heat and remain stable.

If you're cooking at high temperatures, use the following oils:

- Coconut oil
- Butter/ghee
- Animal fats (beef, pork, and duck)

For very low heat cooking, use the following:

- Avocado oil
- Macadamia oil
- Olive oil

Stay away from industrial and seed oils. They're billed as naturally occurring, but they're not. They require a lot of processing and are prone to turning rancid. When they're rancid oils, they create inflammation in the body. Following is a list of fats and oils to avoid altogether:

- Margarine
- Vegetable shortening
- Trans fats
- Soybean oil
- Safflower oil
- Sunflower oil
- Partially hydrogenated oil
- Corn oil
- Canola oil
- Cottonseed oil
- Palm kernel oil
- Peanut oil

Don't fear fat!

Fat, including saturated fat, is essential to your health and, as it turns out, to building a lean, strong body. To access the fat stored in your body for energy, you need to consume fat in your meals.

Dietary fat is also crucial in helping your body absorb fat-soluble vitamins like A, S, E, and K. And honestly, a little fat makes food more palatable, so you feel more satisfied after eating. A diet that's too low in fat can lead to food cravings that compel you to overeat or make poor food choices. Additionally, when your body doesn't regularly receive high-quality fat in meals, it can retaliate with dry skin, hair loss, bruising, intolerance to cold, and in extreme cases, loss of menstruation.

Choose high-quality fats from the "Selecting fabulous fats for a nourishing kitchen" section to make your meals taste great while doing good things for your body.

Adding in kitchen staples for eating well

Outside from ideal choices of proteins, produce, and fats, you can amp up your menu with some healthy and tasty staples. These foods are instrumental in keeping you from going head first into the cereal bowl!

✔ Shredded coconut

✔ Coconut milk, almond milk, and flax milk (instead of dairy)

✔ Canned chilies

✔ Salsa

✔ Fish sauce (Red Boat brand is good)

✔ Hot sauce (gluten free)

✔ Mustard (gluten free)

✔ Vinegar: Red wine and apple cider

✔ Pickles

✔ Apple sauce

✔ Beef jerky (gluten and soy free)

✔ Artichoke hearts

✔ Nut butters (with no added sugar)

✔ Olives

✔ Dried unsweetened fruits (in moderation)

✔ Sun-dried tomatoes

✔ Nuts and seeds (due to the toxin level, peanuts are off the menu)

✔ Tomato sauce

✔ Arrowroot powder (substitute for flour and cornstarch)

✔ Coconut flour (instead of flour)

✔ Almond meal (instead of flour)

✔ Coconut aminos (instead of soy sauce)

✔ Broth: Chicken, beef, and vegetable

✔ Canned tomatoes, tomato paste, and tomato sauce

✔ Canned fish (in water): Tuna, salmon, and sardines

Because of the high mercury levels found in tuna, we suggest using a company, such as Vital Choice (www.vitalchoice.com), that uses a third party to test for heavy metals in smaller fish.

A great way to add a splash of flavor is to familiarize yourself with lots of herbs and spices. We cover superfood herbs and spices in Chapter 10. Experiment with as many as you can, or make a salt/herb blend. Use a ratio of 1:1 dried herbs to sea salt. Coarse Celtic sea salt works best.

Shopping for Healthy Foods

If you're ready to get started on your immune-boosting lifestyle but are at a loss as to where to get the healthiest foods, this section gives you some tips on making healthy shopping simple — and even fun.

Getting food straight from the farm

Community Supported Agriculture (CSA), farmers' markets, picking up farm fresh vegetables at your favorite farm, and online shopping are all ways you can purchase some of the freshest, high-quality food. You may even save some money compared to shopping at traditional grocery stores.

- **Farmers' market:** Find a farmers' market in your area and visit the local vendors. A *farmers' market* is where a community of farmers gets together on a weekly basis and sells their products. You can build relationships or talk about growing conditions, organic, and seasonal foods. At a farmers' market, you'll find great seasonal produce, and, often times, you can get great prices. In addition to produce, some of the farmers may sell eggs or other meats and poultry.

- **CSAs:** At a CSA, you pay a fee to the farm to buy into a share. You visit the farm once a week to get your share of produce from the current grow. Often, you can even pick your own produce at the farm, from whatever's in season, of course.

  CSAs are a great way to try new vegetables. You may have a week where you get some produce in your box that you've never had before. Because you've already paid for it and it's in your box, trying is easy!

  To find a CSA near you, check out these online sources: LocalHarvest (www.localharvest.org) or the Rodale Institute Farm Locator (www.rodaleinstitute.org/farm_locator).

- **Farm stands:** To get fresh produce on your own schedule, you can visit farm stands and pick things out yourself. The way this works is a farm has market hours when you can pick up your very fresh foods. Shopping at a farm stand is a great option because you get to pick exactly what you want, as opposed to a CSA, where it's decided for you every week. Inquire with local farms to find out whether they have farm stand hours.

✔ **Meat share:** Meat shares are a great way to save money while getting high-quality meat. A local farm may offer a meat club in which a supply of grass-fed, pasture-raised meat is for sale on a regular basis (this may include home delivery options), or you can go in on a *meat share* with friends or family, where you organize the purchase of a portion of or even an entire cow. Just make sure you have the extra freezer space to accommodate your share! Visit Eatwild (www.eatwild.com) for a directory of farms organized by state.

Most people have a more difficult time finding healthier meats than produce. If you can't get grass-fed, organic meats locally, here are some online sources:

✔ Gourmet Grassfed: www.gourmetgrassfedmeat.com

✔ U.S. Wellness Meats: www.grasslandbeef.com

✔ Rocky Mountain Organic Meats: www.rockymtncuts.com

✔ Lava Lake Lamb: www.lavalakelamb.com

Exploring traditional grocers and health food stores

Equipped with your list of healthy proteins, vegetables, and staple foods, you're ready to shop. You may be surprised what you can find at your local grocers. Many grocery stores are getting higher quality meats and eggs. Some conventional grocers stock grass-fed and pasture-raised meat, so it's definitely worth checking.

Because most areas have had an increased demand for organic produce, many stores are carrying at least some organic options for fruits and vegetables. If your local store doesn't stock what you're looking for, make a request; often, stores will make an effort to carry what their customers need.

Make sure you don't leave out buyers' clubs and large-scale retailers. They often carry healthy foods at a great price. At these stores, you can get many good finds and can stock your freezer or pantry.

Health food stores can be a great option, but don't assume anything just because it's a health food store. You still have to check the labels and stick to your immune-boosting plan. Go in with your shopping list so you won't get caught in the trap of buying a lot of "healthier" snacks and "healthier" treats. A cheese curl is still a cheese curl, no matter how you bag it!

You can, however, find great produce and pantry items, and some health food stores carry great protein options. You'll eventually find what you like to purchase and where.

Buying organic: Do's and don'ts

Buying locally and seasonally is always healthiest for your immune system. However, you don't always have to shell out the extra bucks for organic, thanks to the research by the Environmental Working Group (EWG). They rated foods based on their pesticide exposure. If the food has a lot of pesticides used in the growing process, they're considered the *Dirty Dozen,* and you should try to buy organic versions. If low pesticide exposure occurs, they're considered the *Clean 15,* and you can buy conventional versions. If your budget just won't allow you to buy organic, buy local and rinse your produce well before eating. Table 13-3 presents the Dirty Dozen and the Clean 15 for quick reference.

Table 13-3	The Dirty Dozen and the Clean 15
Dirty Dozen: Buy Organic	*Clean 15: Conventionally Grown Is Okay*
Apples	Asparagus
Bell peppers	Avocado
Blueberries	Cabbage
Celery	Domestic cantaloupe
Cucumbers	Corn (non-GMO)
Grapes	Eggplant
Lettuce	Grapefruit
Nectarines	Kiwi
Peaches	Mango
Potatoes	Mushrooms
Spinach	Onions
Strawberries	Pineapple
	Sweet peas
	Sweet potatoes
	Watermelon

Preparing Food the Right Way for Wellness

Many people are used to their food tasting good because of more traditional methods of cooking, like frying or breading or using grains, sugary carbohydrates, and other additives to flavor their foods. These methods and ingredients won't get you well, keep you well, or help you live a longer, stronger life.

You certainly don't have to be a gourmet chef to use healthy cooking techniques. Anyone can use these simple methods to prepare foods, which lock in high-octane flavor and provide deep nutrition. In this section, we explain some immune-boosting cooking methods that are simple and still preserve the natural nutrition in your foods.

No matter what method you use to cook your food, using spices and herbs is one of the best ways to add color, flavor, and aroma to your meals. Choose fresh herbs that are bright and aren't wilted. Always add them toward the end of cooking. If you're using dried herbs, you can add them to the earlier stages of cooking. Go ahead and experiment!

Baking

When you think of baking, you may think of traditional breads and other baked goods. Well, a whole other side to baking exists. Your immune-boosting health habits will redefine your thinking of baking. By using lean meats, seafood, poultry, vegetables, or even fruits in a pan or dish either uncovered or covered, you can bake wonderful, immune-boosting dishes The hot, dry air of your oven turns these foods into something special — without the extra calories or fat. You can use chicken or beef broth (try Pacific brand, which is MSG-free and flavorful) to keep your food moist. Also adding in sweet potatoes, carrots, and onions with water adds extra taste and moisture. The heat caramelizes the natural sugars, making for a delicious side dish.

When you bake muffins or other treats, using immune-boosting ingredients, you say goodbye to sugary carbohydrates and hello to grain-free almond flours, coconut meal, and other healthy ingredients.

Braising

When braising meats, first brown them on high heat to caramelize the outside and then slowly cook them in flavored liquid, like water or broth, to make the meat tender and lock in all its flavors. You can even use this liquid afterward for a flavorful, nutrient-rich sauce. You can braise meat in a covered pan in the oven or on the stovetop in a heavy pot with a tight-fitting lid. You can simmer the meat in water, or you can even add herbs, spices, and vegetables. Braising is a fantastic method to use for inexpensive, tougher cuts of meat, because you can turn them into tender meats just by this easy cooking method.

Sautéing and stir-frying

Sautéing is a great method for adding flavor to thinly sliced, uniformly sized meat and vegetables. With just a little fat and a skillet, you pan-cook meat and vegetables until they're browned. When the ingredients brown, this means they've caramelized, adding a burst of natural flavors to your dish. Simply by adding olive oil, some of your favorite seasonings, and herbs tossed in at the end, you can create a hearty, unbelievably tasty dish.

Roasting

Three words describe roasting: *Simple, healthy,* and *delicious.* Place chicken or beef roast in a pan, surrounding it with hearty vegetables, and put it in the oven for a few hours. The meat cooks in its natural juices, and you can simmer and strain the drippings in the bottom of the pan to create a sauce. Roasting is the perfect no-frills, super-nutritious way to prepare a meal for your family in a snap.

Slow cooking

Slow cooking may be the most perfect way of cooking on the planet. If you're busy and like warm, hearty meals, you'll love the magic of the slow cooker. You can make just about anything you can think of in a slow cooker while you're running around with kids, at work, or just relaxing. Meats and vegetables cook on low temperatures over longer periods of time than other cooking methods, so the meat gets tender and the flavors blend together, creating that slow cook magic.

Steaming

Steaming is as basic at it gets and is how you really get the nutrition locked in your vegetables. The steam holds the nutrients into the vegetables, brightening their color and making them inviting to eat. You can even flavor the liquid by adding seasonings to the water, which brings out even more flavor as they cook.

Poaching

To poach foods, slowly simmer ingredients in either water or a broth until they're cooked thoroughly and tender. The food retains its shape and texture with the benefit of not drying the food, leaving it tender and delicious. Poaching is a great way to cook fish so it's tender and flavorful.

Batch cooking

Batch cooking helps you organize your time so you always have healthy food and family staples on hand. Batch cooking also saves you time and money because you always know exactly what you need at the grocery store, which means you make fewer trips and you buy less food that you don't use or need.

Here's how it works: You devote one or two days a week to spend a little time in the kitchen preparing foods that you can use in cooking and that your family eats on a regular basis. Precook as many staple or convenience foods as you can. Prepare foods like hard-boiled eggs, cut and chop veggies, precook meats, make salads, and prepare dips or sauces, such as guacamole.

Schedule your batching days as a routine part of you week. When you do, your cooking become so much less of a chore — it may even be fun. After a couple of times, you get super quick, and it becomes no big deal.

The more access you have to real foods, the better you'll feel and the more you'll get done regardless of time crunches. You can organize your way into more time and a healthier immune-boosting life.

Skipping the grill

Grilling cooks food over direct heat by placing the foods on a grill rack above a bed of charcoal or gas-heated rocks. Although grilling is certainly a warm weather favorite and the center of many fun gatherings, go easy on grilling and don't make it your everyday cooking method. Here's why: When you grill food, the proteins are damaged and carcinogens are produced. Evidence shows that *heterocyclic amines* (HCAs) produced in meat when cooked at high temperature are carcinogenic. This risk is increased when the meat is cooked well done. When you add refined oils in marinades and directly on the grill, you can suppress the immune system and initiate cancer even more.

You can take action to minimize your exposure by using the following tips:

- ✔ **Don't use grilling as your go-to cooking method:** Incorporate other cooking methods mentioned in this section to your cooking repertoire.

- ✔ **Ditch the processed vegetable oils:** On marinades or directly on the grill, opt for saturated fats, which can withstand high heat without becoming rancid. Coconut oil or grass-fed butter are great options. (See the section "Selecting fabulous fats for a nourishing kitchen," earlier in this chapter.)

- ✔ **Veggie up:** When you eat grilled foods, pile on the vegetables. The anti-oxidants and the phenols in them soften the impact of the mutations caused by the grilled meats.

- ✔ **Don't overheat:** Keep meat away from direct heat or let juices fall on the heat source. Make sure you don't overcook or char the food, which greatly increases the carcinogens.

Chapter 14

Breakfasts to Start Your Day in a Healthy Way

. . . .

In This Chapter

▶ Clearing the breakfast confusion and getting some healthy ideas — finally!

▶ Discovering how *easy* breakfast options can be

. . . .

> **Recipes in This Chapter**
>
> ↻ Apple and Cabbage Sauté with Walnuts
> ▶ Egg Crumble with Sausage and Tomato
> ▶ Primal Breakfast Casserole
> ▶ Omelet Muffins
> ↻ Spinach-Filled Deviled Eggs
>
>

*T*he question we're asked more than any other in our practices is, "What should I have for breakfast?" Addressing this concern is important to us, and we know it's vital to you! Clear the breakfast confusion and have a ball with these delicious, easy ways to start your day. These breakfasts really are the breakfasts of champions.

How you begin your day creates the tone for the entire day, so start your day on the right track by deciding on breakfast *the night before*. Success happens when opportunity and preparation meet.

Thinking beyond Traditional Breakfast Foods

Converting patients to a healthier lifestyle almost always brings on the concern, "What in the world can I eat for breakfast?" Food marketers try to convince people that their choices include cereal, granola, oatmeal, creamy wheat cereal, breakfast bars, bagels, grits, or toast and jelly topped off with juice. In fact, these breakfast foods are so deeply ingrained in society that thinking beyond traditional breakfast foods can be difficult; however, if

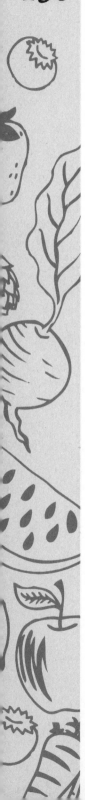

you want to have energy, perform better, and boost immunity, you have to. Don't worry; we show you how. The breakfasts we recommend are made with ingredients low in sugar and high in vitamins and minerals. Ingredients like eggs, nitrite- and hormone- free sausage, apples, cabbage, and spinach or other veggies can create tasty, immune-boosting breakfasts. Using these ingredients may take a little more preparation than a bowl of cereal, but if you try these immune-boosting breakfasts for 30 days, you'll look and feel so much better that the extra time will be so worth it!

Apple and Cabbage Sauté with Walnuts

Prep time: 5 min • **Cook time:** 5 min • **Yield:** 2 servings

Ingredients	*Directions*
1 red apple	*1* Core the apple by cutting it in half and removing the core from each half, using a melon baller or a spoon. Thinly slice, keeping the peel intact.
1 tablespoon coconut oil	
1 cup thinly sliced cabbage (green or Napa)	*2* Heat the coconut oil in a medium saucepan. Add the sliced apple, cabbage, and onion to the oil, and sauté until the cabbage is wilted and the apple is slightly browned.
¼ medium onion, thinly sliced	
½ cup chopped walnuts	
	3 Top with chopped walnuts and serve.

Per serving: Calories 330 (From Fat 243); Fat 27g (Saturated 8g); Cholesterol 0mg; Sodium 8mg; Carbohydrate 18g (Dietary Fiber 1g); Protein 6g.

Note: Like kale, cabbage is a cruciferous vegetable, which is known to reduce your risk of cancer and inflammation. What a way to start the day!

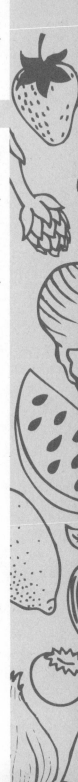

Egg Crumble with Sausage and Tomato

Prep time: 30 min • **Cook time:** 12 min • **Yield:** 2 servings

Ingredients	Directions
4 eggs	*1* Place the eggs in a pot and cover with cold water. Bring to a gentle boil, and then turn off heat and cover pot with lid. Let eggs sit for 10 to 12 minutes.
2 chicken or turkey sausage links (nitrite-, gluten-, and hormone-free), sliced	*2* Transfer the eggs to a separate bowl filled with ice water until the eggs are completely cooled, about 10 minutes. Roll each egg to crack the shell, and peel the eggs. Dice the eggs and set aside in a medium bowl.
1 tomato, diced	
Juice from 1 lemon	
Celtic sea salt to taste	*3* Heat a small skillet over medium heat. Sear sausages on each side until browned.
Ground black pepper to taste	
	4 Add enough water to cook sausage and continue until cooked through and water has evaporated; remove sausages.
	5 To the hard-boiled eggs, add the tomato, lemon juice, sliced sausage links, and salt and pepper to taste. Mix well.
	6 You can spoon the mixture over ½ cup sautéed or raw spinach per serving or just scoop the mixture on a plate and enjoy as is.

Per serving: Calories 202 (From Fat 108); Fat 12g (Saturated 4g); Cholesterol 390mg; Sodium 480mg; Carbohydrate 5g (Dietary Fiber 1g); Protein 18g.

Tip: Preparing the eggs and sausage ahead of time makes your morning a breeze! Simply reheat the sausage before adding it to the egg mixture in Step 5, and this dish will quickly become one of your morning favorites.

Primal Breakfast Casserole

Prep time: 10 min • **Cook time:** 30–40 min • **Yield:** 4 servings

Ingredients	Directions
1 pound ground breakfast sausage or other ground meat	**1** Preheat the oven to 375 degrees and grease an 8-x-8-inch baking pan with grass-fed butter.
4 eggs	**2** In a large skillet, sauté the sausage over medium-high heat, breaking it into small pieces with a spoon or spatula, until almost cooked through.
3 turnips, peeled and grated (a food processor works well for this)	**3** In a large bowl, beat the eggs. Add the grated turnip, scallions, and cooked sausage, and stir to combine.
3 scallions, chopped	**4** Pour the egg mixture into the greased baking pan. Bake for 30 to 40 minutes, until the egg is set. Let cool for 15 minutes before serving.

Per serving: Calories 274 (From Fat 126); Fat 14g (Saturated 4g); Cholesterol 259mg; Sodium 841mg; Carbohydrate 7g (Dietary Fiber 2g); Protein 27g.

Tip: You can easily double this recipe for a larger crowd and use a 9-x-13-inch pan.

Tip: To make your mornings easier, prepare the casserole ahead of time, cover the pan with foil, and freeze it; the dish can go directly from the freezer to the oven.

Note: Make sure to keep boosting your immunity by using only gluten-free, free-range sausage. If you can't, substitute for another healthier meat.

Recipe courtesy Mark Sisson, www.marksdailyapple.com

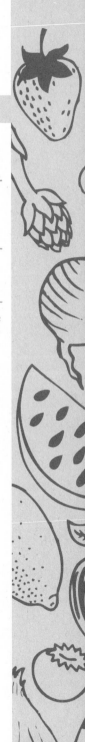

Omelet Muffins

Prep time: 10 min • **Cook time:** 18–20 min • **Yield:** 6 servings

Ingredients	*Directions*
½ **cup ground breakfast sausage**	*1* Preheat the oven to 350 degrees. Generously grease 6 muffin tin cups with grass-fed butter or coconut oil.
6 eggs	
⅛ **cup water**	*2* In a medium skillet, sauté the sausage over medium-high heat, breaking it into small pieces with a spoon or a spatula, until almost cooked through.
½ **cup diced mixed vegetables**	
¼ **teaspoon Celtic sea salt**	*3* In a large bowl, beat the eggs with the water.
⅛ **teaspoon ground black pepper**	*4* In a separate bowl, mix the meat, vegetables, salt, and pepper, and stir to combine. Spoon or scoop into the muffin cups.
	5 Pour the egg over the top of the meat and vegetable mixture in each muffin cup.
	6 Bake for 18 to 20 minutes or until a knife inserted into the center of a muffin comes out almost clean. (The omelets will cook for a minute or two after removed from the oven.)
	7 Remove the omelets from the muffin cups and serve, or cool and store for another day.

Per serving: Calories 95 (From Fat 54); Fat 6g (Saturated 2g); Cholesterol 192mg; Sodium 232mg; Carbohydrate 2g (Dietary Fiber 1g); Protein 8g.

Vary It! Make a Mexican Omelet Muffin by adding ¼ cup diced onions and slightly drained salsa to the eggs. Or replace the ground breakfast sausage with a different meat; just be sure to cook it completely before mixing it with the other ingredients. You can also add Olive Oil Mayo (see recipe in Chapter 17) for a creamier, richer taste.

Recipe courtesy Mark Sisson, www.marksdailyapple.com

Spinach-Filled Deviled Eggs

Prep time: 15 min • **Cook time:** 12min • **Yield:** 12 servings

Ingredients	Directions
12 eggs **One 10-ounce package frozen chopped spinach** **¼ cup Olive Oil Mayo (see recipe in Chapter 17)** **2 tablespoons olive oil** **½ teaspoon garlic powder** **Celt sea salt and ground black pepper to taste**	*1* Place the 12 eggs in a large pot and cover with cold water. Bring to a gentle boil, and then turn off heat and cover pot with lid. Let eggs sit for 12 to 15 minutes.
	2 Drain the water from the pot and transfer eggs into a separate bowl filled with ice water until the eggs are completely cooled. Roll each egg to crack the shell, and peel the eggs.
	3 Defrost the spinach in the refrigerator before using or gently defrost in the microwave according to the package directions. Drain and squeeze dry.
	4 Slice each egg in half and remove yolks, placing them in a large bowl.
	5 To the egg yolks, add the spinach, mayo, oil, and garlic powder. Add salt and pepper to taste, and mix well to combine.
	6 Fill each egg white half with yolk mixture. Cover with plastic wrap and refrigerate before serving.

Per serving: Calories 125 (From Fat 90); Fat 10g (Saturated 2g); Cholesterol 191mg; Sodium 106mg; Carbohydrate 1g (Dietary Fiber 1g); Protein 7g.

Tip: Incorporating spinach into your meals provides great immune-boosting qualities. Loaded with vitamins A and C, iron, and folate, you can't go wrong with this nutrient-dense food!

Recipe courtesy Mark Sisson, www.marksdailyapple.com

Chapter 15

Lunches for a Midday Energy Burst

- -

In This Chapter

▶ Knowing the keys to making healthy lunches

▶ Recharging with energy-boosting meals

- -

Have you ever experienced that midday slump when you feel like you could fall asleep standing up? A major cause of your drop in energy is that you aren't eating the right foods at lunchtime. When you eat energy-boosting foods, you won't even feel a dip in your day!

In this chapter, we share recipes that pack three punches: They're healthy, delicious, and easy. These energy-producing meals help you create a healthy, healing internal environment that's essential for good immunity and good health. Try some of these lunch options, and you won't feel like you need a daily afternoon coffee run!

Saying Goodbye to the Midday Slump

The most important part of lunchtime is to eat foods that balance your blood sugar to carry you through the day. When you eat an immune-boosting combination of good protein, healthy fats, and non-starchy carbohydrates, you avoid the afternoon slump. You tame the craving for midday sugar when you give yourself the right midday fuel. You can also say goodbye to headaches, frequent illnesses, sluggishness, and weight gain.

The immune-boosting recipes in this chapter are satisfying and energizing. When you use ingredients such as peppers, tomatoes, avocados, mushrooms, onions, garlic, healthy spices, lean proteins, and healthy fats — and even chocolate — it's got to be good! These ingredients are truly immune-boosting superfoods.

But there's more: With these superfood lunches, you provide your body with deep nutrition and, before long, you start craving healthier foods.

Chicken Club Wrap

Prep time: 5 min • **Yield:** 2 servings (4 wraps)

Ingredients	*Directions*
4 large lettuce leaves	*1* Wash and pat dry the lettuce leaves.
1 cup chopped cooked chicken	*2* In the center of each leaf, layer the chicken, red pepper, tomato, and avocado slices.
½ cup sliced red pepper	
1 plum tomato, sliced	*3* Top with a dab of mayo.
½ avocado, sliced	
1 tablespoon Olive Oil Mayo (see recipe in Chapter 17)	

Per serving: Calories 396 (From Fat 189); Fat 21g (Saturated 4g); Cholesterol 69mg; Sodium 294mg; Carbohydrate 28g; Dietary Fiber 13g; Protein 31g.

Vary It! Crumble cooked nitrite-free, gluten-free bacon on top to add another layer of flavor and more protein to your wraps.

Recipe courtesy Mark Sisson, www.marksdailyapple.com

Stuffed Bell Peppers

Prep time: 15 min • **Cook time:** 30–40 min • **Yield:** 6 servings

Ingredients	Directions
6 firm red or yellow bell peppers	**1** Preheat the oven to 350 degrees.
1 small eggplant	**2** Cut the tops off the peppers, scoop out the seeds and ribs, and discard. Set the hulled peppers in a baking dish that allows each pepper to fit snugly and remain upright without too much crowding. If needed, shave off a little from the bottom of each pepper so it stands up in the dish.
20 Crimini mushrooms	
1 medium onion	
3 cloves garlic	
½ pound ground beef	**3** Chop the eggplant, mushrooms, and onion, and mince the garlic. Set aside.
One 15-ounce can tomato sauce	
3 teaspoons olive oil	**4** In a large skillet over medium heat, brown the ground beef; drain to remove the fat, and remove the beef to a bowl.
1 tablespoon chopped fresh oregano (or ½ teaspoon dried oregano)	
Celtic sea salt to taste	**5** In the same skillet, sauté the reserved vegetables with the olive oil until softened. Mix in the beef and sauce. Add oregano and salt and pepper to taste.
Ground black pepper to taste	
	6 Fill each pepper with the beef and vegetable mixture and replace it upright in the baking dish.
	7 Bake peppers for 30 to 40 minutes and serve.

Per serving: Calories 241 (From Fat 126); Fat 14g (Saturated 6g); Cholesterol 29mg; Sodium 407mg; Carbohydrate 20g; Dietary Fiber 7g; Protein 10.

Tip: Wrap any leftover peppers individually and place them in the fridge. You can reheat them in the oven for 10 to 15 minutes at 350 degrees, or in the microwave for 1 minute (keeping in mind microwave times vary) for a quick and delicious lunch.

Tip: Batch cooking and preparing staple foods a couple of times a week allows you to whip up dishes in minutes. Avoiding the "nothing to eat" syndrome and always having something healthy on the ready is the key to healthy eating. These peppers fit the bill beautifully! Even if you just prepare the sauté ahead of time while you're cooking other foods, it makes your life easier.

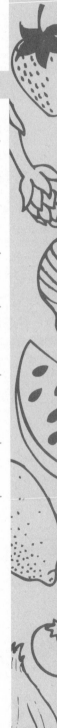

Butter Lettuce Wraps

Prep time: 10 min • **Yield:** 12–14 wraps

Ingredients	Directions
1 head butter lettuce	*1* Carefully peel and separate the leaves of the butter lettuce. Soak them in cold water to rinse (doing so helps them remain crisp) and let them dry.
2 boneless chicken breasts, cooked and shredded or diced	
2 celery stalks, diced	*2* In a medium bowl, combine the chicken, celery, cilantro, and basil and mix. Then add the olive oil and lemon juice and mix again. Finally, add the avocado, and gently mix one last time.
¼ cup chopped fresh cilantro	
⅓ cup chopped fresh basil	
2 tablespoons olive oil	
2 tablespoons lemon juice	*3* Scoop the mixture into the butter lettuce and enjoy!
1 avocado, diced	

Per serving: Calories 107 (From Fat 63); Fat 7g (Saturated 1g); Cholesterol 28mg; Sodium 31mg; Carbohydrate 2g; Dietary Fiber 1g; Protein 10.

Tip: You can roll up the lettuce, tucking in the ends as you go and making sure the filling doesn't spill out. These wraps hold for several hours in the refrigerator. Place them in a flat container or wrap them tightly in parchment paper so they don't unravel.

Vary It! You can change the taste up a bit by using salsa in the mixture or as a dipping sauce.

Chocolate Chili

Prep time: 20 min • **Cook time:** 2–3 hr • **Yield:** 8 servings

Ingredients

2 tablespoons coconut oil

2 medium onions, diced (about 2 cups)

4 cloves garlic, minced (about 4 teaspoons)

2 pounds ground beef

1 teaspoon dried oregano

2 tablespoons chili powder

2 tablespoons ground cumin

1½ tablespoons unsweetened cocoa powder

1 teaspoon ground allspice

1 teaspoon Celtic sea salt

One 6-ounce can tomato paste

One 14.5-ounce can fire-roasted, chopped tomatoes

One 14.5-ounce can beef broth

1 cup water

Directions

1 Heat a large, deep pot over medium-high heat, and add the coconut oil. When the oil is melted, add onions and, stirring with a wooden spoon, cook until they're translucent, about 7 minutes.

2 Add the garlic and, as soon as it's fragrant (about 30 seconds), crumble the ground beef into the pan with your hands, mixing with the wooden spoon to combine. Continue to cook the meat, stirring often, until it's no longer pink.

3 In a small bowl, crush the oregano between your palms to release its flavor. Add the chili powder, cumin, cocoa powder, allspice, and salt. Mix with a fork and then stir into the ground beef. Add tomato paste and stir until combined, about 2 minutes.

4 Add the tomatoes with their juice, beef broth, and water to the pot. Stir well. Bring to a boil, and then reduce the heat and simmer uncovered for at least 2 hours.

Per serving: Calories 472 (From Fat 342); Fat 38g (Saturated 16g); Cholesterol 88mg; Sodium 1056mg; Carbohydrate 14g; Dietary Fiber 3g; Protein 20.

Recipe courtesy Well Fed: Paleo Recipes For People Who Love To Eat *by Melissa Joulwan* (www.theclothesmakethegirl.com)

Tex-Mex Scotch Eggs

Prep time: 15 min • **Cook time:** 30 min • **Yield:** 8 servings

Ingredients	Directions
2 pounds ground beef	**1** Preheat the oven to 375 degrees. Cover a baking sheet with parchment paper.
2 teaspoons Celtic sea salt	
1 teaspoon ground black pepper	**2** Place the ground beef in a large mixing bowl. Add salt, black pepper, cumin, chili powder, parsley, and garlic. Knead with your hands until well mixed.
1 tablespoon ground cumin	
1 tablespoon chili powder	
1 tablespoon minced fresh parsley	**3** Divide the beef mixture into 8 equal servings. Roll each piece into a ball, and flatten it into a pancake shape. Wrap the meat around a hard-boiled egg, rolling it between your palms until the egg is evenly covered.
2 cloves garlic, minced (about 2 teaspoons)	
8 eggs, hard-boiled and peeled	**4** In a shallow bowl, beat the raw eggs. Place the pork rinds (if desired) in a food processor and process until they resemble bread crumbs; pour them onto a plate or in a shallow bowl. Gently roll each meat-wrapped egg in pork rind crumbs (you want just a thin dusting). Then roll each egg in the raw egg and roll a second time in the crushed pork rinds to evenly coat. If you choose to skip the pork rinds, just roll each egg in the raw egg. Place on the baking sheet.
2 eggs, raw	
One 2-ounce bag fried pork rinds (optional)	
	5 Bake for 25 minutes; then increase the temperature to 400 degrees and bake an additional 5 to 10 minutes, until the eggs are golden brown and crisp.

Per serving: Calories 518 (From Fat 387); Fat 43g (Saturated 16g); Cholesterol 328mg; Sodium 884mg; Carbohydrate 2g; Dietary Fiber 1g; Protein 29.

Recipe courtesy Well Fed: Paleo Recipes For People Who Love To Eat *by Melissa Joulwan (*www.the clothesmakethegirl.com*)*

Chapter 16

Dinners and Side Dishes to Strengthen Your System

- -

In This Chapter

▶ Fitting healthy family dinners into a busy life

▶ Checking out tasty recipes that will have you saying "wow!"

- -

*W*e understand that your dinners need to fit into a busy family life. The dinner and side dish recipes in this chapter are well balanced and highly nutritious and help strengthen your body for robust immunity. They have the healthiest ingredients, which are big on flavor and high in nutrients, and help all the functions of your body work at their best! Both tasty and easy, you'll find these recipes to be a great addition to your weekly rotation schedule. We also get you going with some great slow cooker recipes for the ultimate in convenience and health. Talk about a win-win!

In this chapter, we present some of our favorite dinner and side dish recipes to get you in the healthy groove! No matter how crazy your schedule is, you'll have time for these winning dishes.

Before you grab your seafood for these recipes, make sure it comes from a clean source that's low in heavy metals and contaminants. A great resource is the Monterey Bay Aquarium Seafood Watch; check out www.montereybay aquarium.org/cr/SeafoodWatch/web/sfw_search.aspx?s=shrimp. Also, be sure to eat shrimp and shellfish in moderation.

Making Time for Healthy Family Meals

Try to make time for family meals. Our goal in selecting the dishes in this chapter is to provide simple recipes that you can squeeze into your busy life, where your whole family can sit down and eat at the same time. Eating together as a family helps your family values stay intact. And research shows that family meals lead to everyone eating healthier meals, fewer cases of childhood obesity, and even improvement in school grades.

Pull out the calendar, and pick a couple of non-optional family dinner nights a week. Scheduling family dinners creates a rhythm, or pattern, that helps your family dynamics. Everyone knows what to expect, and your family functions smoother as a result.

If you're making meals for only one or two people, you can make the dinners and side dishes for the serving sizes listed in the recipes in this chapter and put leftovers aside for another meal, or freeze them. One of the best strategies for implementing a healthy diet long term is to have healthy food on the ready. When you're hungry and nothing is available, you know what happens! Avoid that trap by having leftovers on hand.

Easy Skillet Shrimp and Kale

Prep time: 10 min • **Cook time:** 10 min • **Yield:** 5 servings

Ingredients	*Directions*
4 tablespoons coconut oil, divided 1 bunch kale, stems removed	*1* In a large skillet, heat 2 tablespoons of coconut oil, and sauté the kale for about 3 or 4 minutes. Remove from the skillet and set aside.
¼ teaspoon fresh grated ginger 2 tablespoons cilantro, chopped 1 medium red onion, sliced 1 red bell pepper, sliced into long strips	*2* In the same skillet, heat the other 2 tablespoons of coconut oil and sauté the ginger, cilantro, red onion, and red bell pepper for 2 minutes.
2 pounds shrimp, peeled and deveined Celtic sea salt and ground black pepper to taste	*3* Add the shrimp, salt, and pepper and cook until the shrimp turns pink, about 2 minutes in a hot pan and 3 minutes if the pan isn't screaming hot. Finish with lemon juice.
Juice of 1 lemon	*4* Serve the shrimp on a bed of the sautéed kale.

Per serving: Calories 261 (From Fat 117); Fat 13g (Saturated 10g); Cholesterol 382mg; Sodium 1046mg; Carbohydrate 10g; Dietary Fiber 2g; Protein 27.

Vary It! If you're not real keen on the taste of coconut, replace the coconut oil with macadamia oil — another immune-boosting oil!

Tip: Two pounds of shrimp is a lot! You can reduce the recipe down to 1 pound, but using 2 pounds gives you a great opportunity to create leftovers, and leftovers = tomorrow's lunch!

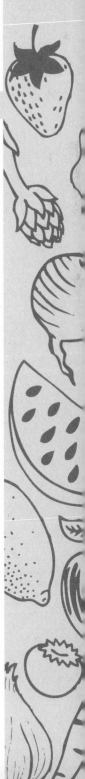

Grilled Spiced Halibut

Prep time: 10 min • **Cook time:** 8 min • **Yield:** 4 servings

Ingredients	Directions
Four 8-ounce halibut fillets	**1** Pat the fish fillets so they're dry.
1¼ teaspoons Celtic sea salt	**2** Heat the grill (either gas or charcoal) to medium heat.
½ teaspoon cayenne pepper	
¼ teaspoon turmeric	**3** In a small bowl, mix all the ingredients except the oil. Then add enough coconut oil to make into a paste (typically, it takes about 2 tablespoons).
1 teaspoon fennel	
1 teaspoon mustard seeds	
1 small onion, finely diced	**4** Place the halibut on a large sheet of tin foil. Fold the sides up to create a "shelf" so nothing can drip off the sides.
3 garlic cloves, minced or pushed through a garlic press	
2 teaspoons ground cumin	**5** Rub the pasty mixture on top of the halibut and place the tin foil on the rack of the grill. Cover loosely with another piece of foil, and close the grill.
¼ teaspoon garam masala	
2 tablespoons coconut oil	
	6 Cook for about 10 minutes; however, because all grills cook differently, and thicker cuts of fish cook differently than thinner cuts, keep your eye on the halibut while cooking so it doesn't overcook.

Per serving: Calories 293 (From Fat 99); Fat 11g (Saturated 7g); Cholesterol 111mg; Sodium 238mg; Carbohydrate 5g; Dietary Fiber 1g; Protein 43.

Note: With this dish, you get so many of the healing spices in one pop! Garam masala is a blend of Indian spices usually used in a powdered form. They're warming, healing, and nutritious spices that not only add a zing but also help you feel grounded and keep you feeling warm on those cold winter days.

Stuffed Spicy Eggplant

Prep time: 15 min • **Cook time:** 15 min • **Yield:** 4 servings

Ingredients	*Directions*
2 large eggplants	*1* Preheat the oven to 400 degrees. Wash the eggplants and cut in half lengthwise. Carve out the pulp, and set aside so you're left with a scooped shell that's about ½-inch thick.
5 tablespoons coconut or macadamia nut oil	
1 onion, chopped	
2 garlic cloves, minced	*2* Chop the reserved eggplant pulp coarsely and set aside.
One 14.5-ounce can diced tomatoes, drained	*3* In a large skillet, heat half of the coconut or macadamia nut oil. Place the eggplant shells cut side down and cook for about 5 minutes.
½ teaspoon dried thyme	
½ teaspoon ground cayenne pepper	*4* With tongs, transfer eggplant shells to a shallow oven-proof dish.
Celtic sea salt and ground black pepper to taste	*5* Add remaining oil to skillet and sauté onion and garlic for 2 minutes over medium heat.
8 ounces cooked ground beef or bison	*6* Add eggplant pulp, tomatoes, thyme, cayenne pepper, and salt and pepper to taste and cook over medium heat until the majority of the moisture evaporates and becomes a stew-like mixture.
¼ cup almond flour	
2 tablespoons fresh chopped parsley	*7* Remove from heat and mix in cooked meat.
	8 Stuff the eggplant shells with the stew-like mixture, top with almond flour (a stand-in for bread crumbs), and bake for 15 minutes. Remove from the oven and top with parsley.

Per serving: Calories 415 (From Fat 270); Fat 30g (Saturated 19g); Cholesterol 40mg; Sodium 204mg; Carbohydrate 26g; Dietary Fiber 12g; Protein 16.

Tip: When choosing eggplant, check the base to determine whether it's male or female (not in the biological sense). "Male" eggplants have a shallow and round indentation on the base, while "female" eggplants have a deep groove or dash. The male eggplant has fewer seeds and is therefore less bitter than the female version, making it more desirable.

Recipe courtesy Mark Sisson, www.marksdailyapple.com

Slow Cooker Italian Gravy

Prep time: 15 min • **Cook time:** 6–8 hr • **Yield:** 8 servings

Ingredients	Directions
2 tablespoons olive oil	**1** Preheat the slow cooker on low.
2 medium onions, chopped	
2 large garlic cloves, minced or pushed through garlic press	**2** In a large skillet, heat the olive oil and sauté the onions, garlic, and oregano until the onions are soft but not browned. Transfer to the slow cooker.
2 tablespoons dried oregano	
One 28-ounce can whole peeled tomatoes with juice	**3** Stir into the slow cooker the whole peeled tomatoes and the crushed tomatoes. Nestle the pork ribs, flank steak, and sausage into the slow cooker.
Two 28-ounce cans organic crushed tomatoes	
1½ pounds pork ribs (bone in)	**4** Cover and cook on low for 6 to 8 hours, until meat is tender.
1½ pounds flank steak	
1 pound Italian sausage, casing removed	**5** Remove the pork, flank steak, and sausage onto cutting board. After slightly cooled, shred pork and flank steak into bite-sized pieces. Slice sausage into ½-inch rounds.
3 tablespoons fresh basil, minced	
Celtic sea salt and ground black pepper to taste	**6** Using a large spoon, remove the fat from the surface of the sauce. Then stir the meat back into the sauce and let sit for about 5 minutes.
	7 Just before serving, add in basil and season with salt and pepper to taste.

Per serving: Calories 742 (From Fat 441); Fat 49g (Saturated 18g); Cholesterol 163mg; Sodium 1173mg; Carbohydrate 21g; Dietary Fiber 6g; Protein 52g.

Tip: This sauce is absolutely fabulous on top of a baked Portobello mushroom!

Easy Slow Cooker Roasted Chicken

Prep time: 15 min • **Cook time:** 4–5 hr • **Yield:** 6 servings

Ingredients	*Directions*
1 tablespoon extra-virgin olive oil	*1* Preheat the slow cooker on high. Add olive oil to the bottom of the slow cooker.
One 4-pound roasting chicken	
1 large garlic clove, minced	*2* Using a sharp knife, cut small slits into the breasts and thighs of a chicken and insert the minced garlic.
Celtic sea salt and ground black pepper to taste	
2 tablespoons grass-fed butter	*3* Season the chicken with the salt, pepper, and parsley.
3 tablespoons chopped parsley	
	4 Heat the butter in a large skillet and brown chicken well on all sides. Transfer the chicken to the slow cooker.
	5 Cook on high for 4 to 5 hours.
	6 Remove from slow cooker, and let sit for 10 minutes before carving.

Per serving: Calories 708 (From Fat 486); Fat 54g (Saturated 16g); Cholesterol 230mg; Sodium 207mg; Carbohydrate 0g; Dietary Fiber 0g; Protein 52.

Vary It! This meal is a great addition to your regular rotation. Steam up a quick vegetable when you come home, and you have a winning, immune-boosting meal!

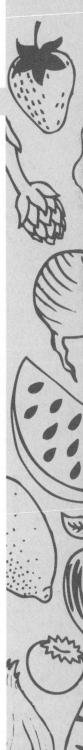

Moroccan Salmon

Prep time: 35 min • **Cook time:** 7 min • **Yield:** 6 servings

Ingredients	*Directions*
1 tablespoon coconut oil, melted	**1** In a small bowl, mix together the oil, orange juice, ginger, cumin, coriander, paprika, salt, and cayenne pepper to form a paste the consistency of thick salad dressing.
1 tablespoon fresh orange juice	
1½ teaspoons dried ginger	**2** Place the salmon in a glass dish, massage the marinade over the salmon, and then cover and refrigerate for 30 minutes.
1½ teaspoons ground cumin	
1½ teaspoons ground coriander	**3** Preheat a gas grill on high with the lid closed for about 10 minutes.
½ teaspoon paprika	
1½ teaspoons Celtic sea salt	**4** Place the salmon skin-side down on the grill, close the lid, and cook for about 3 minutes (the skin should be a little blackened and starting to separate from the pink flesh). Flip the salmon, close the lid, and cook another 3 minutes.
¼ teaspoon ground cayenne pepper	
1½ to 2 pounds wild Alaskan salmon fillets	
	5 Remove from the grill and cut into serving pieces.

Per serving: Calories 340 (From Fat 207); Fat 23g (Saturated 7g); Cholesterol 83mg; Sodium 408mg; Carbohydrate 1g; Dietary Fiber 0g; Protein 31.

Recipe courtesy Well Fed: Paleo Recipes for People Who Love to Eat *by Melissa Joulwan (*www.theclothesmakethegirl.com*)*

Ginger-Lime Grilled Shrimp

Prep time: 25 min • **Cook time:** 6 min • **Yield:** 4 servings

Ingredients	Directions
Juice of 1 lime (about 2 tablespoons)	*1* In a small bowl, squeeze lime to extract the juice, and then add the red pepper flakes, garlic, ginger, salt, black pepper, and cilantro. Mix well with a fork, and then drizzle in the oil, stirring constantly.
¼ teaspoon crushed red pepper flakes	
3 garlic cloves, minced (about 1 tablespoon)	*2* With a small, sharp knife, pierce the back of the shrimp at the head end and carefully cut along the back toward the tail; remove the dark vein that this cut exposes. Rinse in running water and then pat dry.
2 teaspoons freshly grated ginger (about a 2-inch piece)	
¼ teaspoon Celtic sea salt	*3* Place the shrimp in a medium bowl and mix with the marinade. Cover tightly and refrigerate for 20 minutes.
¼ teaspoon ground black pepper	
2 tablespoons fresh cilantro, minced (about 1 tablespoon)	*4* Preheat a gas grill on high heat with the lid closed, about 10 minutes.
1 tablespoon extra-virgin olive oil	
1 to 2 pounds large shrimp	*5* Thread the shrimp on skewers, leaving a little room between them so they don't steam. Grill 2 to 3 minutes per side with the lid closed until cooked through and firm.

Per serving: Calories 199 (From Fat 54); Fat 6g (Saturated 1g); Cholesterol 286mg; Sodium 1363mg; Carbohydrate 4g; Dietary Fiber 0g; Protein 31.

Recipe courtesy Well Fed: Paleo Recipes for People Who Love to Eat *by Melissa Joulwan (*www. theclothesmakethegirl.com*)*

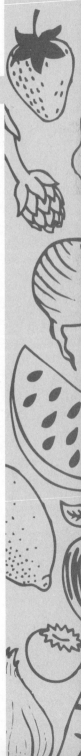

Meatza Pie

Prep time: 15 min • **Cook time:** 30 min • **Yield:** 4 servings

Ingredients	*Directions*
1 pound ground beef	*1* Preheat the oven to 400 degrees. Mix the ground beef and oregano until combined.
2 teaspoons dried oregano	
1 teaspoon olive oil	*2* Divide the meat in half, roll into a ball, and press evenly into an 8- or 9-inch round pie pan. Cover only the bottom of the pan and smooth the meat with damp hands until it's an even thickness. Repeat with the remaining meat and another 8- or 9- inch pie pan to make the second crust.
1 garlic clove, minced (about 1 teaspoon)	
1 teaspoon Italian herb blend	
6 ounces tomato paste	
¼ cup water	*3* Bake for 10 to 15 minutes, until the meat is cooked through and the edges are brown. Leaving the oven on, remove the meat crusts from the oven, drain off any excess fat, and allow to cool in the pan.
¼ cup steamed broccoli florets	
¼ cup steamed red bell pepper strips	
10 black olives, pitted and sliced	*4* Heat a small saucepan over low heat; add the olive oil, garlic, and Italian herb blend, stirring with a wooden spoon until fragrant, about 20 seconds.
Handful of fresh baby spinach leaves	
	5 Add the tomato paste and stir until combined, and then stir in the water. Bring to a boil and reduce heat to simmer for 5 minutes, until thickened.
	6 Spread about ¼ cup sauce on each meat crust, leaving a ½-inch border around the edges. Arrange the vegetables on top, pressing them gently into the sauce. Bake for 10 to 15 minutes, until hot and browned to your liking.

Per serving: Calories 443 (From Fat 333); Fat 37g (Saturated 13g); Cholesterol 88mg; Sodium 500mg; Carbohydrate 11g; Dietary Fiber 3g; Protein 19.

Recipe courtesy Well Fed: Paleo Recipes for People Who Love to Eat *by Melissa Joulwan (*www.theclothesmakethegirl.com*)*

Mashed Cauliflower

Prep time: 5 min • **Cook time:** 5 min • **Yield:** 4 servings

Ingredients	*Directions*
2 garlic cloves **One 16-ounce bag frozen cauliflower florets** **1½ tablespoons coconut oil** **½ cup coconut milk** **2 teaspoons dried thyme** **Celtic sea salt and ground black pepper to taste**	*1* Peel the garlic and cook along with the cauliflower, following the package directions. Transfer the cauliflower and garlic to a food processor or blender and purée, scraping down the sides in between pulses as needed. *2* In a microwave-safe bowl or small saucepan, heat the coconut oil, coconut milk, thyme, salt, and pepper for about 1 minute. *3* Add the coconut milk mixture to the puréed cauliflower and process about 10 seconds. Taste and adjust seasonings.

Per serving: Calories 145 (From Fat 117); Fat 13g (Saturated 11g); Cholesterol 0mg; Sodium x39mg; Carbohydrate 8g; Dietary Fiber 3g; Protein 3.

Note: You can make this recipe with fresh cauliflower, but frozen packs the same nutritional punch and reaches a creamy texture faster and easier than fresh.

Vary It! Try substituting parsley or chives for the dried thyme. You may also use chicken broth in place of the coconut milk.

Recipe courtesy Well Fed: Paleo Recipes for People Who Love to Eat *by Melissa Joulwan (*www. theclothesmakethegirl.com*)*

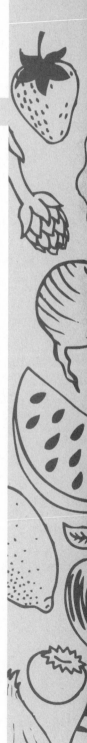

Greek Broccoli

Prep time: 10 min • **Cook time:** 15 min • **Yield:** 4 servings

Ingredients	*Directions*
½ cup water	*1* In a large sauté pan, bring the water to a boil over high heat. Add the broccoli, cover with a tight-fitting lid, and steam the broccoli until tender, about 4 to 5 minutes.
1 pound fresh broccoli, broken into florets	
2 tablespoons extra-virgin olive oil	*2* Drain the broccoli in a colander and rinse with cold water to stop the cooking process.
1 medium onion, diced (about 1 cup)	
3 garlic cloves, minced (about 1 tablespoon)	*3* Dry the pan and heat the olive oil over medium heat. Add the onion, garlic, tomatoes, parsley, and oregano. Sauté until the onions are translucent and the tomatoes begin to pop.
1 cup fresh grape or cherry tomatoes	
½ cup fresh parsley leaves, minced (about 2 tablespoons)	*4* Add the broccoli, tomato paste, paprika, salt, and pepper; stir well to combine. Simmer 5 to 7 minutes until heated through. Taste and adjust seasonings.
½ teaspoon dried oregano	
2 tablespoons tomato paste	
½ teaspoon paprika	
Celtic sea salt and ground black pepper to taste	

Per serving: Calories 132 (From Fat 72); Fat 8g (Saturated 1g); Cholesterol 0mg; Sodium 110mg; Carbohydrate 15g; Dietary Fiber 5g; Protein 5.

Recipe courtesy Well Fed: Paleo Recipes for People Who Love to Eat *by Melissa Joulwan (*www . theclothesmakethegirl.com*)*

Cumin-Roasted Carrots

Prep time: 5 min • **Cook time:** 20 min • **Yield:** 4 servings

Ingredients	Directions
10 fresh carrots	*1* Preheat the oven to 400 degrees. Cover a large baking sheet with parchment paper.
½ tablespoon ground cumin	
¼ teaspoon ground cinnamon	*2* Wash and peel the carrots, and cut them lengthwise into thin strips, about ¼-inch wide. Toss them into a large bowl.
¼ teaspoon Celtic sea salt	
¼ teaspoon ground black pepper	*3* With a fork, mix the cumin, cinnamon, salt, and pepper in a small microwave-safe bowl. Add the coconut oil and microwave until melted, about 15 to 20 seconds.
1½ tablespoons coconut oil	
Juice of ½ lemon (optional)	*4* Pour the seasoned coconut oil over the carrots and toss with two wooden spoons until the carrots are evenly coated. Adjust the seasonings to taste.
Garnish: A few leaves of fresh parsley and mint, chopped (optional)	
	5 Spread the carrots in a single layer on the baking sheet and roast for 15 to 20 minutes, until tender and slightly browned. Remove from the oven and, if desired, squeeze the fresh lemon juice over the top and sprinkle with the chopped herbs.

Per serving: Calories 109 (From Fat 54); Fat 6g (Saturated 4g); Cholesterol 0mg; Sodium 185mg; Carbohydrate 15g; Dietary Fiber 4g; Protein 2.

Recipe courtesy Well Fed: Paleo Recipes for People Who Love to Eat *by Melissa Joulwan (*www.theclothesmakethegirl.com*)*

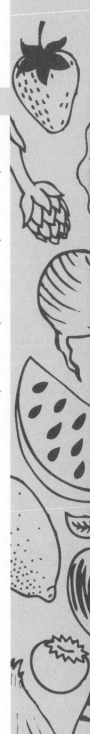

Creamy Cucumbers

Prep time: 30 min • **Cook time:** 60 min • **Yield:** 8 servings

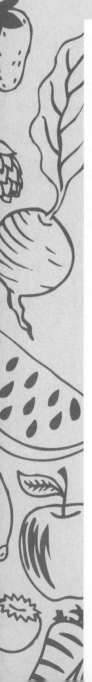

Ingredients	Directions
2 medium cucumbers, very thinly sliced into rounds	**1** Place the cucumbers, onion, and parsley in a large mixing bowl. Stir with a rubber scraper to combine.
½ medium onion, very thinly sliced (about ½ cup)	
⅔ cup fresh parsley leaves, minced	**2** In a small bowl, mix the vinegar, mayo, and garlic lightly with a fork until combined. Pour over cucumbers and gently fold until evenly coated. Season with salt and pepper.
1 teaspoon cider vinegar	
¼ cup Olive Oil Mayo (see recipe in Chapter 17)	
1 garlic clove, minced (about 1 teaspoon)	
Celtic sea salt and ground black pepper to taste	

Per serving: Calories 60 (From Fat 45); Fat 5g (Saturated 1g); Cholesterol 8mg; Sodium 33mg; Carbohydrate 4g; Dietary Fiber 1g; Protein 1g.

Recipe courtesy Well Fed: Paleo Recipes for People Who Love to Eat *by Melissa Joulwan (*www . theclothesmakethegirl.com*)*

Simple Cooked Greens with Fruit

Prep time: 10–15 min • **Cook time:** 10 min • **Yield:** 4 servings

Ingredients	*Directions*
1 bunch Swiss chard, cleaned and dried	**1** Chop the Swiss chard, separating the stems from the leaves.
2 tablespoons olive oil	
1 large garlic clove, minced or put through garlic press	**2** Heat olive oil in large skillet over medium heat; add garlic, chard stems, red pepper flakes, cherries, and orange juice. Stir for 30 seconds, until fragrant.
Pinch red pepper flakes	
2 to 3 tablespoons dried cherries	**3** Add chard leaves, salt, and orange zest; stir until chard is wilted and tender, just a few minutes. Remove the mixture from the pan with a slotted spoon and set aside in a bowl.
¼ cup freshly squeezed orange juice	
Pinch Celtic sea salt	
Zest from the orange (about ½ teaspoon)	**4** Bring the liquid in the pan to a boil and let it thicken. Stir the greens back in. Add maple syrup, if desired. Serve right away.
¼ teaspoon maple syrup (optional)	

Per serving: Calories 101 (From Fat 63); Fat 7g (Saturated 1g); Cholesterol 0mg; Sodium 256mg; Carbohydrate 9g; Dietary Fiber 2g; Protein 2g.

Vary It! You can use other dried fruit here if you don't have cherries. If you have fresh cherries, pit them, cut in half, and you're good to go. Also, any other greens, such as kale or collards, work here as well. If not using chard, don't include the stems of the greens.

Tip: Taking the time to reduce the pan liquids is important to the flavor of this dish. Don't skip it!

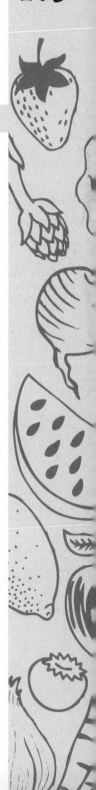

Chapter 17

Soups, Salads, and Sauces for Deep Healing and Cleansing

In This Chapter

▶ Enjoying the phyto-blasting benefits of soups

▶ Discovering how easy cleansing can be with nutrient-dense salads

▶ Creating delectable, fresh sauces

Soups and salads are great for when you want to make an easy meal for a big crowd or when you feel like you just need a pick-me-up. Soups are packed with nutrient-dense ingredients, and salads flood your body with the essential fiber and nutrition it needs. Also cleansing by nature, salads are a great way to get the rainbow greens that are so vital to your immunity.

Making your own sauces takes little time but gives you the opportunity to add taste without empty calories and preservatives. In this chapter, we present recipes for soups, salads, and sauces so tasty you won't believe they can also be healthy!

Taking Charge of Your Health by Cooking for Yourself

Sometimes, a big meal isn't warranted, or perhaps a main course needs the boost of a salad or soup. Focusing on your health is still possible, even in these circumstances. Put as much care into these dishes as any other.

Soup is perhaps one of the simplest ways to add immune-boosting foods to your diet. Soups require a bit of chopping and some time on the stove, and a meal is ready usually with enough leftovers for tomorrow's lunch. Chicken soup has long been called *Jewish penicillin,* because it's full of healing properties. Our version adds even more healing veggies. For a soup with the benefit of cruciferous veggies, we give you a cauliflower curry (and a bonus is that it freezes well).

Salad should be more than just plain lettuce with a few tomatoes drowned in fatty dressing. Salads are a place for veggies to shine; they're an opportunity to either add more produce to the meal or serve as a main, veggie-based course. The Sautéed Mushroom Salad recipe in this chapter also provides a chance to add medicinal, tasty, wild mushrooms to the meal, which taste meaty enough that steak-and-potato lovers won't even miss the meat.

Store-bought sauces can be a real problem in a clean diet because many are filled with unhealthy fats and preservatives, pre-made salad dressings usually contain more sugar than you really need, and cream sauces and traditional mayo are filled with more fats and dairy than you may want to take in. This chapter provides some healthier alternatives; just give them a try and see how easy they are to pull together.

Washing away toxins

If you choose not to buy organic, be sure to wash away toxins that could leave you feeling achy and exhausted and cause brain fog, especially if you have a condition where you're immune compromised. Follow these steps, as recommended by the National Pesticide Information Center (www.npic.orst.edu/health/foodprac.html):

1. Thoroughly wash all vegetables under running water (don't soak or dunk in water), and dry with a paper towel.

2. Scrub fruits and vegetables that are firm enough to handle the scrubbing (like root vegetables, such as carrots).

3. Discard the outer portion of produce anytime you can (such as the case of cabbage or lettuce).

4. Peel fruits and vegetables when possible.

5. Trim the fat and skin from meat, poultry, and fish to minimize residue that may be found in the fat.

Eating a variety of produce reduces your exposure to single pesticides and gives you a variety of nutrients.

When your budget allows, buy organic produce, which are processed without synthetic pesticides or fertilizers. Growing some of your own vegetables or building a relationship with your local farmers' market are also great options to make organic vegetables affordable!

Chicken Vegetable Soup

Prep time: 20 min • **Cook time:** 50 min • **Yield:** 6 servings

Ingredients	*Directions*
2½ pounds chicken breast fillets	*1* Fill a small pot with filtered water and bring to a boil. Drop chicken breasts in and cook for 5 minutes. Remove pot from heat, drain water, and cool the chicken breasts, cutting them into bite-size chunks.
6 cups chicken stock	
1 teaspoon parsley	
1 teaspoon garlic powder	*2* In another pot, add the chicken stock and all herbs and spices, and heat until mixture comes to a boil. Add all vegetables besides cabbage. Reduce heat to medium, and cover and simmer for 30 minutes.
¼ teaspoon oregano	
¾ cup chopped celery	
¾ cup mushrooms	*3* Add the cabbage shreds and chicken. Cover and simmer again for an additional 15 minutes.
½ cup chopped broccoli	
½ cup chopped onion	
½ cup chopped zucchini	*4* Add salt and pepper to taste and adjust seasonings as desired. Serve piping hot!
2 cups shredded cabbage	
Celtic sea salt and ground black pepper to taste	

Per serving: Calories 277 (From Fat 36); Fat 4g (Saturated 1g); Cholesterol 107mg; Sodium 760mg; Carbohydrate 14g (Dietary Fiber 2g); Protein 46g.

Note: What's so great about this dish is that it relies on its natural flavors for taste, so you get a good ol' wholesome bowl of homemade soup. No one has to know it was this easy!

Recipe courtesy Mark Sisson, www.marksdailyapple.com

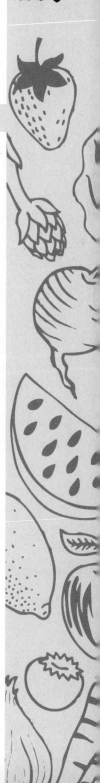

Hearty Vegetable Broth

Prep time: 15 min • **Cook time:** 2 hr 15 min • **Yield:** 6 servings

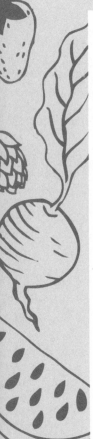

Ingredients	*Directions*
6 carrots	*1* Wash the vegetables well; put all ingredients in a large stockpot and cover with filtered water. Place a lid on the pot and bring to a boil.
2 onions, unpeeled and cut into chunks	
1 bunch celery, including leafy part; chopped	*2* Remove the lid, turn the heat to low, and simmer uncovered about 2 hours. If the veggies start to show above the water line, add more filtered water.
1 bunch cilantro, including stems; chopped	
2 sweet potatoes, unpeeled and quartered	*3* Strain the broth through unbleached cheesecloth into a large bowl to cool. Once cool, check the seasoning; add salt or lemon juice as needed. Make sure to cool completely before refrigerating or freezing.
1 garnet yam, unpeeled and quartered	
6 to 10 garlic cloves	
½ bunch flat leaf parsley	
One 8-inch piece of kombu (seaweed)	
12 to 15 peppercorns	
4 allspice berries	
2 bay leaves	
8 quarts filtered water	
Sea salt to taste	
Lemon juice to taste (about 1 teaspoon)	

Per serving: Calories 124 (From Fat 5); Fat 0.5g (Saturated 0g); Cholesterol 0mg; Sodium 116mg; Carbohydrate 28g (Dietary Fiber 6g); Protein 3g.

Tip: This broth is loaded with minerals and healing agents and is perfect for when you have a cold or when you feel one coming on. You can use this broth as your base for all your soups to keep your immune system humming.

Vary It! If you or a loved one are sick, make this broth with some ginger or turmeric for a nice tonic. Rosemary and oregano are nice, too. Make a big batch of broth and store in small containers in your freezer; you never know when you'll need some!

Coconut Cilantro Soup

Prep time: 10 min • **Yield:** 4 servings

Ingredients	*Directions*
1½ cups lightly packed spinach	**1** Place all ingredients in a blender (Vitamix is a great brand) and blend until well combined.
1 cup lightly packed kale	
One 16-ounce container coconut water	**2** Adjust the ingredients to taste.
One 14-ounce can coconut milk	
Juice of 1 lime	
¼ cup olive oil	
¼ cup coconut aminos	
½ avocado	
1 jalapeño	
2 cloves garlic	
½ to 1 tablespoon chile peppers, depending on desired heat	
Celtic sea salt and ground black pepper to taste	

Per serving: Calories 397 (From Fat 342); Fat 38g (Saturated 21g); Cholesterol 0mg; Sodium 496mg; Carbohydrate 16g (Dietary Fiber 3g); Protein 4g.

Vary It! You can alter the taste quite a bit by adjusting how much lime juice you use.

Tip: Spicy superfoods, like peppers, are called *mucolytics,* and they naturally thin mucus. So this soup will help you when you have congestion of any kind. Also, the coconut is filled with good minerals and healthy fats, and the greens have a high nutrient density. This soup recipe brings powerful healing!

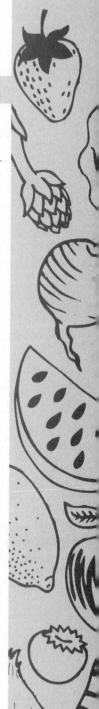

Curried Cauliflower Soup

Prep time: 10 min • **Cook time:** 35 min • **Yield:** 6 servings

Ingredients	*Directions*
1 head cauliflower, cut into florets	*1* Preheat the oven to 400 degrees; line baking sheet with parchment paper.
3 tablespoons olive oil, divided	*2* Toss cauliflower with 1 tablespoon olive oil and ¼ teaspoon salt; spread in an even layer in the pan. Bake until tender, about 25 minutes.
¼ teaspoon plus 2 pinches Celtic sea salt	
1 cup finely diced onion	*3* While cauliflower is roasting, heat the remaining oil in a sauté pan over medium heat and add onion. Add pinch of salt and cook until onions are soft, about 3 minutes.
2 carrots, scrubbed and finely diced	
1 cup finely diced celery	*4* Add carrots, celery, and another pinch of salt; sauté until vegetables begin to brown, about 10 to 12 minutes.
1 teaspoon curry powder	
¼ teaspoon ground cumin	*5* Add curry powder, cumin, coriander, and cinnamon to pan and stir until veggies are coated. Pour in ½ cup broth or water, stir to deglaze the pan (scrape up any browned bits), and let liquid reduce by half. Remove from heat.
¼ teaspoon ground coriander	
⅛ teaspoon ground cinnamon	
6 cups vegetable broth or water, divided	*6* Pour 3 cups broth or water into a blender, and then add half the sautéed veggies along with the roasted cauliflower. Blend until smooth, and then pour the mixture into a soup pot. Repeat with remaining broth and veggies. Add additional water or broth to reach the consistency you like.
Celtic sea salt and/or lemon juice to taste	
	7 Gently reheat the soup and check the flavors. You may need to add a bit more salt or lemon juice.

Per serving: Calories 107 (From Fat 63); Fat 7g (Saturated 1g); Cholesterol 0mg; Sodium 137mg; Carbohydrate 10g (Dietary Fiber 3g); Protein 2g.

Note: This soup is even easier to make with an immersion blender. Just put the veggies, broth, and cauliflower into the soup pot and blend away. You save time, and it's easier to clean up.

Tip: A nice garnish for this soup is finely diced red pepper and chopped cilantro, but the flavor is good without it. This soup freezes well, so make extra!

Purple Slaw Salad

Prep time: 10 min • **Yield:** 2 servings

Ingredients	Directions
2 cups purple cabbage, shredded	**1** Mix everything in a big bowl and let sit for 20 to 30 minutes before serving.
1 cucumber, diced	
¼ cup shredded onion	
1½ cups ground cumin	
3½ to 4 teaspoons freshly squeezed lime juice (to taste)	
½ cup diced tomato	
1 teaspoon Celtic sea salt	
1 tablespoon minced garlic	

Per serving: Calories 91 (From Fat 9); Fat 1g (Saturated 0g); Cholesterol 0mg; Sodium 662mg; Carbohydrate 17g (Dietary Fiber 3g); Protein 3g.

Vary It! This salad is also great with some slivered almonds on top.

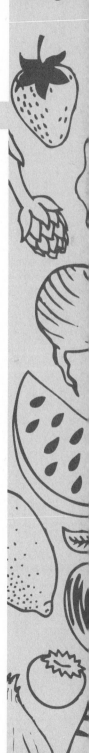

Tuscan Spinach Salad with Egg, Olive, and Avocado

Prep time: 10 min • **Yield:** 4 servings

Ingredients	Directions
2 cups spinach	*1* Combine ingredients in a large bowl. Mix and serve!
2 hard-boiled eggs, chopped	
1 cup fresh basil, chopped	
3 tablespoons olive oil	
1 red onion, chopped	
1 tablespoon fresh oregano	
⅓ cup lemon juice	
1 handful black olives, chopped	
1 avocado, cubed	

Per serving: Calories 234 (From Fat 171); Fat 19g (Saturated 3g); Cholesterol 93mg; Sodium 147mg; Carbohydrate 12g (Dietary Fiber 6g); Protein 7g.

Vary It! You can substitute the hard-boiled eggs for any protein you love.

Sautéed Mushroom Salad

Prep time: 20 min • **Cook time:** 25 min • **Yield:** 4–6 servings

Ingredients	*Directions*
1 pound oyster mushrooms	*1* Clean and trim all mushrooms. If mushrooms are large, cut into ½-inch slices.
½ pound fresh shiitake mushrooms	
2 tablespoons olive oil	*2* Heat olive oil and sesame oil in skillet. Add garlic and ginger and stir about 1 minute. (Don't let garlic get too brown.)
1 teaspoon sesame oil	
4 to 6 cloves garlic, minced or put through garlic press	*3* Add mushrooms and toss over medium heat until they give up moisture. Continue cooking on low until tender and starting to brown in spots. Stir frequently.
2 tablespoons minced fresh ginger	
2 tablespoons fresh lemon juice	*4* Meanwhile, clean all greens and tear into bite-size pieces. Toss in large bowl. Add green onions.
2 teaspoons tamari	
12 packed cups salad greens, including frisée, red romaine, butter lettuce, arugula, and spinach	*5* Dress greens very lightly with olive oil, touch of sesame oil, and lemon juice. Toss to coat and divide among salad plates.
⅓ cup thinly sliced green onions	*6* When mushrooms are tender, add lemon juice and tamari and toss. Place on top of salad greens. You can also garnish with more cilantro leaves.
1 cup cilantro leaves	
Dressing: Additional olive oil, dark sesame oil, and lemon juice to taste	

Per serving: Calories 150 (From Fat 63); Fat 7g (Saturated 1g); Cholesterol 0mg; Sodium 190mg; Carbohydrate 19g (Dietary Fiber 7g); Protein 6g.

Tip: When it comes to which salad greens to choose, be sure to include something delicate like the butter lettuce and something peppery like the arugula. And definitely include the cilantro!

Vary It! Use whichever mushrooms you like the most. Fresh morels, portabellas, and lobster mushrooms all work well here. If you have fresh maitake mushrooms (also known as hen of the woods), definitely include them, because they have amazing healing properties and taste as hearty as meat!

Note: This salad can stand on its own as a light lunch, but it pairs well with meat or fish entrees, too.

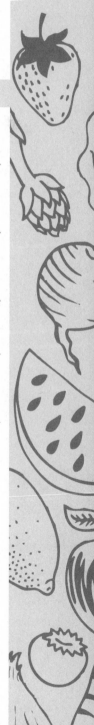

Creamy Nut Sauce

Prep time: 5 min • **Yield:** 3½ cups

Ingredients	*Directions*
2 cups raw cashews	*1* Place cashews in a mini food processor or nut grinder and grind fine. (You can skip this step if you're using a Vitamix; other blenders usually don't get the nuts fine enough.)
2 cups water	
2 teaspoons freshly squeezed orange or lemon juice	
Dash nutmeg	*2* Put cashews, water, orange or lemon juice, nutmeg, and salt into blender and process until creamy. (It may take several minutes to get it creamy, so don't rush this step.)
½ teaspoon Celtic sea salt	
	3 Serve over veggies, such as broccoli, cauliflower, and cooked greens.

Per serving: Calories 108 (From Fat 81); Fat 9g (Saturated 2g); Cholesterol 0mg; Sodium 48mg; Carbohydrate 6g (Dietary Fiber 1g); Protein 4g.

Vary It! Other nuts, such as almonds, walnuts, or pecans, work great in this recipe as well. You can also add in herbs; try 1 cup fresh basil or mint.

Best Stir-Fry Sauce Ever

Prep time: 5 min • **Cook time:** 10 min • **Yield:** ¼ cup

Ingredients	*Directions*
1 clove garlic, minced (about 1 teaspoon) **½ teaspoon crushed red pepper flakes** **2 teaspoons Chinese five-spice powder** **½ teaspoon rice vinegar** **2 tablespoons fresh orange juice** **3 tablespoons coconut aminos**	*1* In a small bowl, mix the garlic, red pepper flakes, five-spice powder, and rice vinegar with a fork to form a smooth paste. Stirring continuously with the fork, pour in the orange juice, and then add the coconut aminos. *2* Use this sauce in stir-fries to coat veggies and proteins; add to wok and stir just before serving.

Per serving: Calories 63 (From Fat 0); Fat 0g (Saturated 0g); Cholesterol 0mg; Sodium 1018mg; Carbohydrate 13g (Dietary Fiber 0g); Protein 0g.

Recipe courtesy Well Fed: Paleo Recipes for People Who Love to Eat *by Melissa Joulwan (*www.the clothesmakethegirl.com*)*

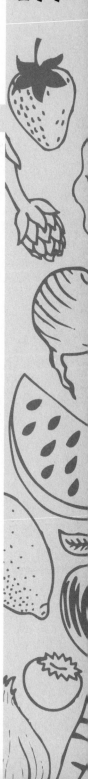

Olive Oil Mayo

Prep time: 10 min • **Yield:** 1½ cups

Ingredients	*Directions*
2 large egg yolks 2 tablespoons water 2 tablespoons fresh lemon juice 1 teaspoon dry mustard 1 teaspoon Celtic sea salt 1 cup olive oil	*1* Heat the egg yolk, water, and lemon juice in a small saucepan over very low heat, stirring constantly.
	2 At the first sign of thickness, remove saucepan from heat and submerge in a large pan of cold water (continue stirring to avoid creating citrusy scrambled eggs — trust us!).
	3 Scoop the mixture into a food processor (or blender), add dry mustard and salt, and blend for a few seconds.
	4 Drizzle the oil slowly into the mixture until all the ingredients are combined. Scoop into a large glass container and chill immediately. Mayo should keep for one week if stored correctly.

Per serving: Calories 169 (From Fat 171); Fat 19g (Saturated 3g); Cholesterol 31mg; Sodium 112mg; Carbohydrate 0g (Dietary Fiber 0g); Protein 0g.

Note: This recipe is great for those folks who are weary of using raw eggs in their mayonnaise! The best place to store mayonnaise is in a Mason jar (or other glass preserving jar).

Recipe courtesy Mark Sisson, www.marksdailyapple.com

Creamy Italian Dressing

Prep time: 5 min • **Yield:** ¼ cup

Ingredients	Directions
½ teaspoon dried Italian herb blend or dried oregano	**1** In a small bowl, crush the dried herbs with your fingers, and then add the mayo and garlic. Blend well with a fork.
¼ cup Olive Oil Mayo (see previous recipe)	
½ clove garlic, minced (about ½ teaspoon)	**2** Drizzle in the vinegar, mixing with the fork, and then taste and season with salt and pepper.
2 tablespoons balsamic, wine, or cider vinegar	
Celtic sea salt and ground black pepper to taste	

Per serving: Calories 191 (From Fat 171); Fat 19g (Saturated 3g); Cholesterol 31mg; Sodium 112mg; Carbohydrate 5g (Dietary Fiber 0g); Protein 1g.

Tip: If the dressing is too thick, add additional vinegar or water ¼ teaspoon at a time, until it's the right consistency. Keep in mind that it will thin slightly as you toss it with your salad ingredients.

Recipe courtesy Well Fed: Paleo Recipes for People Who Love to Eat *by Melissa Joulwan (*www.the clothesmakethegirl.com*)*

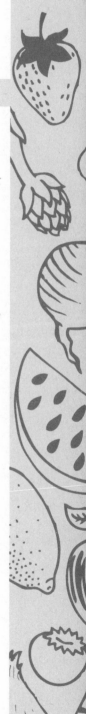

Chapter 18

Desserts and Snacks to Keep You on Track

In This Chapter

▶ Redefining desserts

▶ Discovering how fantastic healthy desserts and snacks can taste

Yes, dessert can actually help you live longer and stronger! With the recipes in this chapter, you can make desserts that taste good enough to rival any bakery yet are packed with that immune-building punch. Also, the grab-and-go snack recipes are great options for when you want something with some taste, a little crunch, or just something simple to pick up your blood sugar. They're vitally nutrient and practical for work or school or to throw in your bag. Enjoy an immune-boosting bite!

This chapter will make your mouth water with the easy desserts and snacks that are good just about any time of the day.

No, Eating the "Extras" Isn't Cheating

When you choose to eat the "extras," like desserts and snacks, you may as well make them foods that feed your cells with the good stuff and help give you energy — because you can get all of that and simplicity and taste to boot!

Many people get caught up worrying about calories, so they avoid desserts and snacks. **_Remember:_** Not all calories are equal. Nutrient-rich foods, like the recipes in this chapter, impart nourishment as well as comfort and convenience, so including them in your diet is okay. The same can't be said about typical snacks and desserts, which give you calories but without any nutrients to speak of! If you plan to eat these extras, keep them in mind as you decide how much of other foods you plan to eat that day. Overeating, even if the food is good for you, isn't good for your immune system!

When choosing ingredients for the recipes in this chapter, keep the following in mind:

- Sweeteners should be organic sucanat or local, raw, unpasteurized honey. *Sucanat* comes from dried sugar cane juice, which is sugar but still includes minerals and B vitamins. It has the same calories as white sugar but has less processing and more nutrients. Honey also includes a host of immune-boosting nutrients, but be sure to use local, raw, organic varieties. Many brands found in supermarkets have been adulterated, and most are pasteurized so the nutrients have been destroyed.

- Chocolate is okay! In fact, chocolate contains polyphenols and other nutrients that are good for your immune system and are anti-inflammatory. But not all chocolate is created equal. Look for dark chocolate, at least 70 percent cocoa or more. Less than that, and it contains too much sugar. You can use *cocoa nibs* — chunks of cacao beans that have been chopped and roasted, no sugar added — in these recipes, but the final result won't be as sweet and will have a slightly different taste.

- Coconut oil is a good choice when looking for an oil that withstands higher heat, and it works well in most of the recipes in this chapter. Coconut oil contains medium chain triglycerides, which are anti-inflammatory and immune boosting. In choosing coconut flakes, look for unsweetened varieties, which should be specified on the package.

Chocolate Chip Cookies

Prep time: 15 min • **Cook time:** 15 min • **Yield:** 12 cookies

Ingredients	*Directions*
4 dates	*1* Preheat the oven to 350 degrees. Grind dates in a food processor until a paste forms, about 40 seconds.
1½ cups walnuts	
½ cup pecans	
1 teaspoon baking soda	*2* Add walnuts and pecans and blend until very finely chopped, about 35 seconds. Add baking soda and salt and pulse a few more times.
⅛ teaspoon Celtic sea salt	
2 tablespoons coconut oil	*3* Warm the coconut oil so it's in a liquid form. With the food processor running, drizzle the coconut oil into the date paste and add the egg and vanilla. Stop mixing as soon as the egg and the oil are blended in.
1 egg	
1 teaspoon vanilla	
¼ to ½ cup chopped dark chocolate	*4* Scrape the batter into a bowl and stir in the chocolate and coconut chips by hand. The dough will be sticky and wet. Drop 12 portions of the dough onto a cookie sheet, and flatten with your fingers. Bake 15 minutes or until nicely browned.
¼ cup unsweetened shredded coconut	

Per serving: Calories 142 (From Fat 108); Fat 12g (Saturated 5g); Cholesterol 16mg; Sodium 126mg; Carbohydrate 7g (Dietary Fiber 2g); Protein 1g.

Note: These cookies are moister than some but hold their shape after baking. Lining the cookie sheet with parchment paper and letting them rest for a minute before removing them to a cooling rack helps.

Vary It! If you want to change this recipe up, you can skip the chocolate chips and use fresh blueberries or sulfite-free dried cranberries.

Recipe courtesy Mark Sisson, www.marksdailyapple.com

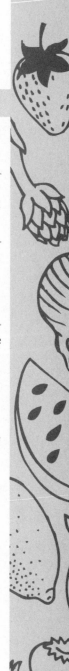

No-Bake Almond Butter Ball Cookies

Prep time: 15 min • **Yield:** 15 cookies

Ingredients	Directions
16 ounces crunchy organic almond butter	**1** Mix together all the ingredients except the coconut flour.
¾ cup honey (organic, raw, local, and unpasteurized)	**2** Slowly add the coconut flour in and keep mixing (by hand is fine) until the mixture isn't as sticky and can be formed into a ball.
½ bag dark chocolate chips (about 5 to 6 ounces)	
½ cup coconut flour	**3** Line a glass pan with unbleached parchment paper and form small balls with the almond butter mixture and place in the glass pan.
	4 Refrigerate for 2 hours for best consistency. Otherwise, just enjoy as is!

Per serving: Calories 312 (From Fat 189); Fat 21g (Saturated 4g); Cholesterol 1mg; Sodium 5mg; Carbohydrate 29g (Dietary Fiber 6g); Protein 7g.

John's Banana Whips

Prep time: 10 min • **Yield:** 2 servings

Ingredients	*Directions*
3 large frozen bananas without the peels **Large handful of frozen strawberries or blueberries (about ½ cup)**	*1* Feed frozen bananas through a juicer that homogenizes (like a Champion juicer), or use a food processor and blend until super smooth.
	2 Put the frozen berries through the juicer or in the food processor as well.
	3 Catch the whip in a container and enjoy!

Per serving: Calories 175 (From Fat 9); Fat 1g (Saturated 0g); Cholesterol 0mg; Sodium 2mg; Carbohydrate 45g (Dietary Fiber 5g); Protein 2g.

Tip: If using a food processor, process the berries first, remove from bowl, and add to the bananas after they're processed to get a smoother consistency.

Vary It! You can jazz up these whips by adding chocolate chips or shredded or flaked coconut. Simply stir them in by hand after the fruit is processed.

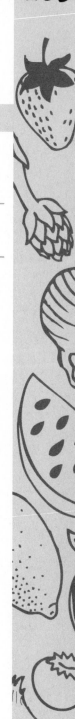

Caramelized Coconut Chips

Prep time: 2 min • **Cook time:** 3 min • **Yield:** 4 servings (about 1 cup)

Ingredients	*Directions*
¼ teaspoon Celtic sea salt ¼ teaspoon cinnamon **1 cup unsweetened coconut flakes**	*1* Mix the salt and cinnamon with a fork in a small bowl and set aside. Heat a cast iron or stainless steel skillet over medium-high heat, about 2 minutes.
	2 Add the coconut flakes to the skillet and distribute evenly to form a single layer in the bottom of the pan. Cook, stirring frequently, for about 3 minutes, but watch closely for desired toastiness. Remove the pan from the heat.
	3 Sprinkle the hot coconut flakes with the salty cinnamon and toss until evenly seasoned. Transfer to a plate and allow to cool in a single layer for maximum crunch. Store at room temp in an airtight container — if they last that long.

Per serving: Calories 147 (From Fat 117); Fat 13g (Saturated 12g); Cholesterol 0mg; Sodium 86mg; Carbohydrate 5g (Dietary Fiber 3g); Protein 1g.

Tip: The coconut flakes will continue to brown a bit even after the pan is off the heat, so stop cooking just before they get too toasted.

Recipe courtesy Well Fed: Paleo Recipes for People Who Love to Eat *by Melissa Joulwan (*www.theclothes makethegirl.com*)*

Roasted Rosemary Walnuts

Prep time: 5 min • **Cook time:** 20 min • **Yield:** 20 servings (about 5 cups)

Ingredients	Directions
5 cups walnut halves ¼ cup olive oil	*1* Heat the oven to 350 degrees. Place unbleached parchment paper on a baking sheet.
¼ cup fresh rosemary, chopped 4 teaspoons Celtic sea salt 1 teaspoon raw, organic honey or sucanat	*2* Place all ingredients in bowl and mix. (Easiest to do this with your hands, because it's sticky.) Transfer mixture to baking sheet.
2 teaspoons ground black pepper	*3* Bake until beginning to brown, about 20 minutes. Stir occasionally. Remove from oven and let cool in pan.

Per serving: Calories 218 (From Fat 198); Fat 22g (Saturated 2g); Cholesterol 0mg; Sodium 254mg; Carbohydrate 5g (Dietary Fiber 2g); Protein 5g.

Tip: These nuts will last about ten days in an airtight container at room temperature. Remember that although nuts are healthy for you, you need to eat them in moderation due to caloric value. The rosemary makes this recipe especially nice for someone recovering from a cold.

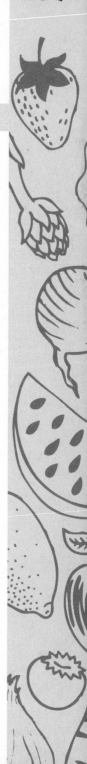

Vegetable Latkes

Prep time: 15 min • **Cook time:** 4–6 min • **Yield:** 5 servings

Ingredients	*Directions*
3 cups of grated carrot, turnip, daikon radish, or zucchini	*1* Wrap a light dish towel around grated vegetables, 1 cup at a time, and squeeze out as much water as possible.
2 eggs, beaten	
Pinch Celtic sea salt	*2* In a bowl, mix grated vegetable with eggs, salt, and pepper. (After frying a few latkes, add more egg as binder only if necessary.)
Pinch ground black pepper	
½ cup organic grapeseed oil	
	3 Heat oil in skillet over medium to high heat. Toss a pinch of the grated vegetable mixture into the pan — the oil is hot enough if it sizzles immediately.
	4 Scoop ¼ or less of the grated vegetable mixture into your hand and form into a very loose patty. Set the patty into the hot pan and press it down gently with a fork.
	5 Cook at least 2 to 3 minutes on each side, until nicely browned. To keep the latkes warm while you cook the rest of the batch, place them in a 250-degree oven.

Per serving: Calories 250 (From Fat 216); Fat 24g (Saturated 3g); Cholesterol 74mg; Sodium 79mg; Carbohydrate 7g (Dietary Fiber 2g); Protein 3g.

Vary It! You can add cinnamon to the carrot latkes, curry powder to the turnip, or fresh herbs to the zucchini.

Tip: If the oil starts to smoke or becomes dark in color, carefully toss out the oil, clean the pan, and start fresh before frying any more latkes. Burnt oil is definitely not immune building!

Recipe courtesy Mark Sisson, www.marksdailyapple.com

Jicama Sticks with a Kick

Prep time: 25 min • **Cook time:** 35 min • **Yield:** 24 servings

Ingredients	Directions
1 jicama, sliced into long thick strips	**1** Mix all the ingredients except the jicama in a bowl.
¼ cup raw organic honey	**2** Marinate the jicama in this mixture overnight.
¼ cup olive oil or macadamia oil	**3** Drain and serve.
⅛ teaspoon chili powder	
⅛ teaspoon cayenne pepper	
⅛ teaspoon ground black pepper	
½ lemon, juiced	
½ lime, juiced	

Per serving: Calories 41 (From Fat 18); Fat 2g (Saturated 0g); Cholesterol 0mg; Sodium 2mg; Carbohydrate 5g (Dietary Fiber 1g); Protein 0g.

Tip: You can whip up a quick jicama dip to add some flavor by mixing 2 avocados, 2 tomatoes, ¼ red onion, chopped, ½ serano chile, chopped, and garlic powder and Celtic sea salt to taste. Dip the jicama sticks and enjoy!

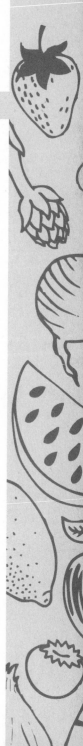

Meat and Spinach Muffins

Prep time: 15 min • **Cook time:** 40 min • **Yield:** 4 servings

Ingredients	Directions
Three 16-ounce bags frozen chopped spinach, defrosted	**1** Preheat the oven to 375 degrees.
½ tablespoon coconut oil	**2** Place all the spinach in a colander and press out the water with a bowl that fits inside the colander; squeeze handfuls of spinach to wring out the remaining water. You should have about 4 cups of spinach.
½ medium onion, diced (about ½ cup)	
1½ pounds ground beef	**3** Heat a large skillet over medium-high heat, about 3 minutes. Add coconut oil and allow it to melt. Add the onion and sauté, stirring with a wooden spoon, until it's crisp-tender and translucent, about 5 minutes.
2 cloves garlic, minced (about 2 teaspoons)	
½ teaspoon Celtic sea salt	
¼ teaspoon ground black pepper	**4** Crumble the meat into the pan, breaking up lumps with the wooden spoon. Add the garlic, salt, black pepper, and cayenne pepper, and cook until the meat is browned. Stir in the spinach until it's combined. Set aside to cool for about 15 minutes.
½ teaspoon ground cayenne pepper	
3 eggs	
	5 Beat the eggs in a small bowl with a fork, and when the meat is cool, add them to the meat; blend well. Using your hands is the easiest way to combine.
	6 Place muffin papers in a 12-count muffin pan. Pack the batter into a ½-cup measure, and then transfer it to the muffin pan, using your hands to pack the mixture tightly into the muffin paper. It should be slightly mounded on top.
	7 Bake for 40 minutes or until the tops are lightly browned. Remove the muffins from the pan, cool, and store covered in the refrigerator.

Per serving: Calories 610 (From Fat 369); Fat 41g (Saturated 16g); Cholesterol 260mg; Sodium 579mg; Carbohydrate 17g (Dietary Fiber 10g); Protein 47g.

Recipe courtesy Well Fed: Paleo Recipes for People Who Love to Eat *by Melissa Joulwan (*www.theclothes makethegirl.com*)*

Sesame-Garlic Nori Chips

Prep time: 10 min • **Cook time:** 15 min • **Yield:** 4 servings (about 42 chips)

Ingredients	Directions
12 nori sheets **Water** **1 tablespoon sesame oil** **3 cloves garlic, minced (about 1 tablespoon)** **Pinch ground cayenne pepper** **Celtic sea salt to taste** **½ tablespoon sesame seeds**	*1* Preheat the oven to 275 degrees. Cover two large baking sheets with unbleached parchment paper or aluminum foil. *2* Place 6 sheets of nori, shiny side up, on the baking sheets. With a pastry brush, lightly brush the shiny side of the nori with water, being sure to reach the edges, then carefully align another sheet of nori on top and press them together. Repeat with the remaining sheets until you have 6 pieces of double-thick nori. *3* Using kitchen shears or a sharp knife, cut the double-thick nori into 1-inch strips, and then cut those strips in half crosswise. You should end up with about 42 chips. Arrange the chips in a single layer on the baking sheets. *4* In a small bowl, combine the sesame oil, garlic, and cayenne pepper. Use the pastry brush to coat the tops of the chips with the oil mixture, and then sprinkle generously with salt. Sprinkle the sesame seeds across the tops of the chips. *5* Place on the middle rack of the oven and bake for 15 to 20 minutes. The chips will crisp and turn a deep, glossy green. Remove from the oven, taste, and sprinkle with more salt if you like; allow them to cool before eating for maximum crunch.

Per serving: *Calories 52 (From Fat 36); Fat 4g (Saturated 1g); Cholesterol 0mg; Sodium 34mg; Carbohydrate 4g (Dietary Fiber 3g); Protein 3g.*

Recipe courtesy Well Fed: Paleo Recipes for People Who Love to Eat *by Melissa Joulwan (*www.theclothes makethegirl.com*)*

Chapter 19

Tonifying Teas and Sensational Smoothies

In This Chapter

▶ Making even your beverages count

▶ Brewing your own probiotics

▶ Mixing up quick liquid breakfasts and snacks

We all know we need to drink more water. But when you're ready to scream at the thought of yet another plain glass of water or when you want to make even what you're drinking count toward your nutrition, this chapter is the place to look.

The collection of teas and tangy beverages in this chapter shows how to easily include immune-boosting ingredients into your life. If you're short on time and need breakfast to be portable, these smoothies are a good alternative. You already know about the benefits of probiotics, so skip the health food store and brew your own. We include the recipes for kefir and kombucha so you can do it yourself. Not only will you have guaranteed live cultures, but you'll also end up with enough to share with friends. What a great way to spread the news and get others on the immune-boosting path!

The kombucha and kefir recipes sound a little intimidating at first, but once you get the hang of it, it takes almost no time at all to make each day. And if you plan to do a smoothie regularly, keep everything you need in the same place in the fridge (such as the fruit drawer), so you don't have to go hunting for it.

Getting Anti-inflammatories and Probiotics in Your Glass

Just as using food to boost immunity is important, so is seizing the opportunity to use beverages for the same thing. It's simple: You need to drink something anyway, so you may as well make it tasty and good for you and skip sugary drinks with empty calories.

Skip supplements and make kefir or kombucha instead as a way of getting the immune-boosting properties of probiotics. You're guaranteed freshness and viability, and these beverages taste good as well! Kefir and kombucha become "self-generating" with just a little attention from you, so you'll have a source of probiotics not only for yourself and your family but also enough to share with others.

Chronic disease is all about inflammation, so finding ways of fighting inflammation is important. The teas and smoothies in this chapter are specifically designed to bring more anti-inflammatory nutrients into your life in tasty, easy ways. When inflammation is at a minimum, your immune system works at its peak, and it's easier to stay healthy. Even better, the flavors in these drinks will help stop the sugar cravings many people have; less sugar means stronger immune systems!

Creamy Turmeric Tea

Prep time: 1 min • **Cook time:** 5 min • **Yield:** 1 cup (1 serving)

Ingredients	*Directions*
8 ounces (1 cup) almond or coconut milk	**1** Gently warm the almond or coconut milk on the stove.
½ teaspoon turmeric	
½-inch round slice ginger root, peeled and finely chopped	**2** In a mug, combine the other ingredients.
Dash cayenne pepper	**3** Drizzle about a teaspoon of the warmed milk into the mug and mix until the liquid is smooth with no lumps. Add the rest of the milk and mix well. Strain out ginger before drinking.
½ to 1 teaspoon raw, organic honey or other sweetener	
Optional additions: small pat of butter, cinnamon, or cardamom	

Per serving: Calories 578 (From Fat 513); Fat 57g (Saturated 51g); Cholesterol 0mg; Sodium 37mg; Carbohydrate 20g (Dietary Fiber 6g); Protein 6g.

Note: Although this beverage isn't technically a tea, it's great as a pick-me-up in the morning or a great wind-down in the evening. It's particularly good when you have sniffles or a cold. Also, this "tea" goes great at the end of a meal instead of dessert!

Recipe courtesy Mark Sisson, www.marksdailyapple.com

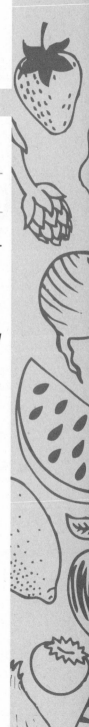

Mulled Cider

Prep time: 5 min • **Cook time:** 20 min • **Yield:** 6 servings

Ingredients	Directions
2 cinnamon sticks, broken into pieces	*1* Combine all ingredients other than cider in a small bowl. Place 6 tablespoons of the mixture in a metal tea ball or wrap in cheesecloth. Place remaining spice mixture in an airtight container for later use (it keeps well in the freezer).
6 whole nutmegs, broken into pieces	
⅓ cup dried orange peel	
⅓ cup dried lemon peel	*2* Put tea ball or cheesecloth in a small saucepan with cider; bring to a simmer. Turn off heat and let it rest for 10 minutes prior to serving.
¼ cup whole allspice	
¼ cup whole cloves	
2 tablespoons coarsely chopped crystallized ginger	*3* Remove spice ball and serve.
6 cups organic apple cider, unpasteurized and unfiltered	

Per serving: Calories 141 (From Fat 18); Fat 2g (Saturated 1g); Cholesterol 0mg; Sodium 16mg; Carbohydrate 12g (Dietary Fiber 4g); Protein 1g.

Tip: Make your own dried orange and lemon peels: Every time you juice a lemon or orange, first peel it with a vegetable peeler, leaving the white part behind. Lay these strips of peel on a paper towel and let dry at room temp overnight. Collect them all in a small jar and put with your spices.

Vary It! Mulling spices are equally good with wine or even lemonade. Chill the lemonade prior to serving.

"The Dr. Oz Show" Special Smoothie

Prep time: 5 min • **Yield:** About 3 cups (1 serving)

Ingredients	Directions
1 tablespoon flax seeds 3 Brazil nuts ½ cup blueberries 1 cup Swiss chard leaves, torn into small pieces (no stems) 1 to 2 cups brewed green tea, cooled	*1* Place all ingredients into blender in order listed. Blend for 1 to 2 minutes. Add filtered water as necessary to achieve desired consistency.

Per serving: Calories 281 (From Fat 126); Fat 14g (Saturated 3g); Cholesterol 0mg; Sodium 104mg; Carbohydrate 39g (Dietary Fiber 6g); Protein 5g.

Note: Coauthor Wendy made this smoothie as a guest on *The Dr. Oz Show*. Dr. Oz liked it so much that he's shared it with others since!

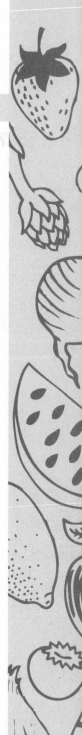

Kombucha

Prep time: 20 min • **Rest time:** 5–7 days • **Yield:** 1 gallon

Items Needed	Directions: First Fermentation
1 gallon filtered water	*1* Heat ½ gallon filtered water to boiling.
10 tea bags (black or green tea)	*2* Add tea bags and keep water near boiling for 5 minutes. Add sucanat and stir to dissolve.
1¼ cup sucanat	
Kombucha SCOBY (symbiotic culture of bacteria and yeast) with small amount of starter liquid	*3* Pour hot tea through a strainer into a 1-gallon container, preferably glass or ceramic. Add remaining ½ gallon filtered water and stir.
	4 After cooled to room temperature, add SCOBY with starter liquid. Cover the container with a permeable top, such as wax paper, parchment paper, or a kitchen towel. Secure with rubber bands.
	5 Set at room temperature in the dark for 5 days. Beginning on Day 5, taste the tea each day for sweetness. It's ready when the healthy bacteria have eaten enough of the sugar, and the sweetness is to your liking.

Second Fermentation (optional)

When the sweetness is to your liking and if you want to develop some fizz, do the following steps.

1 Save 1 to 2 cups of liquid for the next batch.

2 Bottle the remaining liquid into ball jars or bottles with crimp tops.

3 Let the bottles sit for 1 to 2 weeks at room temperature in the dark to develop best carbonation.

Per serving (1 quart): Calories 36 (From Fat 0); Fat 0g (Saturated 0g); Cholesterol 0mg; Sodium 0mg; Carbohydrate 8g (Dietary Fiber 0g); Protein 0g.

Note: You can flavor your kombucha at the bottling step: Add a slice or two of ginger root to each bottle prior to sealing it. You can also add a few dried cherries, raisins, or dried apple slices.

Resources and the inside scoop on SCOBY

You can purchase kombucha SCOBY from a number of online providers or check a local food co-op. Once you have yours going and it starts to grow, you can share with friends. (You'll have more than you need!)

The SCOBY floats around in the liquid; don't misunderstand and think it's mold. Mold *can* occur (it would be thin and white and floating on top of the liquid), so be sure all the containers you use for bottling and brewing are clean and dry.

If you don't like the small bits of SCOBY that sometimes get into the drink itself, strain it through a fine sieve or cheesecloth when you bottle it.

The kombucha will last years and years without refrigeration.

Don't worry about the sugar: The SCOBY eats it all, so you're not really getting much, depending on how sweet you let it be when you consume it.

For support and ideas as you get started making kombucha, check out this great group: http://health.groups.yahoo.com/group/original_kombucha/.

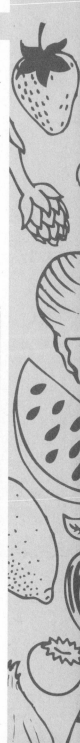

Water-Based Kefir

Prep time: 5 min • **Rest time:** Overnight • **Yield:** 1 quart

Ingredients	*Directions*
1 quart filtered water **⅓ to ¼ cup sucanat** **¼ cup kefir grains** **Few dried cherries, figs, or raisins (optional)**	*1* Fill a quart Mason jar (or similar container) to within 1 to 2 inches from the top with filtered water. Be sure the jar is very clean.
	2 Add sucanat and stir to dissolve. Add kefir grains and fruit, if desired.
	3 Put lid on lightly (don't screw it down). Place the jar out of direct sunlight at room temperature for 12 hours.
	4 Taste the liquid; if not too sweet, it's done. Strain into a clean jar and discard fruit. Enjoy the kefir!
	5 Rinse kefir grains with filtered water. Use them to start a new batch.

Per serving (1 quart): Calories 55 (From Fat 0); Fat 0g (Saturated 0g); Cholesterol 0mg; Sodium 7mg; Carbohydrate 11g (Dietary Fiber 3g); Protein 0g.

Tip: To make this kefir fizzy, tighten down a lid on the jar of completed kefir liquid and leave at room temperature overnight. Also, leave it a bit sweeter than you would if you planned to drink it right away to give the bacteria something to keep eating. If you don't want it fizzy but can't drink it all right away, put it in the fridge to slow the fermentation process and keep it nearly the same sweetness.

Tip: Vary the flavoring of your kefir with a slice of ginger and a slice of lemon as it ferments.

Note: As you continue to make kefir, the grains keep growing and changing. Soon, you'll have more than you need. Don't put more into the jar than you need; stick to the amount listed. But don't throw the extra grains away, because they still have loads of probiotic activity. Give them to a friend, or feed them to your pets.

Kefir Smoothie

Prep time: 5 min • **Yield:** 1 quart (1–2 servings)

Ingredients	Directions
2 cups plain dairy kefir	**1** Place all ingredients into blender or Vitamix. Blend for 1 to 2 minutes. Drink right away or it will separate!
1 cup berries (strawberries, blueberries, raspberries)	
2 tablespoons flax seeds	
½ cucumber, peeled and seeded if large	
1 stalk celery	
½ lime, juiced directly into the blender	
Pinch turmeric	
Pinch cardamom	

Per serving: Calories 511 (From Fat 198); Fat 22g (Saturated 11g); Cholesterol 60mg; Sodium 285mg; Carbohydrate 53g (Dietary Fiber 12g); Protein 25g.

Resources for making kefir

For resources on making water- and dairy-based kefir, check out the following:

✔ Everything you'll ever need to know about kefir: http://users.sa.chariot.net.au/~dna/kefirpage.html.

✔ Sources to purchase kefir starter grains: http://users.sa.chariot.net.au/~dna/kefirpage.html and http://kefirlady.com (dairy and water/sugar grains available).

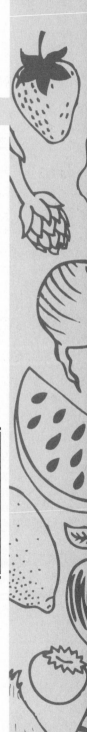

Protein-Packed Morning Smoothie

Prep time: 5 min • **Yield:** About 1 quart (1–2 servings)

Ingredients	*Directions*
2 tablespoons flax seeds	**1** Place all ingredients into blender or Vitamix and blend for 1 to 2 minutes. If your blender has trouble with this recipe, use more liquid and blend after the addition of every few ingredients.
3 Brazil nuts	
3 tablespoons hemp seeds	
¼ large red bell pepper, chopped	
½ orange, peeled	**2** Pour into a jar with lid and take with you to drink throughout the morning.
½ apple, unpeeled, chopped and seeded, or 1 cup berries	
About 1½ cups raw greens (kale, chard, spinach)	
2 cups brewed green or white tea, cooled	

Per serving: Calories 735 (From Fat 351); Fat 39g (Saturated 30g); Cholesterol 0mg; Sodium 92mg; Carbohydrate 84g (Dietary Fiber 18g); Protein 26g.

Note: This recipe is very flexible. Use what you have on hand. You can use sesame seeds or pumpkin seeds; in the winter if fresh fruit is scarce, use frozen (mango chunks are nice!). The basic formula is nuts, seeds, bell pepper, fruit, greens, and tea. That's it!

Part V
The Part of Tens

The 5th Wave   By Rich Tennant

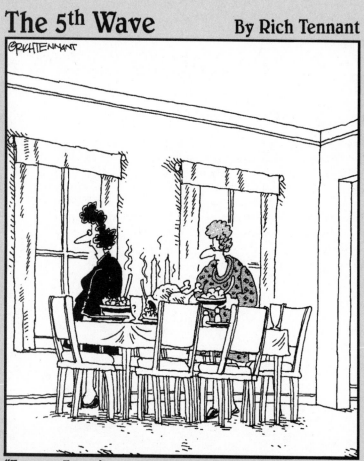

"I guess I can't complain about them being late for dinner. I'm the one who insisted everyone take a walk before meals."

In this part . . .

This part features fun and easy tips to help you drive home your understanding of an immune-friendly life-style! The chapters in this part provide ten tips to keep colds and the flu at bay, ten breathing techniques to keep you healthy, ten exercises that nearly anyone can do at any time and anywhere, and last but certainly not least, ten ways to transition your family to an immune-boosting lifestyle.

Chapter 20

Ten Tips to Avoid Colds and Flu

. . . .

In This Chapter

▶ Keeping yourself and your surroundings clean

▶ Using exercise, vitamins, and herbs to fight illness

. . . .

*I*f you're out in the world, you're exposed to the cold and flu of seasonal changes. In this chapter, we provide some guidelines to help you avoid getting caught by the bug. Boost your immune system and avoid the common ills with these ten tips!

Wash Your Hands

Although this reminder may be obvious to some folks, the reality is that most people don't wash their hands regularly. Hospitals even have to remind doctors and other staff to do it! You know how it goes: You shake someone's hand, and then you pick up your phone — there goes any bugs from that person to your hand and phone. Or worse, you pass it on to someone else.

If you've already developed a cold or flu, wash your hands often, especially because you're probably using your hands to cover your mouth and nose when you sneeze. And to be extra careful, wave your hellos and goodbyes and skip the handshake.

Clean Your Phones and Keyboards

If you share a phone or keyboard with another coworker or use one in a conference room or other open space, definitely wipe it down before and after using it. Assume that someone who is sick has touched the phone or computer before you. Viruses and even bacteria can live on plastic for quite a while, so don't assume you're safe. Simple alcohol wipes are good enough and won't harm the plastic. (Antibacterial wipes can be expensive and actually lead to resistant bacteria; they also don't work on viruses.) Clean your equipment at the beginning and end of each day, even if you think no one else has touched it, just in case.

Air Out Your Workspace

Many people don't have the good sense to stay home and rest when they're sick. Or sometimes employers aren't understanding about illness, so people go in to work and end up coughing all over the place. If that happens in your area, open a window to disperse any viruses or pathogenic bacteria your coworker may be spreading. If that isn't possible, consider getting an air purifier for around your desk to help you avoid direct exposure to airborne particles. We don't suggest using air fresheners because they don't kill any viruses, plus they're made of toxic chemicals, which put more of a burden on your immune system.

If opening a window or using an air purifier is impractical in your space (or forbidden), you can also use essential oils to help purify the air. Rosemary essential oil and tea tree oil have antibacterial and antiviral activity. Put some essential oil on a cotton ball or handkerchief and leave it on your desk in a small dish.

Get a Good Night's Sleep

Your immune system works best when you're well rested. When you skip sleep, your cortisol and DHEA levels (stress hormones) get unbalanced, leading to poor immune function. Breathing deeply and avoiding TV, computers, and e-readers for at least 30 minutes prior to bedtime helps with better sleep. You may also take melatonin, passionflower, or 5-HTP to assist in normalizing sleep patterns. Also, the old home remedy of a glass of warm milk actually works because it contains tryptophan and casein, which can assist in drowsiness and relaxation. Some people even find that writing down all the things on their to-do list that keep running through their head helps calm their mind. Meditating or practicing techniques from the Institute of HeartMath can also lead to better sleep (see Chapter 11 for information about HeartMath).

Take a Walk

Exercise has been shown to be a huge benefit for your immune system. No, not a grueling round on weight machines that you hate, but a brisk walk or fairly active yoga class fits the bill just fine. If you're really in tune with your body, you'll notice that first sniffle, that first mild headache, or that dull throat pain. Start the exercise then, and you'll nip things in the bud. When you're dragging and can't keep your head up easily, it's time to take it easy. The idea here is early intervention — it works wonders.

Eat an Orange Every Day

These days, everyone's pinched for time, and doing everything you "should" do for your health can feel overwhelming. Here's a simple tip: Eat an orange. A real orange (not orange juice), the whole thing, every day. Eating an orange gives you a huge boost of vitamin C and a good bit of fiber and other nutrients. The fiber slows down how much the sweetness in the orange raises your blood glucose (the slower, the better). Big swings in glucose and insulin are detrimental to your immune function. So peel that orange and enjoy it as dessert. Or add it to a smoothie, in a salad, or alongside cooked greens.

Take Oscillococcinum

Homeopathy is a form of healing that uses mild remedies that stimulate the body's own healing properties. Although *how* these remedies exert their effect isn't fully understood, hundreds of years of experience prove their power. One of the best known remedies for the flu and cold symptoms is *Oscillococcinum.* It's made from the highly diluted, fermented liver and heart of a duck and has been shown to resolve symptoms within 48 hours in up to 70 percent of patients. The remedy comes in small vials of tiny pellets that you place under the tongue and allow to dissolve.

Take this remedy at the first sign of cold or flu symptoms and repeat doses every six hours for several days. Although not specifically recommended by the manufacturer, you can also take it prophylactically during flu season: one dose each week. You can find oscillococcinum in health food stores and even some drug stores.

Supplement with Herbal Andrographis

Andrographis paniculata is an herb used in traditional Asian healing systems for thousands of years. It's primarily used for healing infections of various kinds, although traditionally it has also been used for protection of the liver. Recent scientific study has shown that it increases TNF-alpha, interleukin 2, and lymphocyte production, which would clearly boost immune activity. It also decreases inflammation in lungs during upper respiratory infections and has the ability to lower fevers.

During cold and flu season, keep this herb around. Unlike some herbs and remedies, andrographis paniculata will still work well even if you don't start it right as symptoms begin. It usually begins to act within 36 to 48 hours, although you should take it at least one to two days after symptoms stop. Use in pregnancy has not yet been studied, and an interaction with blood thinners, such as Coumadin, can occur, so use it carefully in those circumstances. It often lowers blood pressure, so be aware of this if you take an antihypertensive agent.

Take Echinacea in Root Extract or Tea Form

This herb is one of the most widely used and studied herbs in North America. Interestingly, the published data on its use varies widely, from showing good effects to no effect at all. Some studies used the root of the plant, and some used the leaves and stems; some used small doses of the herb, and some used higher doses; some studies started the herb at the first sign of symptoms, and some started it later. All these variables impact the outcome of the study.

In our practices, we've found that echinacea works well if taken at the first sign of a cold or flu, taken often enough, and taken in high enough doses. Coauthor Wendy usually recommends a tincture made from the root of the plant, used every four to six hours, along with several cups daily of a tea with echinacea as one of its main components. I recommend Echinacea and Roots Tea, which I get from Mountain Rose Herbs, www.mountainroseherbs.com. Because it's made of roots, it needs to be simmered on the stovetop for at least 20 minutes to extract the goodness from the roots. Doing so isn't terribly convenient, so I usually brew up a big pot of this tea, and reheat it as needed throughout the day.

If an echinacea tincture actually includes the root, which it should, the tincture should make your mouth tingle for just a minute when you first take it. If you feel this tingle, you can be assured that you have a quality product. If you don't feel it, the tincture may not include the root, and you can assume it won't work as well as you want.

Up Your Vitamin D Intake

We hope you keep your vitamin D level optimal *all* the time, but if you're exposed to several people with a cold or the flu, take extra vitamin D for a few days or so to prevent getting sick. Several studies show that a rapid increase in vitamin D consumption revs up the immune system enough to ward off a viral attack. If you usually take 5,000 IU daily, increase your intake to 10,000 IU for up to a week at a time. After that, go back to your usual dose so you don't run the risk of overdosing. If you find that you need to increase your dose often during a season, get your blood level checked, just in case. A blood level up to 100 is safe, but if you're close to that, you may want to skip this suggestion and use one of the other tips instead. However, if you've increased your dose several times and your blood level is still pretty low (like 30 to 40), maybe you should take more on a daily basis!

If you have hyperparathyroidism, sarcoidosis, renal disease, or unexplained high calcium levels, be careful about taking large doses of vitamin D. Although vitamin D is safe and has few side effects or contraindications, these three situations and possibly others require close observation when using vitamin D in high amounts. Check with a holistic practitioner for suggestions in your particular case.

Chapter 21

Ten Breathing Exercises for a Better Immune System

In This Chapter

▶ Recognizing how breathing differently can affect your body

▶ Detoxifying, revitalizing, and improving your immune system with breath

*Y*ou breathe every day, all day. It's the one thing you can't live without. But you may not know that how you breathe is essential to your health. There's healthy breathing and not so healthy breathing, and in this chapter, we share ten breathwork techniques that specifically boost the immune system. You don't need any equipment, and you don't have to go anywhere special; it's just you and your breath. It's free and couldn't be more convenient!

Do these breathing exercises in the order in which they appear in this chapter. Each one builds upon the one before it.

Breath Awareness Exercise

How you breathe influences your mood, which ultimately influences your health and immune system. Start with something simple: Notice your breath.

This exercise takes just 5 to 15 minutes. Find a comfortable seated position, either in a chair, on the floor, or leaning against the wall. Your back should be fairly straight, and your hips should be a bit higher than your knees (sitting on a cushion or pillow usually does the trick). If sitting is uncomfortable for any period of time at all, you can also do this exercise lying down, although we don't recommend it if you can avoid it, because you may get so calm that you simply fall asleep!

Settle in to your seat. Try to have as few distractions around you as possible; turn your phone on silent (or off), turn off the TV, maybe put your pets in another room (they'll be curious about what you're up to!). Set a timer for 5 to 15 minutes — however much time you have — so you don't have to watch the clock. Now, close your eyes, and pay attention to how you're breathing. Try not to change it; just observe. Are you breathing quickly? Does the breath feel rushed or anxious or shallow? Or does it feel slow and deep? Is it even, or is it choppy?

Now, notice *where* you feel your body breathing. Some people feel it in their nostrils, some feel it in their throat, and some feel it in their chest. Can you feel it at the tips of the nostrils, just as the air enters the nostril? What does your belly do when you breathe? Does it move at all? What do your ribs do? Do they move? If so, do they all move, even the ones up high by your collarbones?

Spend several minutes just observing what you do when you breathe. Keep your eyes closed until the timer goes off. Try to focus on the breath itself; as thoughts come up, simply put them aside and go back to the breath.

This practice is the foundation for all other breathwork. You need to know how you breathe before you can actively change anything!

Three-Part Breath

This breathwork practice you actually *should* do lying down, because noticing what's happening is much easier in a lying down position. So find a quiet place to lie down with no distractions.

Place one hand on your belly and the other hand on your chest, over your heart. Now, inhale and feel your hands move. First, the hand on your belly moves up as you pull air deep into your chest, expanding the diaphragm. Then, the hand on your chest moves up as your ribs expand. Finally, make sure you take the breath all the way to the top of your lungs, under the collarbones. Pause for just a second. Then, start to exhale. Take the air out of your belly, contracting your diaphragm completely so that all the air is let out and your hand drops. Then notice the air leaving your chest as well as your hand drops there. Pause with the air out. Do the practice again, noting how it feels to fill your belly with air and fill your lungs completely.

Regular practice of this three-part breath leads to improved ventilation of your lungs (always a good thing!) as well as improved control of your diaphragm, which is important for the other breath practices to follow.

Rhythmic Breathing

The primary reason we want you to do this form of breathwork is to stimulate the immune system by stimulating the relaxation response. The same technique, however, can also be used to either rev you up or calm you down. It just depends on what "count" you use as you breathe.

First, get into a comfortable, upright position where your spine is erect. Eliminate external distractions — put your phone on silent, close the door, tell your family you're busy, and so on. Notice your breath, as we instruct you to do in the earlier section "Breath Awareness Exercise." After a moment or so of awareness, it's time to start counting.

Feel for the pulse on your wrist or on the side of your neck. You'll use the time between heartbeats as the length of time for a count. Some people have rapid heart rates; others much slower. Use your own body as a measure.

Using this pulse-time, count as you inhale. Try to inhale for at least 4 counts initially, though it may last much longer as you practice. Then pause, neither inhaling nor exhaling, for 2 to 3 counts. Then exhale to a count of 4 (or however long your inhale lasted). Then pause for a count of 2 to 3. Repeat the cycle.

Doing this rhythmic breathing at an even rate (same time for inhale and exhale) is stabilizing. Many people feel more grounded after this exercise. However, changing the rate of the inhale or exhale can affect your mood. If the inhale is longer than the exhale, you'll feel energized, even anxious. If the exhale is longer than the inhale, you'll feel calmer, more peaceful. So play with this breath practice. Try to lengthen your breaths, especially the exhales. This exercise has been shown to directly change the immune function, and you can create calm and peaceful feelings from the breath you take.

Ujjayi Breath

This exercise is the typical breath used during a yoga asana (posture) practice. It involves breathing in and breathing out through the nose. A slight constriction in the throat causes the breath to form a wave-like sound, like a soft hissing.

First, sit upright without any distractions around you. Some people find it helpful to tilt their chin down just a bit to draw their attention to the back of their throat. Now, using your diaphragm, draw breath in through your nose and deep into your belly. Pause. Let the air out through the nose as well. If you're keeping the throat partially constricted, you should hear a soft hiss, both on the inhale and on the exhale. If you're not sure you're doing this right, simply open your mouth and sigh, and then close your mouth and make the same sound while breathing through your nose.

In yoga, the main benefits of doing this breathing are to focus the mind, to form a smooth breath that's easy to follow (by the sound it makes), and to provide a way to slow the breath down. As for immune-boosting benefits, ancient yogis professed that this technique improved immune function and led to longer lives. No studies have been done to support that specifically, but it's a foundational breathwork practice and one to master before moving on to other, more powerful pranayama.

Breath of Fire

The breath of fire exercise may be a bit more strenuous than the previous breathwork exercises in this chapter, or at least isn't like something you're used to doing. This particular pattern is both easy and complex. You only need to have good control of your abdomen and diaphragm.

Go slowly with this exercise at first, because it's easy to hyperventilate. If you start to feel dizzy, either slow down or stop for a few minutes and then restart.

You may want to try this breath alone the first time. No distractions. Sit upright in a comfortable position. Close your eyes, and take a few calm, deep breaths through your nose. Then, start focusing on your navel: Draw your navel in forcefully to exhale, and then push your navel out forcefully to bring air deep into your lungs. Breathe in and out through your nose, not your mouth. Start slowly, but as you get the hang of it, pick up the pace. Ideally, this breathwork is done fairly rapidly. Don't take breaks between the inhale and the exhale; if you get lightheaded, simply stop.

The benefits of this practice lie primarily in detoxification, which factors into better immune function (see Chapter 12 for information about detoxification). It improves lung capacity and moves out stale air, helping detoxify the respiratory system. The forceful movement of the diaphragm also massages internal organs, which has been shown to improve liver and gallbladder efficiency, also aiding detoxification.

Lion's Breath

The lion's breath exercise stimulates the lymphatics in your neck (because you're contracting the muscles there), and it helps release emotional tension, which in the long run helps stabilize the immune system.

First, kneel on the floor with your ankles crossed. Settle your bottom onto the crossed ankles as well as you can. Place your hands on your knees, with your fingers splayed out like cat claws in action. Lean forward just a bit. Now, take a deep inhalation through the nose. Then simultaneously open your mouth wide and stretch out your tongue, curling its tip down toward the chin, open your eyes wide, contract the muscles on the front of your throat, and exhale the breath slowly out through your mouth with a distinct "ha" sound (see Figure 21-1). The breath should pass over the back of the throat. Do this breathwork several times; work up to about a minute or two.

Some people say you should be looking up toward the spot between your eyes; others say you should be looking down at the tip of your nose. Either way, you'll look pretty funny!

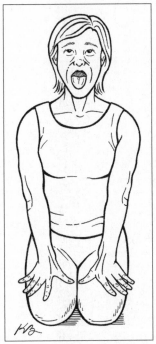

Figure 21-1:
Lion's
breath.

Illustration by Kathryn Born

This breath exercise is one you should definitely share with your kids; they'll have a blast with it and not even realize it's good for them!

Alternate Nostril Breathing

This breathwork pattern aims at balancing. It balances the inhalation with the exhalation and the left and right sides of your nose. It has also been shown to balance the left and right sides of your brain (the analytical with the emotional). The deep breathing alone has been shown to improve mood, but the balancing between the brain hemispheres is likely the real reason this pattern has been shown to improve stress hormone levels. As you recall from other chapters, stress management is vital to an optimal immune system.

Sit in any comfortable sitting posture with the spine erect, eyes closed, and shoulders relaxed. Make the Vishnu Mudra with the right hand: Make a soft fist and lift the thumb and the last two fingers up, keeping the middle two fingers at the base of the thumb (see Figure 21-2a). During the practice using this mudra, you use the thumb to close the right nostril and the ring finger to close the left nostril.

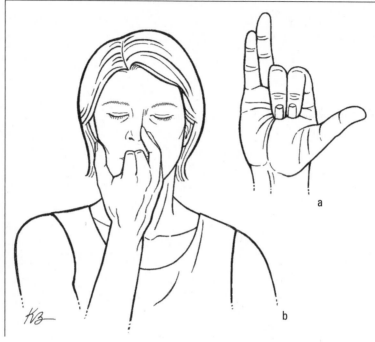

Illustration by Kathryn Born

With the left hand, make the Chin Mudra: Join the tips of the index finger and the thumb, keeping the rest of the fingers open and relaxed. Keep the hand on the left knee, palm facing up.

Use the right thumb to close the right nostril. To get started, exhale through the left. Begin the first round by inhaling through the left nostril. At the end of inhalation, close the left nostril with the ring finger and open the right (see Figure 21-2b). Then exhale through the right nostril. Inhale now through the right. At the end of inhalation, close the right nostril with the thumb again and exhale through the left, completing one cycle of breathing. Continue for about six to seven similar cycles. Make sure to use deep and soft Ujjayi breaths (see earlier section) for each inhalation and exhalation.

Yogi Nerve Revitalizing Breath

In this breathing practice, you get to move your arms! It's designed to increase nerve stimulation and, in yogic belief, to increase energy moving through your whole body. This exercise stimulates lymphatic flow in the arms and upper chest, so that alone improves immune function.

Stand erect. Do a full, three-part breath as discussed earlier in this chapter and hold it while doing the following steps:

1. Extend the arms straight in front of you, letting them be somewhat limp and relaxed, with only sufficient muscular effort to hold them out.

2. Slowly draw your hands back toward your shoulders, gradually contracting the muscles and putting force into them so that when they reach the shoulders, the fists will be so tightly clenched that a tremulous motion is felt.

3. Then, keeping the muscles tense, push the fists slowly out, and then draw them back rapidly (still tense) several times.

4. Exhale vigorously through the mouth. Then take a big breath and let it out with a sigh.

The point here is that you start with loose arms, then tense them as they come back to the chest, then pump them several times back and forth *before you exhale.* This exercise feels amazing and is a great way to start the day on those mornings when you'd rather be in bed. It's also good for the mid-afternoon slump or just after dinner when you still have stuff to do but would rather crash!

Sitali Breath

Sitali breath is designed to aid in detoxification. It's also cooling and is said to help stop cravings for food, alcohol, and so on. It helps regulate digestion (which, as we've discussed, is important for immune function) and can even be used to cool a fever.

Sit comfortably and curl the tongue into a *U* shape, as shown in Figure 21-3. (**Note:** Some people aren't genetically capable of curling their tongue. If you can't, stick your tongue out of your mouth and do the rest of the breath practice, using the same instructions.). Using the tongue almost like a straw, place the tip just at the lips and close the lips around it. Now, sip air in through your tongue and mouth, and exhale slowly through your nose. Continue this for several minutes. When you're done, inhale one last time, pull in the tongue, hold the breath for a few counts then exhale and relax. Repeat this cycle for two to three rounds.

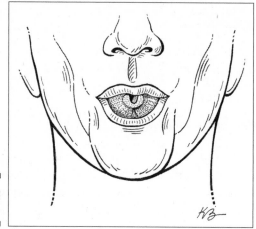

Figure 21-3:
Sitali breath.

Illustration by Kathryn Born

Breath Retention

If you have uncontrolled blood pressure problems, a history of anxiety, or are currently pregnant, skip this exercise. Otherwise, this breath exercise is a fabulous way to improve your energy and may help in lymphatic flow (due to energy movement).

Sit comfortably and take a few slow breaths in and out. Then, as you inhale, slowly contract your pelvic floor muscles (as if you're doing a Kegel exercise or trying to keep from urinating) and hold your breath. Lower your chin to your chest as you hold the breath. Count to 2 or 3, and then slowly raise your head and relax your pelvic floor as you exhale. Take a few more slow breaths in and out. Repeat the breath retention.

You can also do this retention on the exhale. After you exhale completely, contract the pelvic floor and lower your chin. Count to 2 or 3, then release the pelvic floor, raise your head, and inhale slowly. Then take a few slow breaths in and out.

Don't do a lot of these retentions at one time (no more than three or four) and don't hold for longer than a few seconds without guidance from a yoga instructor. If you overdo this practice, it can "stir up" your energy and increase anxiety levels. Done appropriately, however, it is calming and centering.

Chapter 22

Ten Boosting Exercises You Can Do Anywhere

*I*f we were to give you a pill and tell you that taking this pill daily would reduce your chance of almost every disease that exists, including colds, the flu, heart disease, cancer, diabetes, and osteoporosis, would you take it? Well, you *do* have that pill, and it's free. It's called exercise!

Exercising can make all the difference in how you feel and the energy levels you have throughout the day. And exercising can keep you alive and well.

A research study done in 2008 on 1,002 participants found that the frequency of colds among people who exercised five or more days a week was 46 percent less than in people who were mostly sedentary (exercising one time or less per week). The people who exercised got fewer viral infections, and when they did come down with an illness, it was mild. In fact, they experienced 41 percent fewer days of illness. These results are remarkable and show that exercise is certainly worth the effort.

Although extreme exercise may place stress on the body, vigorous exercise that can elevate heart rate is beneficial to your immune system. The gentle exercises in this chapter will wake your body up and turn your brain power on. You'll get the oxygen flowing and even burn some calories.

Thymus Reset

Your thymus gland is a soft, flat tissue located in the upper chest under the breastbone and plays a big part in your immune and hormonal system. If you feel a cold coming on, have some congestion, or feel sluggish or anxious, give the thymus reset a try. Better yet, do this exercise every day as a preventative measure or to wake your thymus for a burst of energy.

You can do this exercise anywhere and in any position (standing, sitting, or even half asleep)!

1. Place your hand on the center of your breastbone, just below the notch on your collarbones, as shown in Figure 22-1.

2. Make a fist and firmly pound on this spot for about 20 seconds while breathing in and out deeply.

You should feel more energized, balanced, and calm.

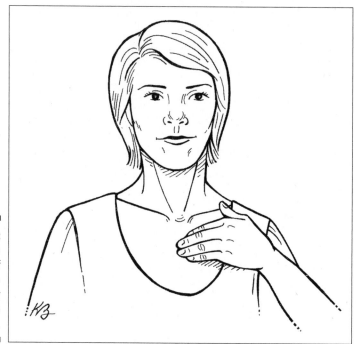

Figure 22-1: Find the center of your breast-bone for the thymus reset.

Illustration by Kathryn Born

K-27 Energy Buttons

K-27 stands for *kidney merdian number 27* and relates to acupressure points along what Chinese medicine calls the kidney meridian. To understand what the meridians are, think about them as a transportation system. You have 12 of these transportation systems throughout the body, and each one carries energy (called *chi,* or *qi*). If one of these transportation systems is blocked, the nourishing effect of the energy stops, and the body suffers. Illness can result until this pathway of energy is unblocked. The kidney meridian harbors much of the body's reservoir of essential energy, and stimulating the K-27 points releases this energy.

The K-27 technique gives you energy and your brain a boost. It's useful when you feel tired, if you have a lowered immune system, or when you're experiencing jet lag. One of the best times for stimulating your energy buttons is right before you have to take a test, for that extra clarity.

Follow these steps to stimulate the K-27 energy buttons:

1. Place your index fingers on the *U*-shaped notch at the top of the breast bone, right where a man knots his tie.

2. With your fingers, follow down over your collarbone out to each side about an inch into the soft tissue to the left and right of the breastbone (see Figure 22-2).

   The depressions you find here are your K-27 points.

3. Massage both K-27 points for 20 seconds, either simultaneously or separately, and take deep breaths, in through the nose and out through the mouth.

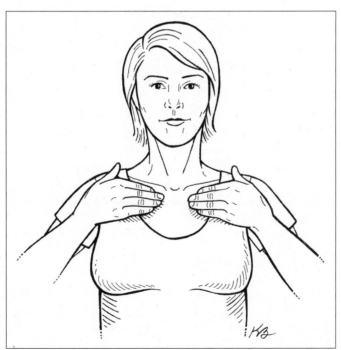

Figure 22-2:
Locate your
K-27 energy
points.

Illustration by Kathryn Born

Knowing where the K-27 points are is easy enough to teach kids — and they get a kick out of learning these acupressure points. They can stimulate their K-27 points before a test or when they feel like they need a little energy.

Spleen Thump

The spleen is central to the immune system. By thumping the spleen point, you can bolster your immune system, lift your energy, and even help balance your blood sugar. Even better, it takes only a minute! Follow these steps to perform the spleen thump:

1. Move your fingers under the center of each breast (under where a women's bra would end).

2. Go down a rib and out about an inch or so to each side, as shown in Figure 22-3.

3. Find the depression between the seventh and eighth rib.

4. Bunch your fingertips together and tap both sides 30 times while breathing deeply.

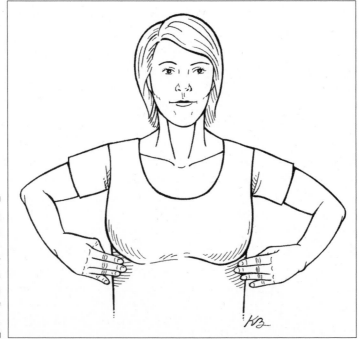

Figure 22-3:
The spleen thump benefits your immune system and energy level.

Illustration by Kathryn Born

TIP

Doing the previously mentioned thymus reset, K-27, and spleen thump every morning to awaken and center your body is a wonderful pattern to put into your daily immune-boosting routine.

Chair Pose

You may be familiar with the chair pose if you've ever done yoga. This pose massages your organs, stretches your spine, and opens up your chest to get your oxygen flowing. This basic yoga posture is also great for strengthening the immune system.

1. Stand up straight with feet hip-width apart.

2. Turn your heels a little outward and let your weight rest on your toes.

3. Hang your arms downward along your body, palms facing inward toward your body.

4. Inhale and stretch your arms up over your head and lengthen your spine.

5. Exhale, bend your knees, and move your upper body forward to 45 degrees. Keep your back straight, and let the weight of your upper body sink into your pelvis, as shown in Figure 22-4.

6. Breathe deeply five times and slowly release the pose.

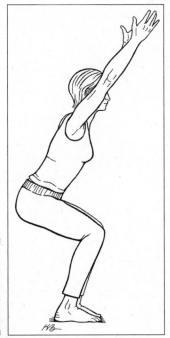

Figure 22-4:
Proper body positioning for chair pose.

Illustration by Kathryn Born

Bound Bridge

If you feel exhausted all the time, your body may be experiencing fatigue from chronic stress. The causes may be from chemical toxicity, nutritional deficiency, emotional stress, sleep deficiency, or one of many factors that may cause your body to feel depleted.

The bound bridge yoga pose combats the burnout from constant stress. This exercise is restorative and can bring balance and energy to your body.

1. Lie on your back with your knees bent, pointing straight up, and feet on the floor. Your feet should be parallel to each other and about 6 inches apart.

2. Press down with your feet and lift your hips off of the ground. Keep pressing your abdomen inward toward your spine for stabilization.

3. Grab your ankles with your hands (see Figure 22-5). Keep your feet, arms, shoulders, and head on the ground.

4. Keep your knees from drifting inward. You may place a yoga block in between them to keep them in place.

Figure 22-5: Bound bridge pose opens up your body and lets energy flow freely.

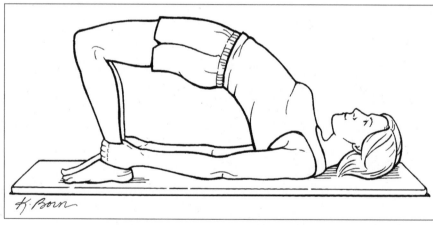

Illustration by Kathryn Born

Rebounding

Rebounding is one of the best movements you can do for your immune system. Rebounding helps keep your *lymphatic system* healthy and in order. Your lymphatic system is a drainage network made up of clear fluid that contains protein molecules, salt, glucose, and other substances. The system has the job of draining extra fluids from the tissues so they don't swell. It also protects the body against germs, bacteria, and viruses through a network called *lymph nodes.* Because your lymph system has no built-in pump (like the circulatory system) to keep things moving along, you must circulate lymph through the lymphatic system by moving. Rebounding does a beautiful job of accomplishing this task.

Rebounding also nourishes and cleanses all your cells every time you bounce for that extra dose of healing. The increased oxygen through deeper breathing also helps you relax, so it's great for stress management as well.

To do this exercise, you need a rebounder. Rebounders look like mini trampolines and measure about 38 to 48 inches in diameter. Most fold up for easy storage. You can buy them in any sporting goods or discount chain.

1. Simply bounce gently on the trampoline's surface.

2. As you get accustomed to jumping and build coordination, balance, and stability, progress to lifting both feet off of the surface at the same time and lifting your knees up high or kicking your feet toward your bottom for a more intense workout.

Start with three times a week for five minutes. You can do this exercise frequently (up to six days a week) because of its low impact. Whether you gently bounce or you progress to a more rigorous workout, you'll get great benefits.

The beauty of rebounding is that you can listen to music or watch TV while jumping. Plus it's a low-impact exercise, so if you have trouble with other weight-bearing exercises (for example, if you have arthritis or knee problems), rebounding may offer you a good alternative.

Walking

Walking may seem like an overly simple exercise, but the value it adds to your health is often surprising. In fact, it adds so much to your health that you simply can't dismiss the power of a good walk.

Your lymphatic system is responsible for removing toxins from your cells, but it needs movement to work efficiently. Walking helps move fluid through your lymphatic system, so your body carries healthier cells. Walking also helps your body release white blood cells at a faster speed, helping you to have more healing power quicker. You also get increased blood flow, all of which helps stimulate your immune system, which may be why you get fewer colds and flu symptoms when you exercise. Regular walks may even strengthen your immune system as you age (which normally declines with age).

Besides boosting your immune system, here are some other important benefits of walking:

- Reduces your risk of or manages Type 2 diabetes
- Improves your mood and may just be the best natural antidepressant
- Manages your weight
- Lowers your blood pressure
- Lowers bad cholesterol and elevates good cholesterol
- Energizes your body
- Acts as a natural detox

 The great thing about walking is that it has no limitations. You can enjoy its benefits in the busiest of cities or in the sprawling countryside. Also, you can easily adjust the intensity to a scale that makes you comfortable. Always start slow and progress as your body gains endurance and strength.

Shaking the Tree

This exercise is a *Qigong* exercise, which is a form of martial art in which you learn to sense the qi (chi) moving in your body. Over time, you gain physical, mental, and even spiritual effects. Qigong exercises can help you relax and feel a sense of balance and focus.

The shaking the tree movement helps to gently loosen your joints, muscles, and internal organs. It's a great way to release tension and awaken the body at the start of a day.

1. Stand with your feet shoulder-width apart, arms at your sides.
2. Start the movement from the bottom of your feet.
3. Shake in an up-and-down motion.
4. You can shake your arms in motion with the rest of the body or let them hang loosely at your sides.
5. Breathe fully and shake for about two minutes, making the motions smaller and smaller until you stand completely still.
6. Feel the continued vibrations throughout your body as your body opens and increases its blood flow.

 Be sure to breathe through the nose, calm your mind, and sense your body, breath, and qi. Keep your shoulders soft, never fully exert yourself, and keep the crown of your head straight up.

Ragdoll Twist

The ragdoll twist is another Qigong exercise to improve your physical, mental, and energetic focus. This gentle movement moves qi through your body to relax and loosen the body, helping you strengthen your health and immunity.

1. Stand with your feet parallel, slightly wider than shoulder-width apart.

2. Turn your torso to the right, and at the same time, swing your arms to the right, allowing them to stay relaxed so they "flop."

3. Let your right hand tap over your kidney (lower back) as your left hand taps over your liver and gallbladder (upper right side, just under your breast).

4. As you twist to the right, pivot your left foot inward on the ball of your foot.

5. Repeat the same on the left side, going from right to left for about two minutes.

Cross-Crawl Pattern

When you perform a walking cross-crawl pattern, you're activating both hemispheres of the brain. Doing this exercise on a regular basis builds stronger nerve networks. The communication between both sides of the brain becomes sharper and faster, providing you with better reasoning (brain power).

1. Start the exercise by stimulating the K-27 energy buttons (discussed earlier in this chapter), just to give your immune system a little extra boost right out of the gate.

2. Bend your right leg at the knee while swinging your left arm in front of you across the centerline of your body. Touch your left elbow to your right knee.

3. Bend your left leg at the knee and touch your right elbow to the left knee.

4. Repeat the exercise, switching back and forth, 20 times for each leg.

Crawling is such a healthy party of a baby's development because the cross-pattern movements build the bridge between the right and left hemispheres of the brain. This movement helps your spinal muscles and coordination and allows your body's systems to work together effectively. When the body's system works together as a team, you prevent health issues. The cross-crawl pattern works in a similar way, helping your body develop its nervous system.

Chapter 23

Ten Ways to Get Your Family on the Immunity Bandwagon

. . . .

In This Chapter

▶ Transitioning your family without the battle

▶ Strategies to make healthy eating simple

▶ Shopping for immune-boosting foods

▶ Getting the basics of building an immune-boosting plate

. . . .

Discovering how to eat and live in a way that boosts your immune system is a wonderful feeling. When you're healthy, you look and feel amazing, and when you start to get big results, you want your family to share in your enthusiasm and good health.

Whether your family needs to make big changes or small ones, we provide useful tips in this chapter. You may find these tips particularly valuable because, as much as you want to enroll your loved ones into your healthy lifestyle, it's not always easy. This chapter is all about having a solid strategy equipped with tips so you can be a strong leader.

Showing kids why being healthy is important, figuring out how to make healthy living fun, setting ground rules at mealtimes without the battle, building a superfood plate for kids, making shopping with kids fun, and discovering how your family can enjoy tasty treats and still build immunity are all up for grabs in these ten tips!

Be a Strong Leader

The first rule in transitioning your family into a healthy lifestyle is to carry a positive and confident attitude about what you're doing and how you're living. Leave no room for doubt or confusion when it comes to your commitment and radiant health.

Kids download everything you do. They learn from an interesting platform called *modeling,* meaning what you do, kids naturally imitate, or mirror. Do you eat vegetables? Do you have healthy foods on the table at mealtimes? Does your family see you eating and preparing nourishing foods? You can't have rules for children that you don't follow yourself.

You can't bully your way into transformation. When someone pursues change with no heart, it's not lasting change. That's where the theory "they'll come to you when they're ready" holds. If you want other members of your household to embrace change, be a great role model. Have healthy foods available and have *your* food values in order. That's how you affect change.

Teach Kids the "Why" of Healthy Living

Have you ever gone through the motions of doing something just because? Maybe someone said to do it, maybe it was a role you had to take on for work, or maybe it was just something you got in the habit of doing. Something is usually missing when you do something just because — *heart.* When you do things with heart, the passion to succeed follows.

No matter what age or stage your kids are in, explain some simple facts about why they should eat healthy foods. You don't have to make a big deal about it; it can even be in passing. As long as you do teach them the *why.* Here are some examples:

- ✔ You should be able to pronounce the ingredients on a food label; otherwise, they're probably chemicals that you don't want in your body.

- ✔ If too many ingredients are on the label, the foods are too processed and aren't going to give you the nutrients you need. You'll get some energy but no nutrition.

- ✔ Fruits and vegetables have antioxidants, which keep your cells super healthy and protect you against getting sick.

- ✔ Fruits and vegetables have vitamins and minerals, which make every structure and function of your body work. When you get too low on these vitamins, you get sick easier, and performing well in all areas of life can be difficult.

- ✔ Fruits and vegetables have fiber in them, which helps move things along your intestines so your body stays cleansed and not clogged.

- ✔ Your body needs healthy proteins to build and repair everything in your body, like strong muscles.

✔ Healthy fats make your brain and all your cells work better so you can do everything better. These fats are super important to have.

✔ Your cells really need water so they're not stuck together, which causes you to get tired and worn out.

Keep your explanations simple — no big words or lengthy lectures — just some simple facts so your children understand why eating healthy foods is important. Explaining the *why* behind the choices you make helps them feel ownership and helps them *want* to have a healthier lifestyle. That's a sure-fire prescription for success.

Recognize Junk Food Marketing

Advertising affects kids' food choices a great deal. It's a tough battle, but parents should be aware that food and beverage companies spend $2 billion annually promoting unhealthy foods to kids, and kids watch more than ten food-related ads every day.

In a study conducted by Stanford University, a group of children were offered two identical meals, one in a plain wrapper and one in a package from a popular fast-food chain. Even young children associated a better taste experience with the name-brand selection, suggesting that marketing and expectation have an impact on perceived taste.

Bring your kids to the store and show them packaging geared toward kids. Explain that many foods are boxed or wrapped in a certain way to entice kids. Read the label with them (or read it to them) and let them discover that just because the food may look attractive on its labeling, it doesn't mean that it's good for them. Teach kids about what's being marketed on the television and Internet, too.

Make Healthier Eating Fun

The best way to transition your family to healthier eating is to remain strong and make it fun! Keeping things light relaxes the body and allows everyone in your family to learn and retain information. If you're too intense about your ambitions, it can cause stress, which usually causes your body to tighten and resist.

Here are some ways to create a healthy learning experience, so your kids discover healthy eating, without the battle:

✔ **Make foods *look* fun.** When food looks appetizing or fun to eat, it triggers the brain to desire the food. Use cookie cutters to make fun shapes; ice cream scoops to make mountains; raisins, olives, baby carrots, or apple slices to make faces — anything creative to make your family excited about the food they're eating.

We love this food face dinner plate, which makes turning healthy foods into fun foods for kids easy. Check it out at www.perpetualkid.com/food-face-dinner-plate.aspx.

✔ **Play food guessing games.** Put out different bowls with healthy foods in them. Have the kids cover their eyes (or blindfold them) and make them guess what food they're tasting. Playing games is a great way to get them to try new foods.

✔ **Let kids pick their own fruits and veggies.** Kids love feeling like they're calling the shots!

✔ **Use toothpicks instead of regular utensils.** Put out healthy snacks and let kids pick them up with a toothpick. Kids find this more fun than a blockbuster movie.

Change Breakfast First

When transitioning your family to healthier eating, switching out with one meal at a time is usually best. Breakfast is one of the best meals to start with because your family's hungriest at this time and most willing to try different foods.

Practicing healthy food principles while transitioning your family is important, and here's a good one to start with: There are no trademarked breakfast, lunch, or dinner foods. Any foods can be eaten at any time. As nutrition evolves, you know that the idea is to eat *real* food — foods that are unprocessed, unpackaged, and filled with nutrients. As long as you're eating these nutrient-rich foods, any meal is the right time for them!

Always keep hard-boiled eggs on hand. You can eat them on their own or chop them with nitrite-free sausage or bacon for a quick and easy breakfast. Check out the breakfast recipes in Chapter 14 for more ideas.

Set Some Dinner Rules

Sometimes as a parent, you have to lay down the law for the greater good of your child. So is the case of dinner rules. They're there to encourage kids to try as many new vegetables as possible. Setting down these two rules will make a big difference because you're creating patterns and pathways in your child (as well as in your spouse or partner) that establish positive eating habits:

- ✔ **Every dinner must follow the 2-plus-1 rule: Offer 2 cooked vegetables and 1 raw vegetable.** This rule anchors into your family's mind that vegetables at mealtimes are standard. Therefore, eating vegetables becomes normal to them. You can use this time to talk about the different kinds of vegetables (or seasonal vegetables) and encourage them to venture out and try new ones.

   If you make a dish that includes a vegetable, that counts; if you make spaghetti squash for dinner, that's one vegetable. Just make sure you include a raw vegetable as well, such as snow peas, sugar snap peas, kohlrabi, jicama, cucumbers, carrots, and crisp bell peppers.

- ✔ **Everyone must try one bite of every vegetable on the table, and that's non-negotiable.** Remember the end game: to familiarize your family to all types of foods, including vegetables, and have their taste buds get accustomed to these tastes.

During mealtimes, try to avoid distractions, include everyone in the conversation, and focus on any positive interactions. Doing so makes your mealtime a good opportunity to touch on appropriate mealtime behaviors and making smart food choices.

Teach Kids the Basics of Building a Healthy Plate

Explain macronutrients — carbohydrates, proteins, and fats — to your kids and make sure they understand that these nutrients are the cornerstones of building a healthy plate. Then show them healthy options for each one. A great way to accomplish this is to involve your kids (and your spouse or partner) in meal planning and cooking.

Explain to your kiddos that when they're away from home and making food choices, they should try to have all these nutrients on their plate. You want to help them develop a healthy mental checklist. Explain that although they may not be able to cover all their bases all the time, they can still do their best.

As far as general guidelines are concerned, the point is to work on building a plate for your child where half of the plate is filled with fruits and vegetables with a small portion of protein and some healthy fat in every meal (see Figure 23-1). When you want a little more nutritionally filling foods, add in a healthy dense source of carbohydrate, like a sweet potato topped with grass-fed butter.

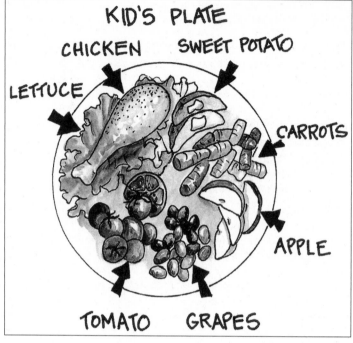

Figure 23-1:
An example of an immune-boosting plate for kids.

Illustration by Elizabeth Kurtzman

Don't *ever* talk about calories with your kids. If your child needs to eat more, the messages from the brain determine hunger. When your children experience a true physiological need for calories and when they're truly hungry, they'll eat. If they need to lose weight, talk to them about eating better for health. Health should *always* be the focus.

Encourage Teamwork in the Kitchen

One of the best ways you can get your kids excited about eating healthier is to enlist them to help in the kitchen. Another bonus when you plan your meals and cook with your kids is that they get time with *you*. Uninterrupted time with you is the best gift you can possibly give your children. Kids want to feel safe, loved, and important, and having some kitchen teamwork time accomplishes this on all accounts.

Take Your Family on a Food Field Trip

One of the best ways you can excite your family about healthy living is to show them where food comes from. Doing so connects them to food in a way that they grow a true appreciation for *real food,* thus immersing them into a healthy living lifestyle that helps make the transition more meaningful and really stick.

Here are some great options to teach your family about where food comes from:

- **Find a farmers' market in your area and visit the local vendors.** You can build relationships and talk about growing conditions and organic and seasonal foods.

- **Join a Community Supported Agriculture (CSA), which allows you to buy into a share of a farm.** You visit the farm once a week and pick up your vegetables. This ritual is also a great way to try new vegetables because you may get a vegetable that you've never had before. When it comes home in your box and you've already paid for it, trying is easy!

- **Go to a farm that has farm-stand days, where you can pick up fresh vegetables.** For example, every Tuesday and Thursday, the farm may have market hours where you can pick up fresh foods. This option lets you pick exactly what you want, as opposed to a CSA, where what you get is decided for you.

If options for a food field trip are limited in your area, get your family involved in growing vegetables in your own garden. Kids love to garden and are always proud to share a tomato that they grew themselves. Even if your kids just pick one or two of their favorites, growing your own vegetables can go a long way to making the connection to where food really comes from.

The important point is to just get kids involved in appreciating good food and its sources. Knowing where food comes from and just how good it will taste will encourage children to have an appreciation for real foods from the start.

Manage Sweets

Kids love treats — and, let's face it, adults do, too! Even if your family shares a deep love and affection for sweets, you can manage these cravings in the following ways:

- If you don't bring it into the house, it can't be eaten. If you decide a treat is in order, load up the family to go out and get it, but don't bring any home.

- Worry about what you *can* control, and don't get crazy about the rest. Teach good food choices at home and provide real foods; your family members will begin to make the connection between the foods and sugars they eat and how they make their body feel. They'll discover these positive and negative associations in time with your guidance.

Some sweets, such as birthday cake at parties or holiday cookies that you bake together, are okay *some of the time*. Make sure everyone in your family understands the line in the sand and the difference between special occasion treats and everyday real foods.

✔ Redefine desserts by making healthier treats with wholesome ingredients, like fresh fruit and almond flour.

✔ Don't reward kids with sweets. Food exists to nourish, not to show love or reward.

✔ Pull the plug on sweet drinks in your home. Sugary drinks have become a huge problem for kids (and adults) and are a factor in the diabetes crisis. Offer water and iced herbal teas if they want something else. Just a pitcher of water with some oranges and lemons is usually enough to keep them happy.

One of the best things you can do when your kids eat sweets is to make sure they're getting real sweets and not a bunch of chemicals or *frankensweets* (fake stuff dressed up to look like cakes and treats). The more refined a sugar is, the worse it is. See Chapter 8 for more on sugar and what to avoid at all costs.

How do I get my significant other onboard?

Just like you have to be a strong leader and lead by example with your kids, you have to do the same with your significant other. First, give your absolute best, most compelling pitch as to why eating healthier is so important. If your partner accepts your pitch, do what you can to support him or her. Be enthusiastic to help during the transition, because you know that with your support and excitement, your partner has a much better chance of success.

If your significant other doesn't even want to try to eat healthier, your only course of action is to keep on being a strong leader. Show by example how much energy you have and how much better you feel. Prepare some healthy recipes from Part IV, and let your partner see how simple it is to stay onboard. Show him or her that eating

healthier *can* be delicious and won't make you heavy, bloated, constipated, or get your blood sugar all out of whack. Eating can actually make you feel better, not worse. *Show,* don't *tell,* how much better you look and feel.

If all else fails, accept your partner for who he or she is — crappy food and all. Don't get resentful or frustrated; the stress hormones counterbalance your great strides and efforts. It simply isn't worth what it does to you internally. Just keep on being positive and realize it's not your issue. Maybe someday, you just may get the question "so this healthy food is really working for you, huh? Do you think it will work for me, too?" We see this in practice more than you may think. So hang tight, and keep doing what you need to do to take care of you!

Appendix

Metric Conversion Guide

• •

*N**ote:* The recipes in this book weren't developed or tested using metric measurements. There may be some variation in quality when converting to metric units.

Common Abbreviations	
Abbreviation(s)	*What It Stands For*
cm	Centimeter
C., c.	Cup
G, g	Gram
kg	Kilogram
L, l	Liter
lb.	Pound
mL, ml	Milliliter
oz.	Ounce
pt.	Pint
t., tsp.	Teaspoon
T., Tb., Tbsp.	Tablespoon

Volume

U.S. Units	Canadian Metric	Australian Metric
¼ teaspoon	1 milliliter	1 milliliter
½ teaspoon	2 milliliters	2 milliliters
1 teaspoon	5 milliliters	5 milliliters
1 tablespoon	15 milliliters	20 milliliters
¼ cup	50 milliliters	60 milliliters
⅓ cup	75 milliliters	80 milliliters
½ cup	125 milliliters	125 milliliters
⅔ cup	150 milliliters	170 milliliters
¾ cup	175 milliliters	190 milliliters
1 cup	250 milliliters	250 milliliters
1 quart	1 liter	1 liter
1½ quarts	1.5 liters	1.5 liters
2 quarts	2 liters	2 liters
2½ quarts	2.5 liters	2.5 liters
3 quarts	3 liters	3 liters
4 quarts (1 gallon)	4 liters	4 liters

Weight

U.S. Units	Canadian Metric	Australian Metric
1 ounce	30 grams	30 grams
2 ounces	55 grams	60 grams
3 ounces	85 grams	90 grams
4 ounces (¼ pound)	115 grams	125 grams
8 ounces (½ pound)	225 grams	225 grams
16 ounces (1 pound)	455 grams	500 grams (½ kilogram)

Length

Inches	Centimeters
0.5	1.5
1	2.5
2	5.0
3	7.5
4	10.0
5	12.5
6	15.0
7	17.5
8	20.5
9	23.0
10	25.5
11	28.0
12	30.5

Temperature (Degrees)

Fahrenheit	Celsius
32	0
212	100
250	120
275	140
300	150
325	160
350	180
375	190
400	200
425	220
450	230
475	240
500	260

Index

• *Q* •

• *R* •

• *S* •

Apple & Mac

iPad 2 For Dummies,
3rd Edition
978-1-118-17679-5

iPhone 4S For Dummies,
5th Edition
978-1-118-03671-6

iPod touch For Dummies,
3rd Edition
978-1-118-12960-9

Mac OS X Lion
For Dummies
978-1-118-02205-4

Blogging & Social Media

CityVille For Dummies
978-1-118-08337-6

Facebook For Dummies,
4th Edition
978-1-118-09562-1

Mom Blogging
For Dummies
978-1-118-03843-7

Twitter For Dummies,
2nd Edition
978-0-470-76879-2

WordPress For Dummies,
4th Edition
978-1-118-07342-1

Business

Cash Flow For Dummies
978-1-118-01850-7

Investing For Dummies,
6th Edition
978-0-470-90545-6

Job Searching with Social
Media For Dummies
978-0-470-93072-4

QuickBooks 2012
For Dummies
978-1-118-09120-3

Resumes For Dummies,
6th Edition
978-0-470-87361-8

Starting an Etsy Business
For Dummies
978-0-470-93067-0

Cooking & Entertaining

Cooking Basics
For Dummies, 4th Edition
978-0-470-91388-8

Wine For Dummies,
4th Edition
978-0-470-04579-4

Diet & Nutrition

Kettlebells For Dummies
978-0-470-59929-7

Nutrition For Dummies,
5th Edition
978-0-470-93231-5

Restaurant Calorie Counter
For Dummies,
2nd Edition
978-0-470-64405-8

Digital Photography

Digital SLR Cameras &
Photography For Dummies,
4th Edition
978-1-118-14489-3

Digital SLR Settings
& Shortcuts
For Dummies
978-0-470-91763-3

Photoshop Elements 10
For Dummies
978-1-118-10742-3

Gardening

Gardening Basics
For Dummies
978-0-470-03749-2

Vegetable Gardening
For Dummies,
2nd Edition
978-0-470-49870-5

Green/Sustainable

Raising Chickens
For Dummies
978-0-470-46544-8

Green Cleaning
For Dummies
978-0-470-39106-8

Health

Diabetes For Dummies,
3rd Edition
978-0-470-27086-8

Food Allergies
For Dummies
978-0-470-09584-3

Living Gluten-Free
For Dummies,
2nd Edition
978-0-470-58589-4

Hobbies

Beekeeping
For Dummies,
2nd Edition
978-0-470-43065-1

Chess For Dummies,
3rd Edition
978-1-118-01695-4

Drawing For Dummies,
2nd Edition
978-0-470-61842-4

eBay For Dummies,
7th Edition
978-1-118-09806-6

Knitting For Dummies,
2nd Edition
978-0-470-28747-7

Language & Foreign Language

English Grammar
For Dummies,
2nd Edition
978-0-470-54664-2

French For Dummies,
2nd Edition
978-1-118-00464-7

German For Dummies,
2nd Edition
978-0-470-90101-4

Spanish Essentials
For Dummies
978-0-470-63751-7

Spanish For Dummies,
2nd Edition
978-0-470-87855-2

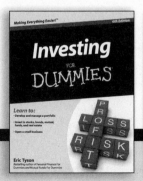

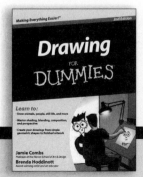

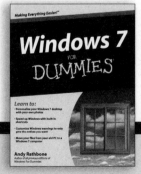

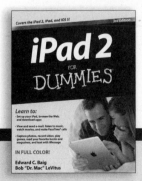

Available wherever books are sold. For more information or to order direct: U.S. customers visit www.dummies.com or call 1-877-762-2974.
U.K. customers visit www.wileyeurope.com or call (0) 1243 843291. Canadian customers visit www.wiley.ca or call 1-800-567-4797.

Connect with us online at www.facebook.com/fordummies or @fordummies

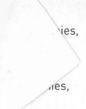
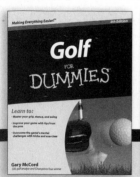
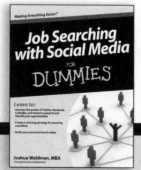
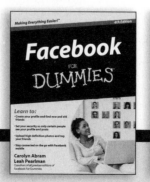
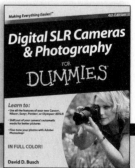

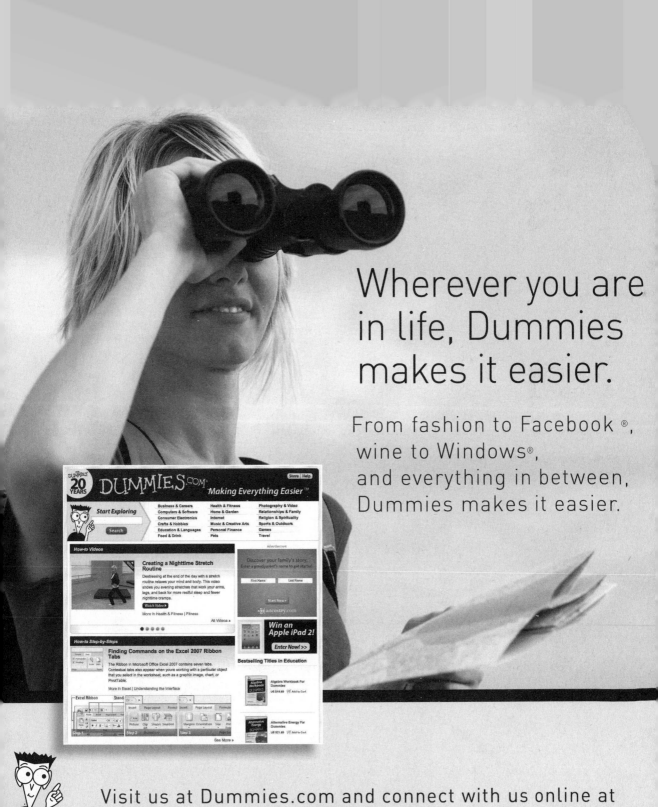

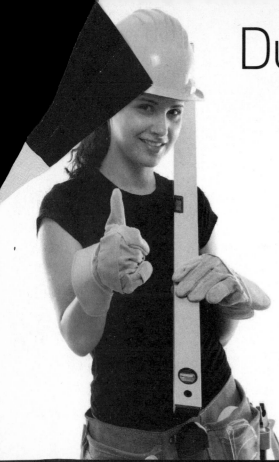
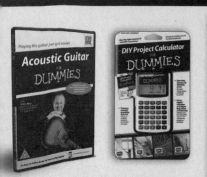
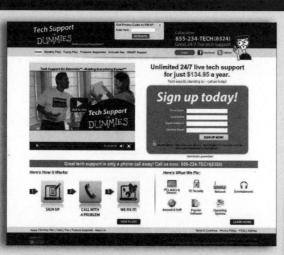
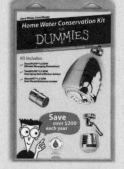
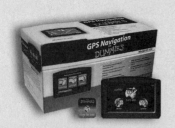
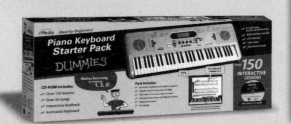
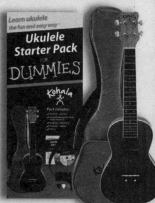
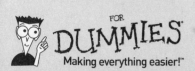